ANATOMY
TO COLOR
AND STUDY

THORAX
ABDOMEN
AND
PELVIS

3rd edition

Ray Poritsky, Ph.D. Emeritus
Department of Anatomy
Case Western University School of Medicine
Cleveland, Ohio

ISBN: 978-0-9835784-3-7
Copyright © 2011 Ray Poritsky
Digitally Reproduced by:
CONVERPAGE
23 Acorn Street
Scituate, MA 02066
www.converpage.com

All rights reserved. No part of this publication may be reproduced, stored in a retrieval system, or transmitted, in any form or by any means, electronic, mechanical, photocopying, recording or otherwise, without the written prior permission of the author.

CONTENTS

Part I: Introduction and Thorax

Cartoon: The Four "Birds" of the Thorax
1 Planes of the body
2 Anatomic position
3 Some common movements
4 Skeletal landmarks (upper anterior)
5 Bones of the skeleton (lower anterior)
6 Skeletal landmarks (upper posterior)
7 Skeletal landmarks (lower posterior)
8 Muscles of anterior trunk
9 Muscles of anterior thorax and abdomen
10 Section through lactating breast
11 Fibrous supporting membranes in the breast
12 Lactating breast
Cartoon: Coracoid process and acromion
13 Skeletal landmarks (thorax and upper arm)
14 Skeletal landmarks (pelvis and hip)
15 Anterior thoracic muscles
16 Muscle attachments of the anterior thorax
17 Anterior thoracic wall seen from inside
18 Contents of thorax with anterior wall removed
19 Intercostal muscles
20 Intercostal muscles
21 Cross section of thoracic wall with intercostal arteries
22 Section of thoracic wall with intercostal arteries
23 Arteries of the thorax and upper arm
24 Thoracic spinal nerve
25 The pericardium
26 The interior of the posterior pericardial sac with the heart removed and the great vessels cut
27 Exterior of the heart
28 Interior of the heart
29 Trace the course of blood through the heart
30 The heart: ventricles exposed
31 Base and diaphragmatic surface of heart
32 Right atrium and right ventricle
33 Left ventricle
34 Heart valves and valve action
35 The four heart valves
Cartoon: Muscle
36 Coronary arteries (most common pattern)
37 Coronary veins
38 Cardiac conducting system
39 Cardiac fibrous skeleton
40 Aortic valve and its fibrous support
41 Nerves to the heart
42 Trachea, bronchi, and mediastinal surface of the lungs
43 Bronchopulmonary segments: left lung
44 Bronchopulmonary segments: right lung
45A Bronchopulmonary segment
45B Bronchopulmonary segment
46 Lungs and pleura
47 The pleura and pleural recesses
48 Trachea, esophagus, and vagus nerve
49 Right mediastinum
50 Left mediastinum
51 Diaphragm
52 Azygos vein and its tributaries
53 Blood flow in the fetus
54 Fetal heart in late development
55 Circulatory changes after birth
56 Thoracic splanchnic nerves
57 Autonomic nervous system
58 Thoracic duct and related structures
59 Mediastinum after removal of heart and pericardium
60 Cross section at thorax level of bifurcation of pulmonary trunk
61 Cross section of thorax just below pulmonary valve
62 Cross section of thorax just below aortic valve
63 Cross section of thorax at level of male nipple
64 Cross section of thorax with right dome of diaphragm and right lobe of liver

Part II: The Abdomen

Cartoon: Duodenum
1. Segmental innervation of the skin of the anterior trunk
2. Muscles of the anterior and lateral abdominal walls I
3. Muscles of the anterior and lateral abdominal walls II
4. Muscles and layers of the anterior abdominal wall
5. External abdominal oblique aponeurosis and superficial inguinal ring
6. Inguinal canal dissection
7. Inguinal ligament and related structures
8. Lower anterior abdomen wall viewed from the inside
9. Thoracic and abdominal viscera after removal of anterior thoracic and abdominal walls
10. Thorax and abdominal viscera in relation to the skeleton, anterior view
11. Frontal (coronal) section of the trunk
12. Thoracic and abdominal viscera, left aspect
13. Thoracic and abdominal viscera, right aspect
14. Thoracic and abdominal viscera in relation to the skeleton, posterior view
15. Midsagittal section of the female peritoneal cavity
16. The stomach
17. Blood supply of the stomach
18. Stomach, duodenum, and pancreas
19. Pancreas, duodenum, and spleen

Cartoon. Some Latin anatomic terms
20. Celiac trunk and its branches
21. Nerve supply of the stomach
22. The liver (hepar)
23. Liver, visceral surface (posterior/inferior aspect)
24A. The intestines I
24B. The intestines II
25. Distribution of the superior mesenteric artery and vein
26. Blood supply of the jejunum
27. Blood supply to the small intestine
28. Mucosa of jejunum and ileum
29. Blood supply of large intestine
30. Ileocecal valve, vermiform appendix, terminal ileum, and cecum
31. Arterial supply of vermiform appendix, terminal ileum, and cecum
32. The hepatic portal system
33. Posterior abdominal wall, peritoneal attachments
34. Posterior abdominal wall, kidneys, and related structures
35. The kidney I
36. The kidney II
37. Posterior abdominal wall, showing principal muscles and nerves

Part III: Pelvis

Cartoon: Testicle, Latin, little witness
1. Hip (coxal) bone, lateral aspect
2. Hip bone, medial aspect
3. Hip bone lines of fusion
4. Male pelvis dissection
5. Male pelvis median section
6. Male reproductive organs
7. The penis
8. Scrotum and spermatic cord
9. The testis
10. Urethral sphincter in the male
11. Male pelvis, frontal section I
12. Male pelvis, frontal section II
13. Pelvis and perineum
14. Muscles of male perineum
15. Nerves and arteries of the male perineum
16. Male pelvis and perineal muscles
17. Arterial supply of male pelvis
18. Male urogenital tract
19. Autonomic ganglia and nerves in the male abdomen and pelvis
20. Female perineum
21. Female erectile tissue
22. Clitoris and vestibular bulb
23. Female pelvis, median section
24. Female superficial perineal muscles
25. Nerves of female perineum
26. Arteries of the female perineum
27. The uterus
28. Female pelvic diaphragm and related structures
29. Female pelvis from the front and above
30. Uterus and related structures
31. Female pelvic diaphragm from above
32. Arterial supply of the female pelvis
33. Muscles on medial surface of pelvis
34. Female urogenital sphincter I
35. Female striated urethral sphincter II
36. Pelvis and ligaments

This book allows the reader to learn human anatomy in a simple and direct manner by coloring and labeling key anatomical structures. Many students will be engaged in anatomical dissection in the gross anatomy laboratory (the word *anatomy* comes from the Greek "to cut").

These plates cover the seven regions of the body. The traditional color scheme of anatomy textbooks and atlases is red for arteries, blue for veins, yellow for nerves, pink to reddish brown for muscles, and white or light tan for bones. The reader will find that good quality sharp color pencils work quite well.

There is very little explanatory text. In a few places, short paragraphs have been added that impart important aspects of applied anatomy. Etymological cartoons are interspersed throughout for a brief change and convey some information about Latin and Greek roots.

Color pencils ready... go!

Ray Poritsky, Ph.D.

ACKNOWLEDGMENTS

Many of the illustrations were drawn by the author, who has had formal training in anatomy and medical illustration. Additional drawings were done by Helen Williams, Susan Weil, Cheryl Owens, and James Bille. The author used the following texts as source materials: Spalteholz and Spanner: *Atlas of Human Anatomy*, 16th ed., Philadelphia, F.A. Davis, 1961; Wolf-Heidegger: *Atlas of Systematic Human Anatomy*, New York, Hafner, 1962; Hollinshead and Rosse: *Textbook of Anatomy*, 4th ed., Philadelphia, Harper and Row, 1985; Netter: *The Ciba Collection of Medical Illustrations*, Summit, NJ, Ciba Pharmaceutical Company, 1959, 1962; Clemente: *Anatomy: A Regional Atlas of the Human Body*, 3rd ed., Baltimore and Munich, Urban & Schwarzenberg, 1987; Rohen and Yokochi: *Color Atlas of Anatomy: A Photographic Study of the Human Body*, New York and Tokyo, Igaku-Shoin, 1984; Moore: *Clinically Oriented Anatomy*, Baltimore, Williams & Wilkins, 1982; Clemente: *Anatomy of the Human Body*, 13th ed., Philadelphia, Lea & Febiger, 1985; Williams and Warwick: *Gray's Anatomy*, 36th British ed., Edinburgh, Churchill Livingstone, 1980; Anson: *Morris' Human Anatomy: A Complete Systematic Treatise*, 12th ed., New York, McGraw-Hill, 1966; Pernkopf: *Atlas of Topographical and Applied Human Anatomy*, Munich, Urban & Schwarzenberg, 1980. I also found certain Somso anatomical models most helpful for several of the drawings.

The following sources were employed for the section on The Upper Limb and The Lower Limb and are gratefully acknowledged. Several figures were drawn by Cheryl Owens and Wayne Timmerman. Illustrations are reworked and updated figures from Eycleshymer and Jones: *Hand Atlas of Clinical Anatomy*, Lea & Febiger, 1925. Other atlases and texts consulted include: Wolf-Heidegger: *Atlas of Systemic Human Anatomy*, Hafner, 1962; Spalteholz and Spanner: *Atlas of Human Anatomy*, 16th ed., F.A. Davis, 1961; Hollinshead and Rosse: *Textbook of Anatomy*, 4th ed., Harper and Row, 1985; Clemente: *A Regional Atlas of the Human Body*, 3rd ed., Urban & Schwarzenberg, 1987; Töndury: *Angewandte und Topographische Anatomie*, Fretz & Wasmuth, 1949; Williams (ed): *Gray's Anatomy*, 38th British ed., Churchill Livingstone, 1995; Netter: *The Ciba Collection of Medical Illustrations*, Ciba Pharmaceutical Company, 1959.

I thank and warmly dedicate this book to my wife Connie.

Part I: Introduction and Thorax

The Four "Birds" of the Thorax
(A Shameless Pun)

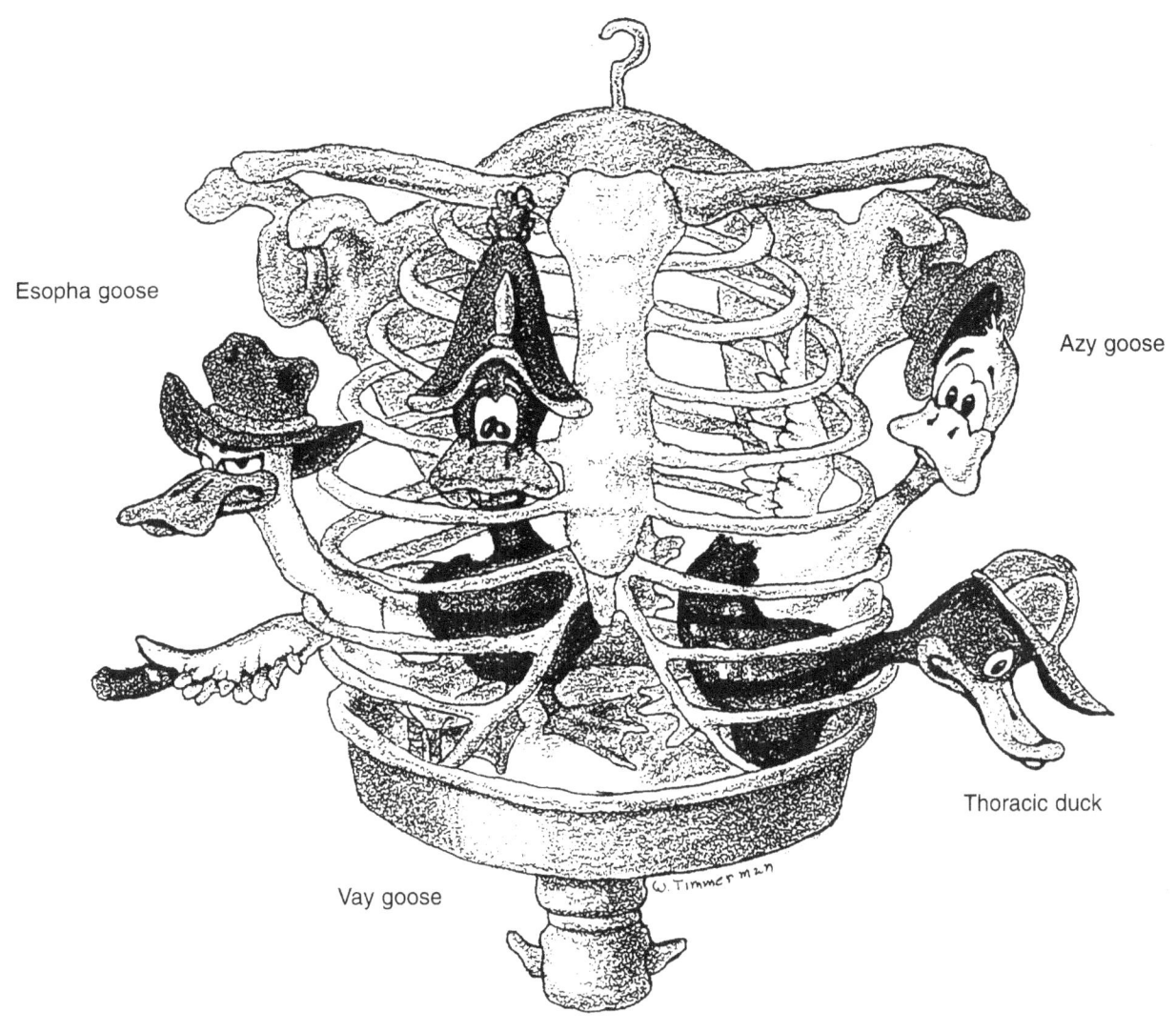

The "Esopha goose" is the esophagus

The "Azy goose" is the azygos vein

The "Vay goose" is the vagus nerve

The "Thoracic duck" is the thoracic duct
(the largest lymph vessel in the body)

Th-1 Planes of the Body

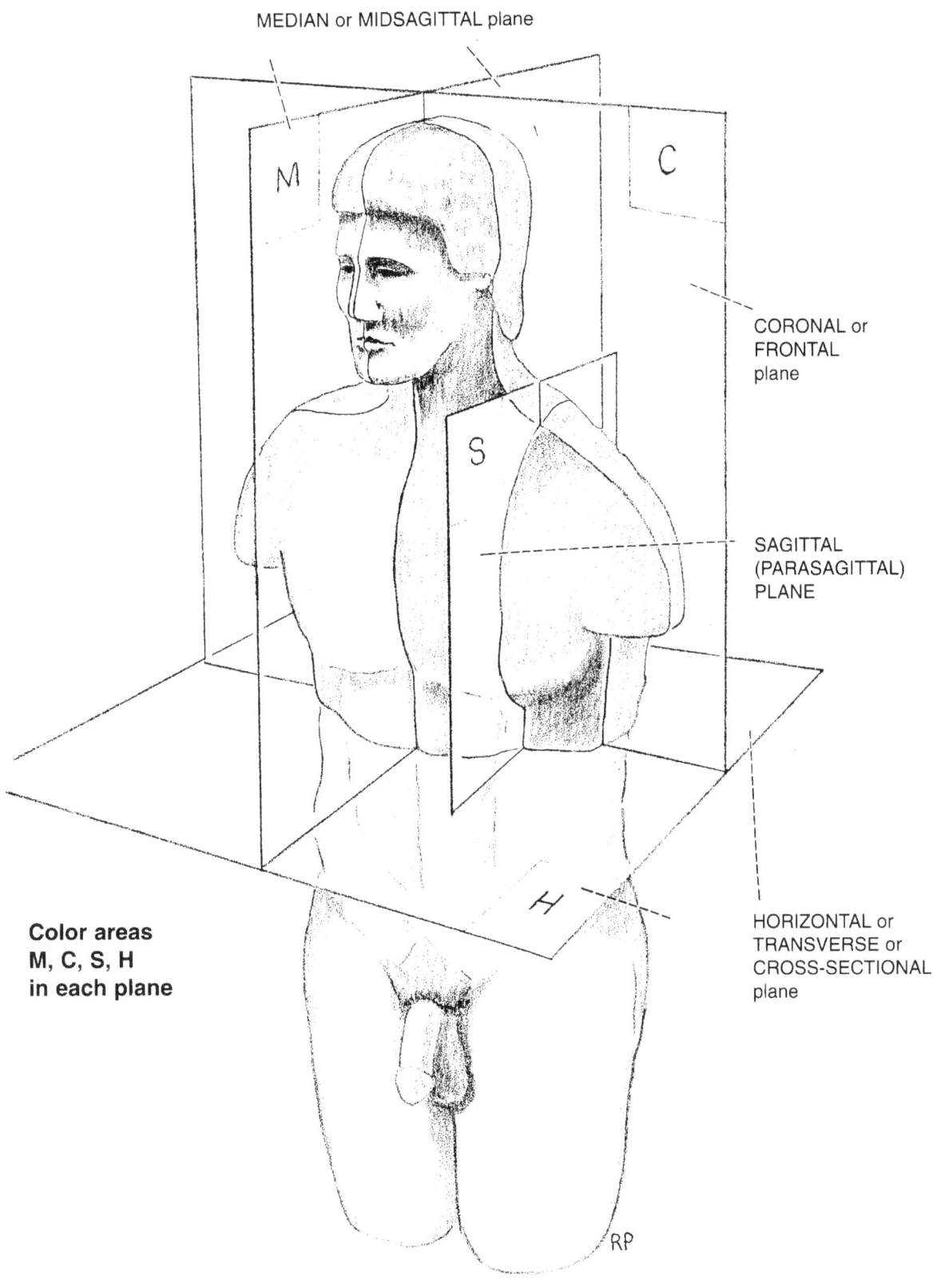

MEDIAN or MIDSAGITTAL plane

CORONAL or FRONTAL plane

SAGITTAL (PARASAGITTAL) PLANE

HORIZONTAL or TRANSVERSE or CROSS-SECTIONAL plane

Color areas M, C, S, H in each plane

Th-2 Anatomic position

Color each arrow

SUPERIOR

PROXIMAL

DISTAL

VENTRAL
ANTERIOR

DORSAL
POSTERIOR

MEDIAL

LATERAL

INFERIOR

CAPUT (HEAD)
CERVIX (NECK)
BRACHIUM (UPPER ARM)
ANTEBRACHIUM (FOREARM)
POLLEX (THUMB)
THUMB LATERAL
GENU (KNEE)
CRUS (LOWER LEG)
SURA (CALF)
RP
HALLUX (BIG TOE)

In the anatomic position the body is erect with the hands at the sides and the palms facing forward. Thus the thumb is lateral and the little finger medial. The head is described as superior and the feet inferior even when the body is horizontal. (After S. R. Peck, *An Atlas of Human Anatomy for the Artist*, New York, Oxford University Press, 1986.)

Th-3 Some common movements

- ARM FLEXED
- ELBOW FLEXED
- WRIST AND FINGERS FLEXED
- WRIST AND FINGERS EXTENDED
- KNEE FLEXED
- HIP (THIGH) FLEXED
- ARM FULLY ELEVATED
- THUMB AND FINGERS EXTENDED
- LEG (THIGH) ABDUCTED
- ARM FULLY ABDUCTED

Color each figure

Th-4 Skeletal landmarks
(upper anterior view)

Color and label

1 Frontal bone
2 Zygomatic bone
3 Maxillary bone
4 Mandible
5 Clavicle
6 First rib
7 Manubrium
8 Sternum (body)
9 Xiphoid process
10 Costal cartilage of rib 7
11 Acromion process of scapula
12 Humerus
13 Radius
14 Ulna
15 Carpal bones (wrist bones)
16 Coracoid process of scapula
17 Scapula (shoulder blade)
18 Fifth lumbar vertebra
19 Ilium of coxal (hip) bone
20 Sacrum
21 Greater trochanter of femur
22 Pubic symphysis

13 _____
14 _____
15 _____
16 _____
17 _____
18 _____
19 _____
20 _____
21 _____
22 _____

1 _____
2 _____
3 _____
4 _____
5 _____
6 _____
7 _____
8 _____
9 _____
10 _____
11 _____
12 _____

Continued on opposite page

Th-5 Bones of the skeleton
(lower anterior view)

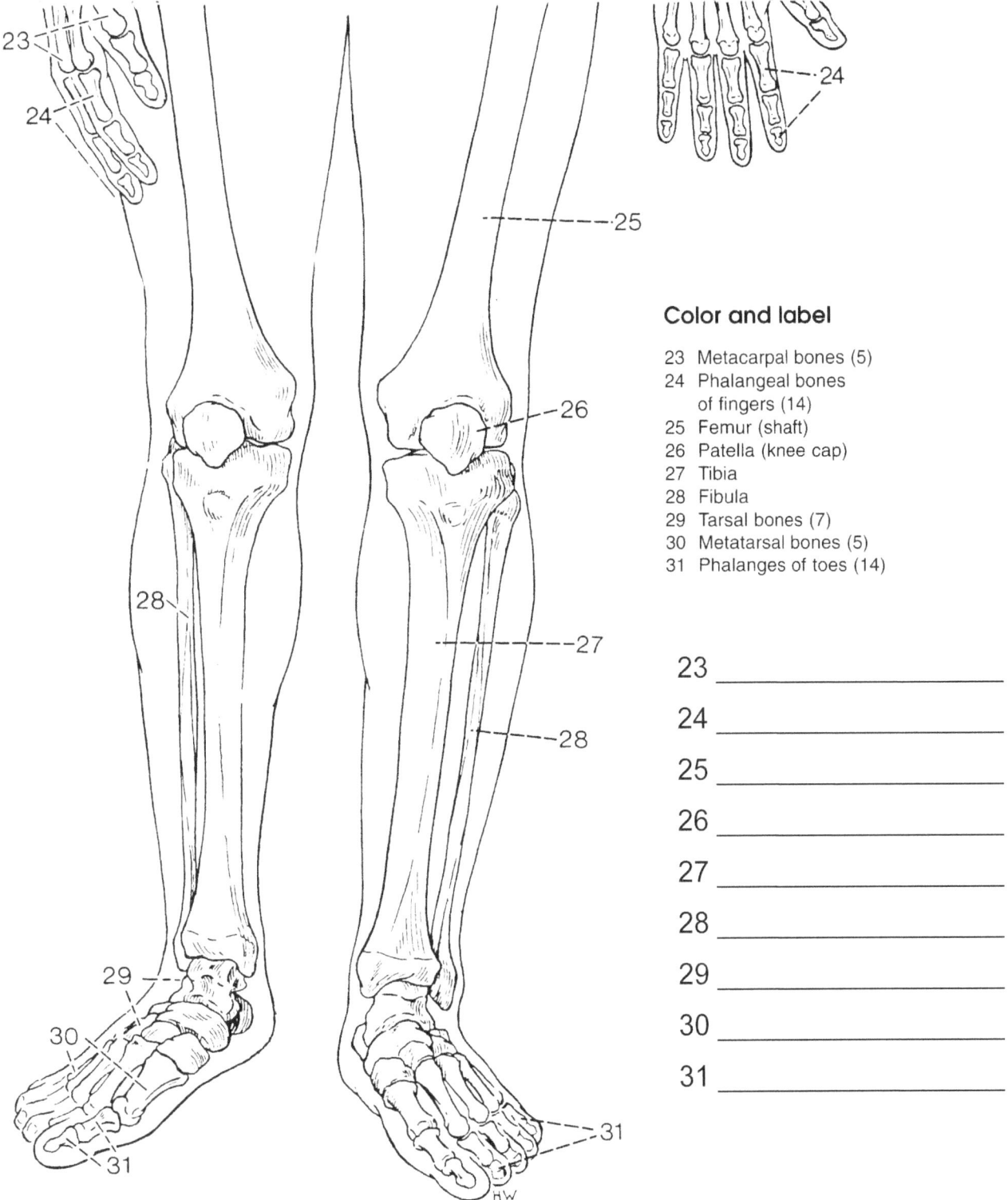

Color and label

23 Metacarpal bones (5)
24 Phalangeal bones of fingers (14)
25 Femur (shaft)
26 Patella (knee cap)
27 Tibia
28 Fibula
29 Tarsal bones (7)
30 Metatarsal bones (5)
31 Phalanges of toes (14)

23 _____
24 _____
25 _____
26 _____
27 _____
28 _____
29 _____
30 _____
31 _____

Th-6 Skeletal landmarks
(upper posterior view)

Color and label these bones

Seven cervical vertebrae (C1-C7)
Twelve thoracic vertebrae (T1-T12)
Five lumbar vertebrae (L1-L5)
Twelve pairs of ribs
Scapula
Humerus
Ulna
Radius

Note that cervical vertabrae C1 and C2, unlike the other 25 vertebrae, have their own names, **atlas** and **axis** respectively.

Label these landmarks

1 Parietal bones
2 Occipital bone
3 Sagittal suture
4 Lamboid suture
5 First cervical vertebra (atlas)
6 Second cervical vertebra (axis)
7 Acromion of scapula
8 Spine of scapula
9 Infraspinous fossa
10 Greater tubercle of humerus
11 Lateral epicondyle
12 Olecranon of ulna
13 Head of radius
14 Ilium of coxal bone

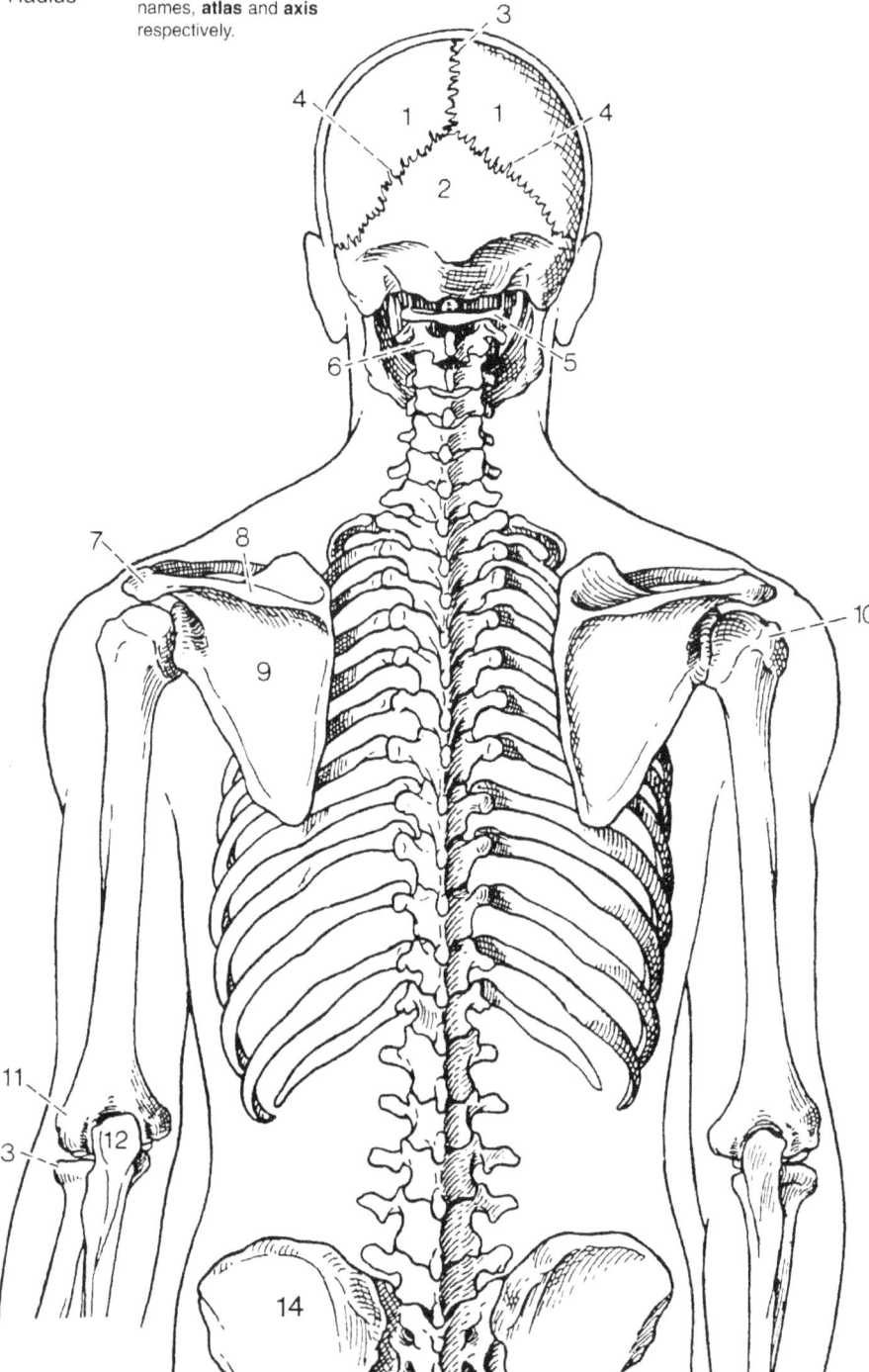

1 _____
2 _____
3 _____
4 _____
5 _____
6 _____
7 _____
8 _____
9 _____
10 _____
11 _____
12 _____
13 _____
14 _____

Continued on opposite page

Th-7 Skeletal landmarks
(lower posterior view)

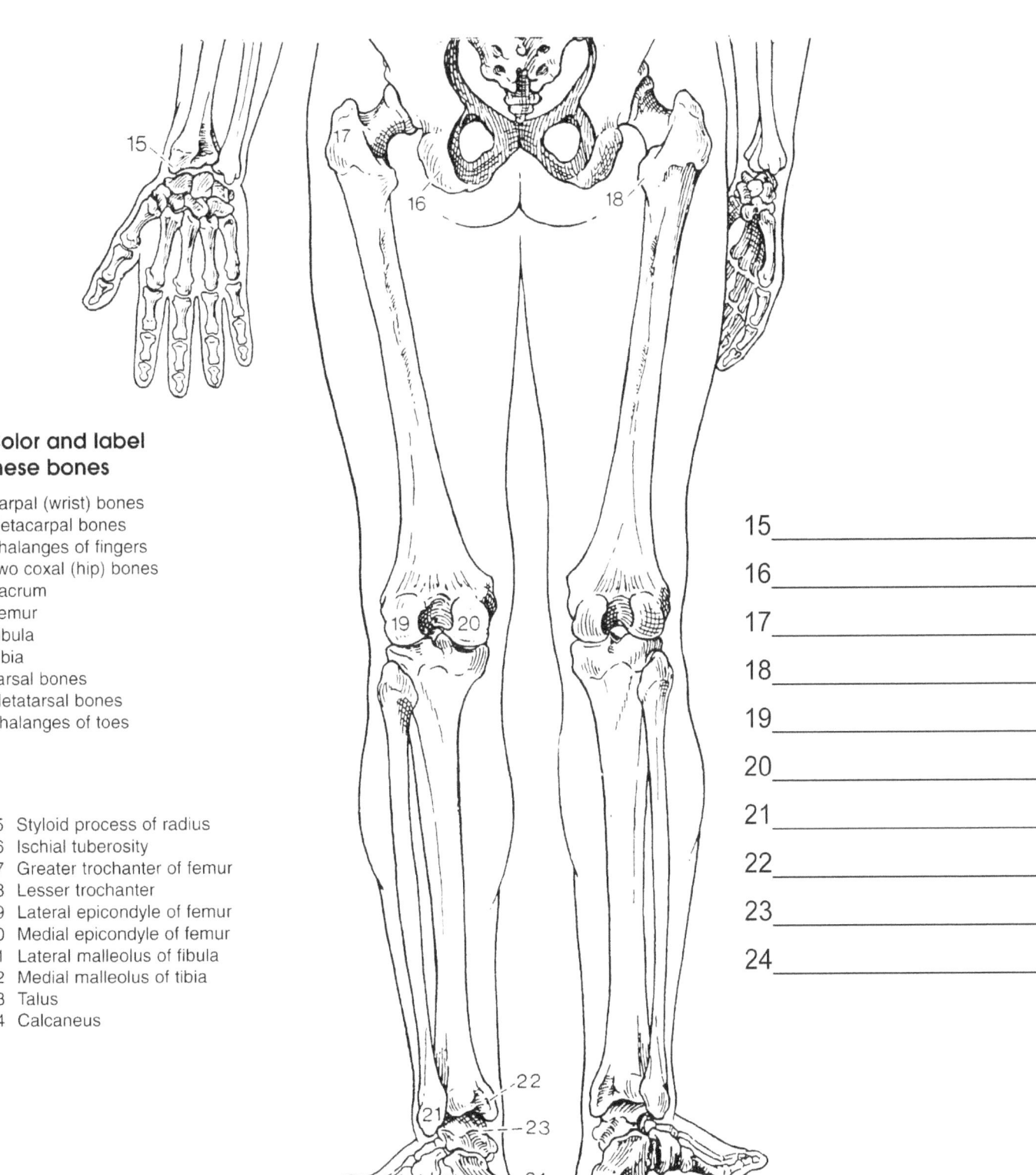

Color and label these bones

Carpal (wrist) bones
Metacarpal bones
Phalanges of fingers
Two coxal (hip) bones
Sacrum
Femur
Fibula
Tibia
Tarsal bones
Metatarsal bones
Phalanges of toes

15 Styloid process of radius
16 Ischial tuberosity
17 Greater trochanter of femur
18 Lesser trochanter
19 Lateral epicondyle of femur
20 Medial epicondyle of femur
21 Lateral malleolus of fibula
22 Medial malleolus of tibia
23 Talus
24 Calcaneus

15 _____
16 _____
17 _____
18 _____
19 _____
20 _____
21 _____
22 _____
23 _____
24 _____

Th-8 Muscles of the anterior trunk
(opposite page)

Color and label

1. Pectoralis major
2. Subclavius
3. Trapezius
4. Coracoid process
5. Deltoid (cut)
6. Tendon of long head of biceps brachii
7. Pectoralis minor
8. Long head of biceps brachii
9. Short head of biceps brachii
10. Latissimus dorsi
11. Internal intercostal seen beneath membrane of external intercostal
12. Rectus abdominis (cut)
13. Rectus sheath (posterior layer)
14. Semicircular line (lower border of posterior layer)
15. Internal abdominal oblique
16. Rectus abdominis (cut)
17. Great saphenous vein
18. Sartorius
19. Femoral vein
20. Margin of saphenous hiatus (falciform margin)
21. Spermatic cord
22. Umbilicus
23. Linea alba
24. Rectus sheath (anterior layer)
25. External abdominal oblique
26. Digitations of serratus anterior
27. Deltoid
28. Sternum
29. Clavicle
30. Trapezius
31. Sternocleidomastoid
32. Sternocleidomastoid sternal clavicular origins (cut)

1 _____
2 _____
3 _____
4 _____
5 _____
6 _____
7 _____
8 _____
9 _____
10 _____
11 _____
12 _____
13 _____
14 _____
15 _____
16 _____
17 _____
18 _____
19 _____
20 _____
21 _____
22 _____

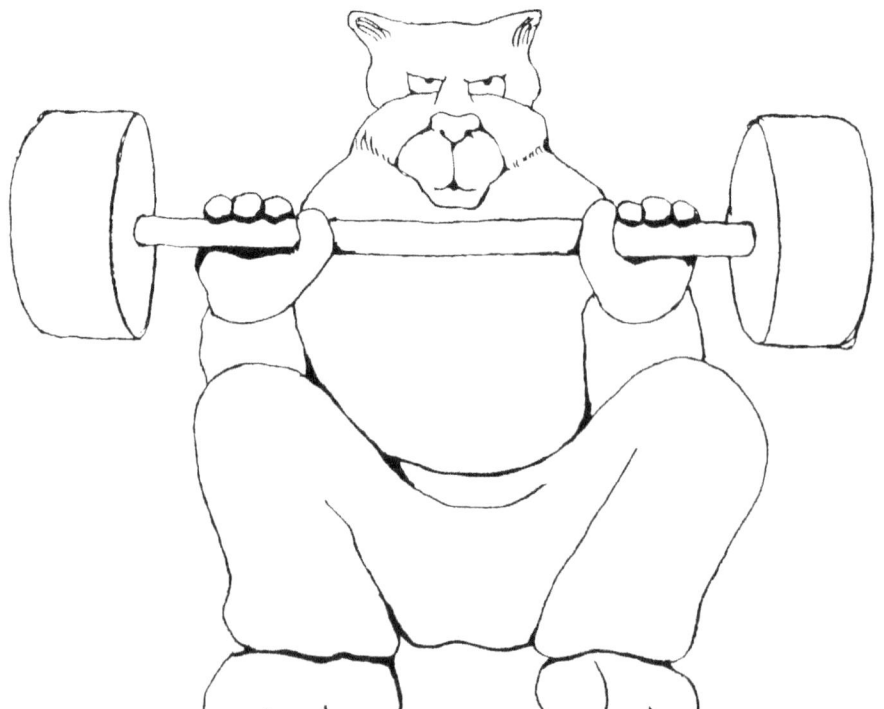

The word muscle originally meant "little mouse"

Th-8 Muscles of anterior trunk

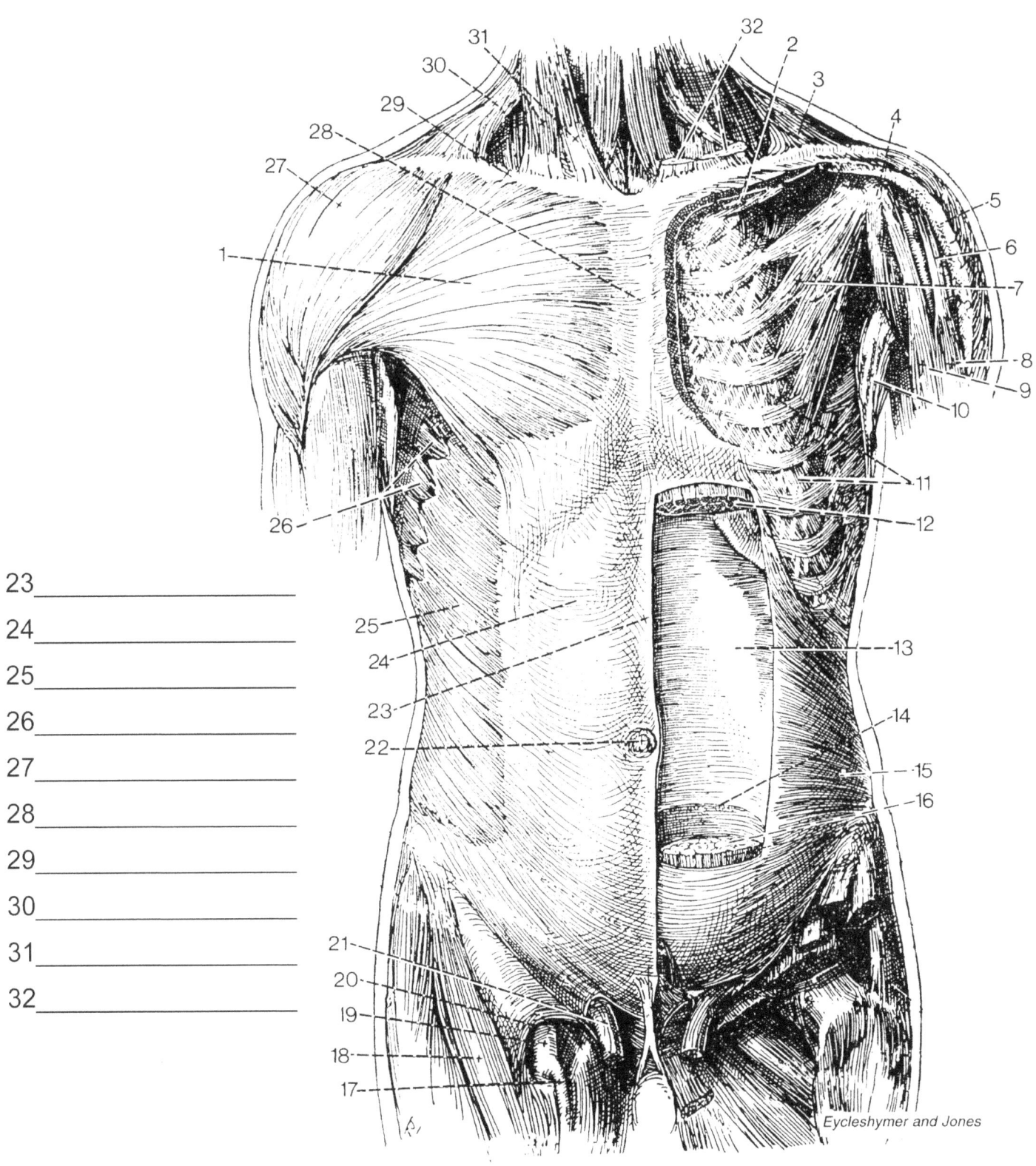

23 _____
24 _____
25 _____
26 _____
27 _____
28 _____
29 _____
30 _____
31 _____
32 _____

Eycleshymer and Jones

11

Th-9 Muscles of anterior thorax and abdomen

1 _____
2 _____
3 _____
4 _____
5 _____
6 _____
7 _____
8 _____
9 _____
10 _____
11 _____

Color and label
1 Pectoralis major
2 Serratus anterior
3 Rectus abdominis
4 Tendinous intersection
5 Rectus sheath (cut)
6 External abdominal oblique
7 Internal abdominal oblique
8 Deltoid
9 Sternocleidomastoid
10 Sartorius
11 Latissimus dorsi

After E. A. Seeman, Fritz Schiders Plastisch-Anatomischer Handatlas (after Duval-Neelsen). Leipzig, M. Averbach and Franz V. Stuck Verlag, 1929.

Th-10 Section through lactating breast

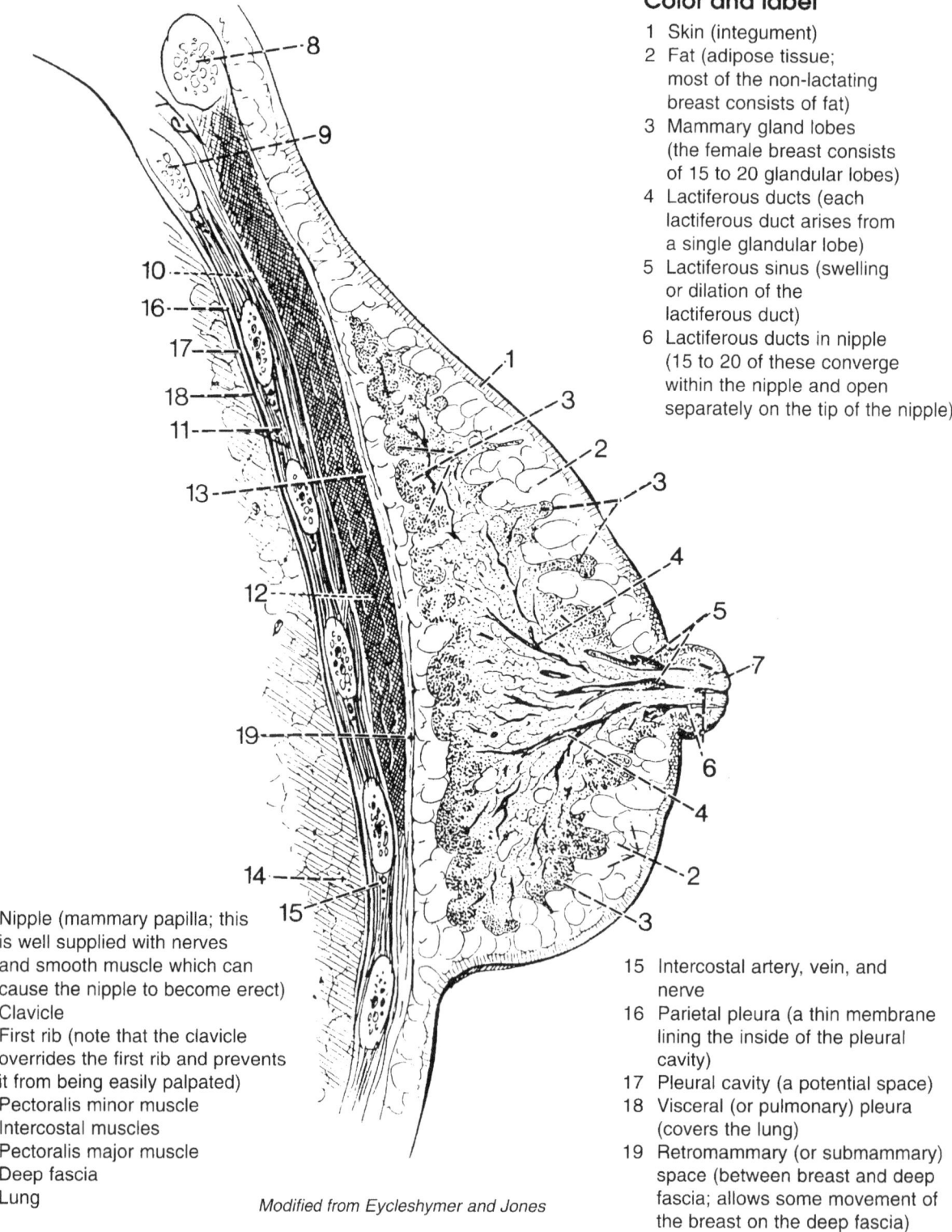

Color and label

1. Skin (integument)
2. Fat (adipose tissue; most of the non-lactating breast consists of fat)
3. Mammary gland lobes (the female breast consists of 15 to 20 glandular lobes)
4. Lactiferous ducts (each lactiferous duct arises from a single glandular lobe)
5. Lactiferous sinus (swelling or dilation of the lactiferous duct)
6. Lactiferous ducts in nipple (15 to 20 of these converge within the nipple and open separately on the tip of the nipple)
7. Nipple (mammary papilla; this is well supplied with nerves and smooth muscle which can cause the nipple to become erect)
8. Clavicle
9. First rib (note that the clavicle overrides the first rib and prevents it from being easily palpated)
10. Pectoralis minor muscle
11. Intercostal muscles
12. Pectoralis major muscle
13. Deep fascia
14. Lung
15. Intercostal artery, vein, and nerve
16. Parietal pleura (a thin membrane lining the inside of the pleural cavity)
17. Pleural cavity (a potential space)
18. Visceral (or pulmonary) pleura (covers the lung)
19. Retromammary (or submammary) space (between breast and deep fascia; allows some movement of the breast on the deep fascia)

Modified from Eycleshymer and Jones

Th-10 Section through lactating breast
(opposite page)

1 _____
2 _____
3 _____
4 _____
5 _____
6 _____
7 _____
8 _____
9 _____
10 _____
11 _____
12 _____
13 _____
14 _____
15 _____
16 _____
17 _____
18 _____
19 _____

Th-11 Fibrous supporting membranes in the breast

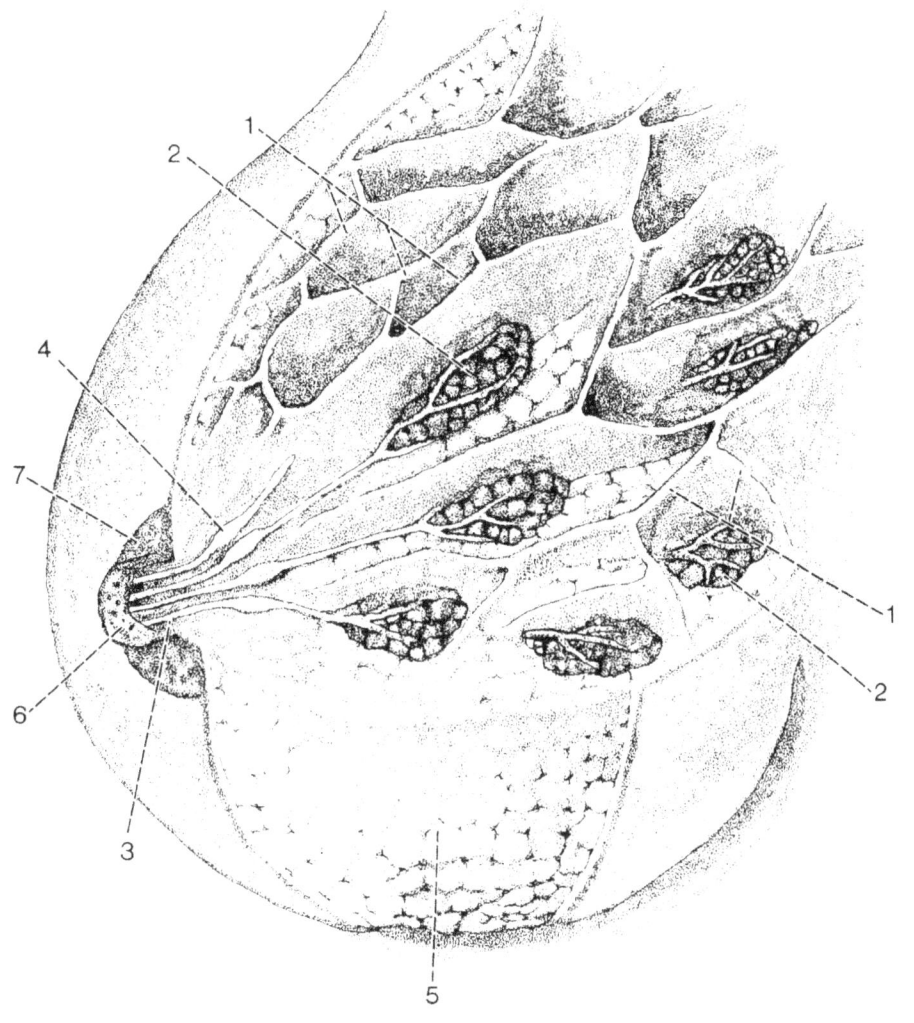

Color and label

1. Fibrous septa (partitions) extend from the fascia around the mammary gland lobes to the skin; they are most prominent in the upper part of the breast where they were once called the suspensory ligaments of Cooper.
2. Mammary gland lobes 15 to 20 in number; these are roughly pyramidal in shape with their apices pointed towards the nipple. Most, but not all, enlarge during lactation and secrete milk.
3. Lactiferous duct; each glandular lobe is drained by its own duct which opens separately as one of 15-20 tiny orifices on the nipple.
4. Lactiferous sinus; swellings in the ducts which accumulate milk during lactation
5. Fat (adipose tissue)
6. Nipple (Latin, *papilla*); note that the nipple is traversed by 15-20 lactiferous ducts.
7. Areola; pigmented area of skin that surrounds the nipple; during pregnancy and lactation, small areolar glands secrete a protective oily substance.

1_____
2_____
3_____
4_____
5_____
6_____
7_____

Th-12 Lactating breast

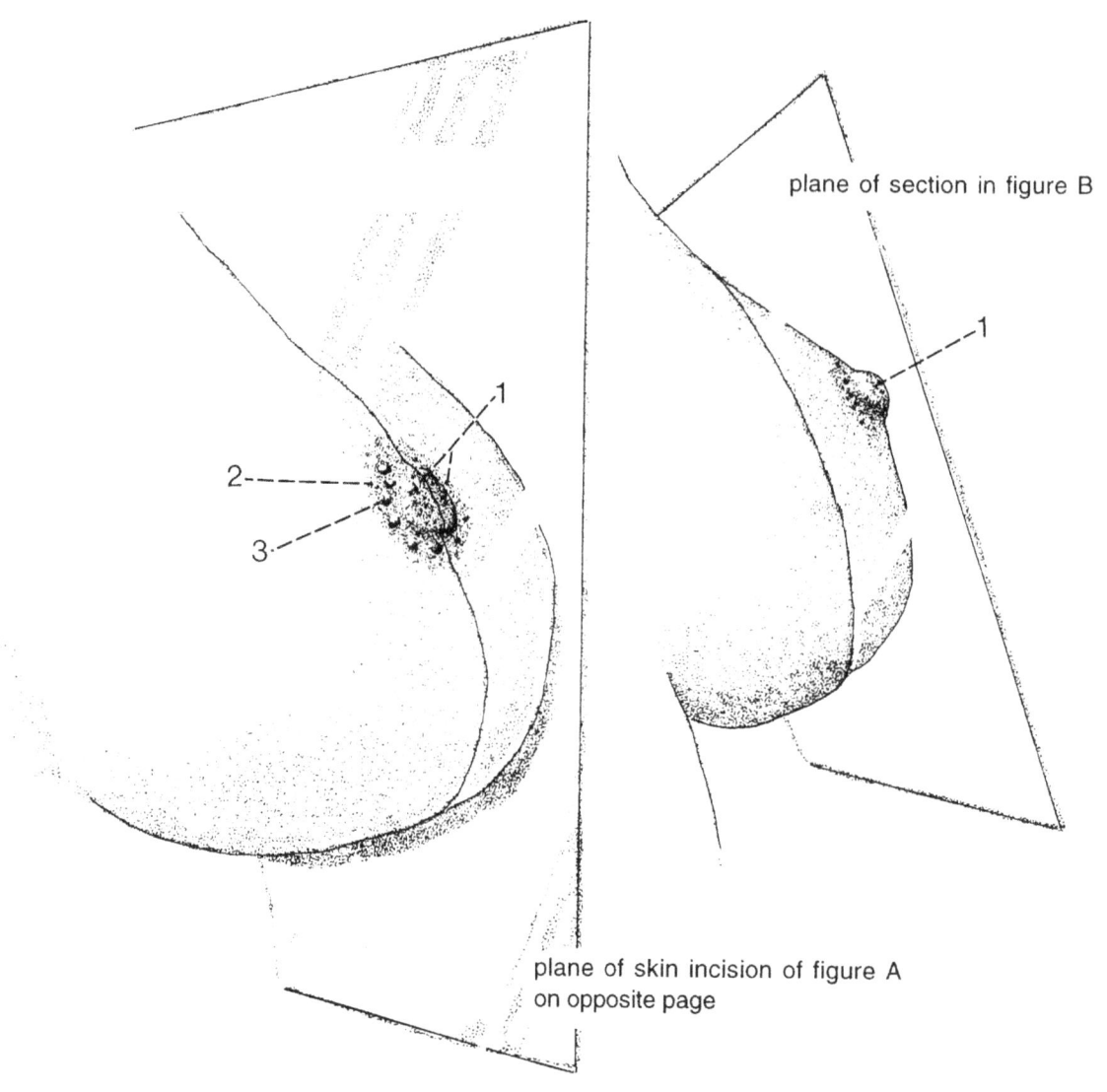

plane of section in figure B

plane of skin incision of figure A on opposite page

Color and label

1 Nipple (papilla)
2 Areola
3 Areolar glands
4 Nipple with 15 to 20 openings (orifices) of main lactiferous ducts
5 Main lactiferous duct (each drains a single glandular lobe)
6 Mammary gland lobes (15 to 20 in number; note their pyramidal shape with their apices directed forward towards the nipple; these are greatly enlarged during lactation)
7 Lactiferous ampulla (sinus or dilation of the lactiferous duct)
8 Fat (fills the spaces between the glandular lobes and smooths out the contour of the breast; fat is metabolically consumed during lactation)
9 Fibrous membranes or septa (these extend from the glandular lobes to the skin; they are most prominent in the upper part of the breast where they are called the suspensory ligaments of Cooper; the fibrous septa also form pockets which hold the fat)

1_____
2_____
3_____
4_____
5_____
6_____
7_____
8_____
9_____

Th-12 Lactating breast

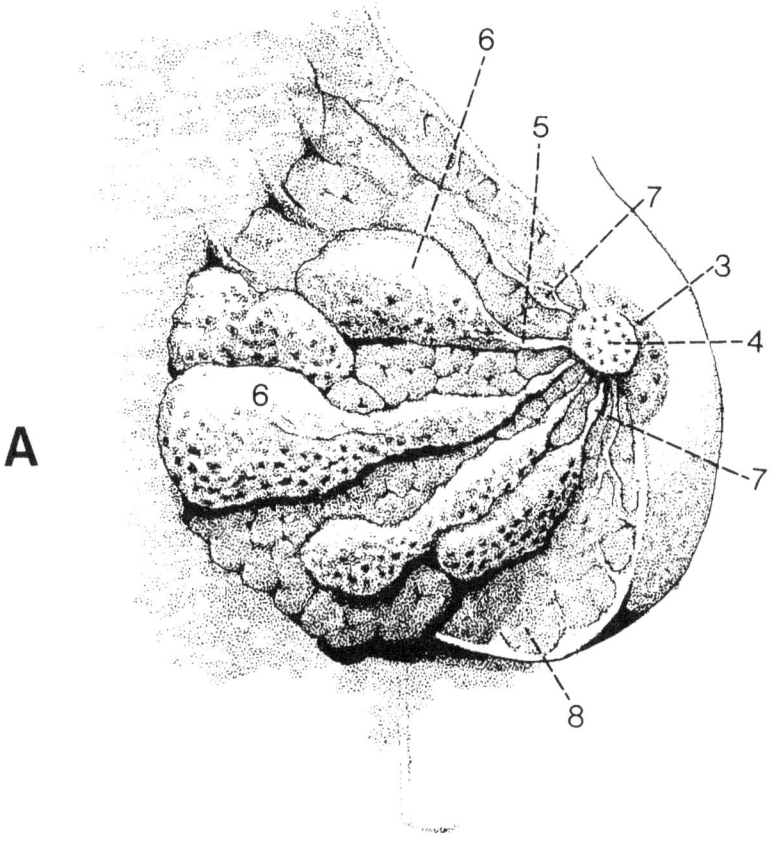

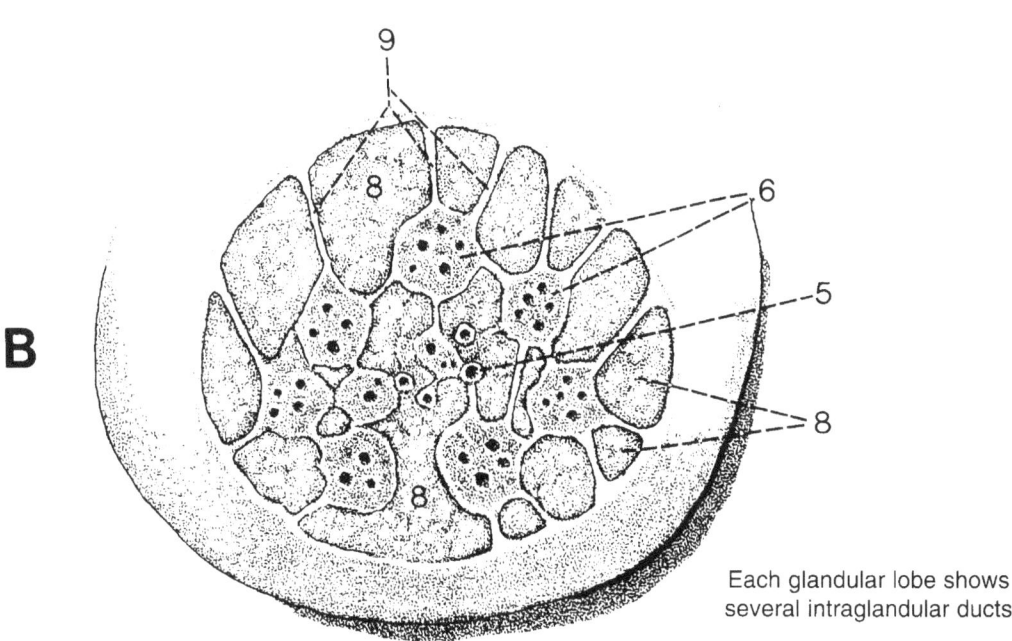

Each glandular lobe shows several intraglandular ducts

Coracoid Process and Acromion

The **scapula**, or shoulder blade, has two bony projections with rather interesting names. One of these projections is the **coracoid process**. Its name is derived from the Greek word for raven, *korax*, and means "shaped like a raven's beak" (*korax*, "raven" + *eidos*, "appearance"). The other bony projection is the **acromion**, and its name is derived from the Greek *akron*, "peak" or "extremity", and *omos*, "shoulder". The acromion can be felt as the bony prominence of the shoulder where it forms the expanded apex of the spine of the scapula.

An *acronym* is a word consisting of the first letters of a series of words. It is derived from *akron*, "first" or "initial" (used here in the sense of the *first* or *initial letter*) + *onyma*, "name". The government is especially adept at alphabetizing the names of government agencies with acronyms. The very early and famous acronym *ichthus* or *ichthys*, Greek for "fish", was used by early Christians as a symbol for "Jesus Christ, Son of God and Savior". The X in Xmas is from the Greek letter *X*, or chi, and stands for the first letter of the Greek word for Christ.

Rostrum means "beak" or "snout". In anatomy *rostrally* means "toward the nose". *Rostrum* also means a "ship's prow". The Roman Forum was ornamented with prows of ships captured from their enemies. These prows were used by orators to make speeches; thus, the word *rostrum* came to mean a stand for a speaker.

Scapula meant shoulder blade in Roman times, as it does today. A winged shoulder blade or scapula results from damage to the serratus anterior muscle often caused by the shoulder rest of a crutch repeatedly rubbing against the long thoracic nerve, which supplies the serratus anterior muscle.

Calcar avis ("bird's spur"; *calcar*, "spur" + *avis*, "bird") is a bump on the medial wall of the posterior horn in both lateral ventricles of the brain.

Pinna, or **penna**, means feather. Muscles are sometimes described as *bipennate* (like a feather with a central tendon) or *unipennate* (all the fibers obliquely attached to a tendon on one side).

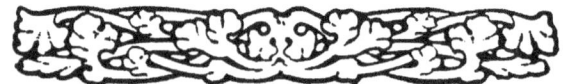

Coracoid process and acromion
An etymological cartoon

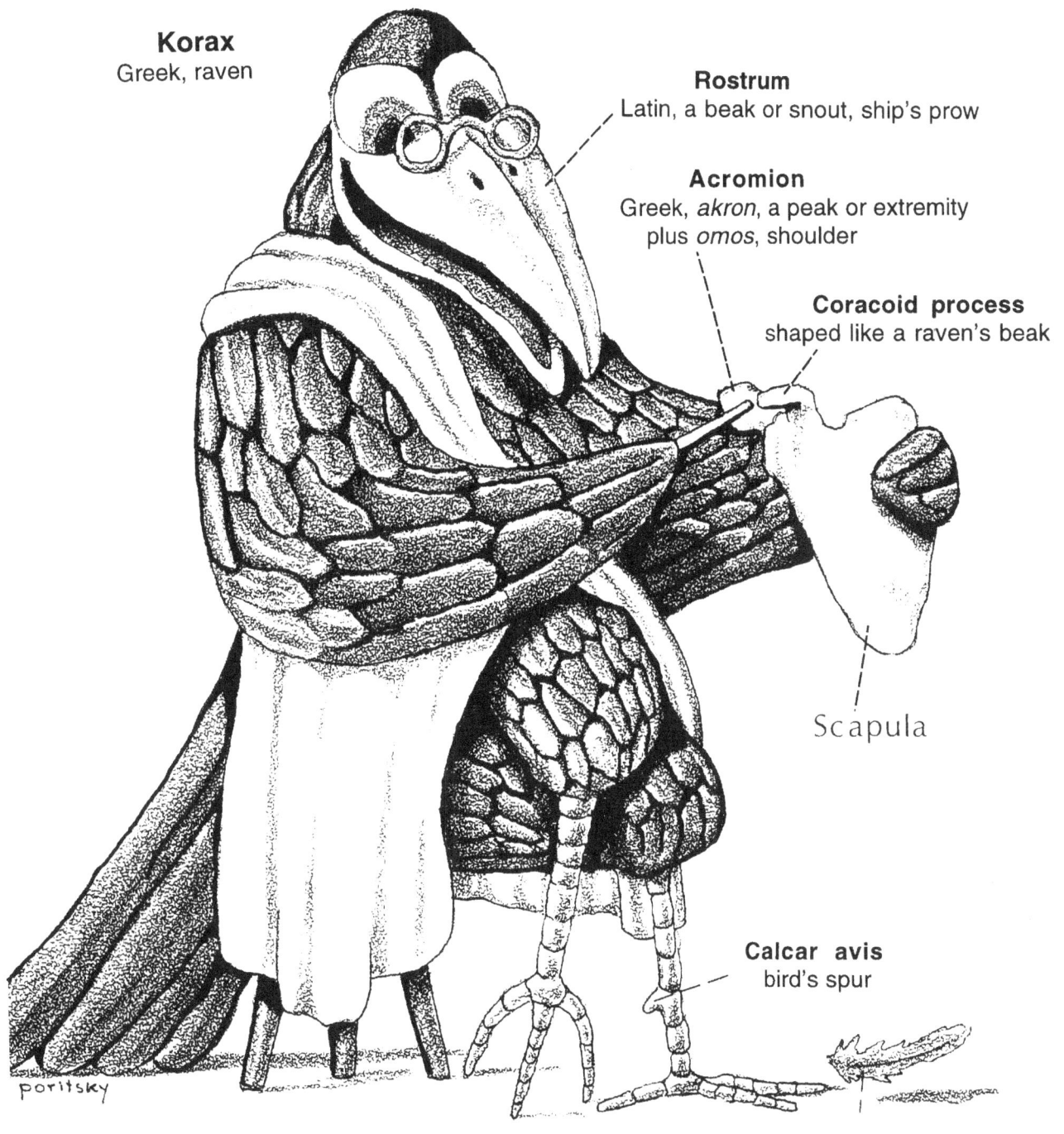

Th-13 Skeletal landmarks (thorax and upper arm)

Color the skeleton and label each of these landmarks

1 Greater tubercle of humerus
2 Lesser tubercle of humerus
3 Intertubercular groove
4 Head of humerus
5 Glenoid fossa of scapula
6 Coracoid process
7 Deltoid tuberosity
8 Clavicle
9 Jugular notch
10 Sternoclavicular joint
11 Acromion of scapula
12 Sternal angle
13 Rib 7; the first 7 ribs are "true ribs" because their costal cartilages attach directly to the sternum.

The bony thorax consists of the sternum (manubrium, body, xiphoid process), the 12 pairs of ribs on each side, and the 12 thoracic vertebrae.

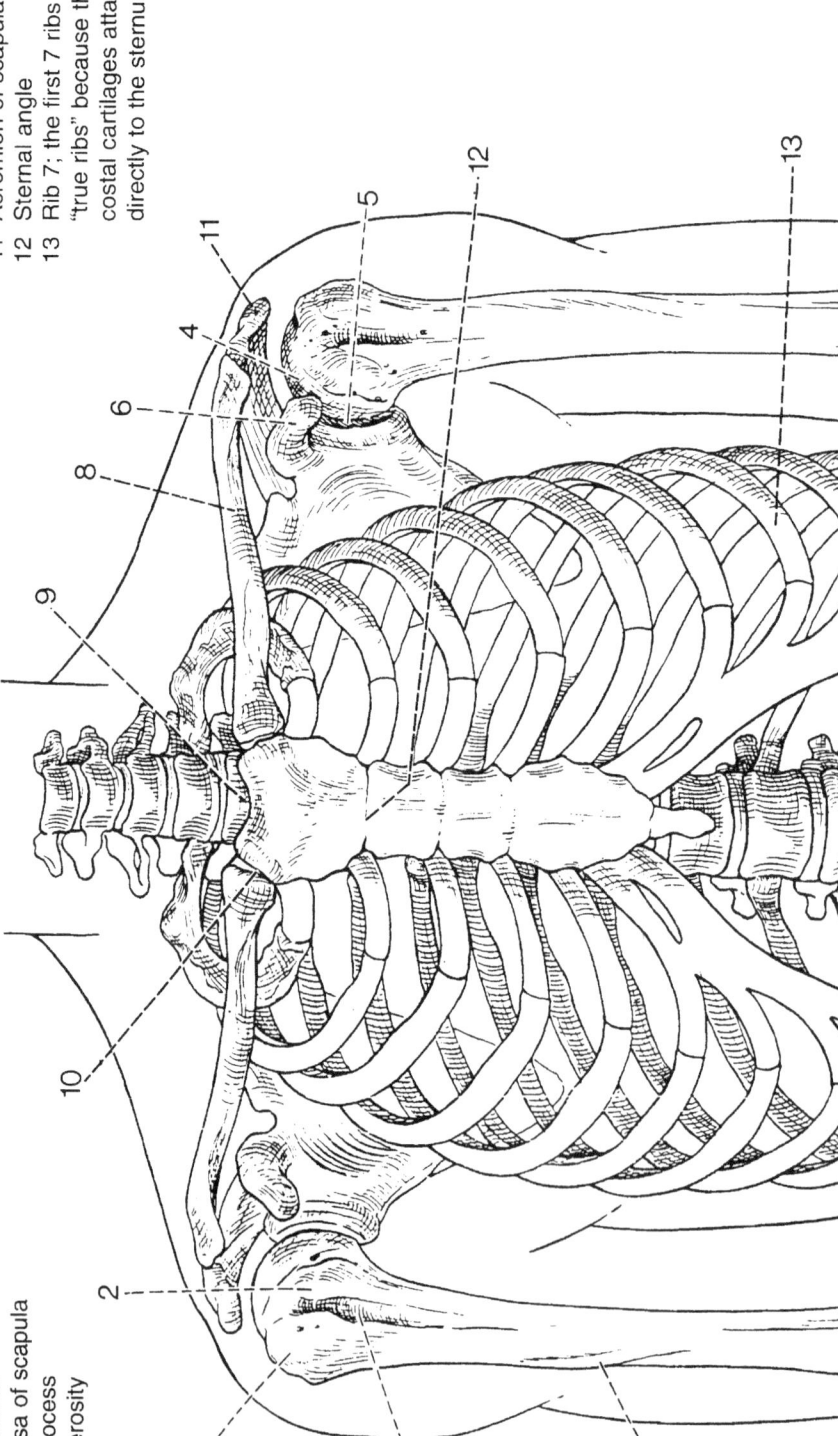

Ribs 8, 9, and 10 are "false" ribs because their costal cartilages do not reach the sternum, but rather attach to the costal cartilage of the rib above.

Ribs 11 and 12 are the "floating" ribs. They are short with very short costal cartilages that end freely. However, they do not float, since they articulate with thoracic vertebrae 11 and 12.

Continued on opposite page

Th-13 Skeletal landmarks (thorax and upper arm)
(opposite page)

1. _____
2. _____
3. _____
4. _____
5. _____
6. _____
7. _____
8. _____
9. _____
10. _____
11. _____
12. _____
13. _____

Th-14 Skeletal landmarks (pelvis and hip)

Color the skeleton and label each of these landmarks

14 Capitulum of humerus
15 Trochlea of humerus
16 Coronoid process of ulna
17 Radial tuberosity
18 Head of radius
19 Styloid process of radius
20 Styloid process of ulna

21 Ala of ilium
22 Iliac crest
23 Anterior superior iliac spine
24 Anterior inferior iliac spine
25 Head of femur
26 Neck of femur
27 Obturator foramen

Th-14 Skeletal landmarks (pelvis and hip)
(opposite page)

14 _____
15 _____
16 _____
17 _____
18 _____
19 _____
20 _____
21 _____
22 _____
23 _____
24 _____
25 _____
26 _____
27 _____

Th-15 Anterior thoracic muscles

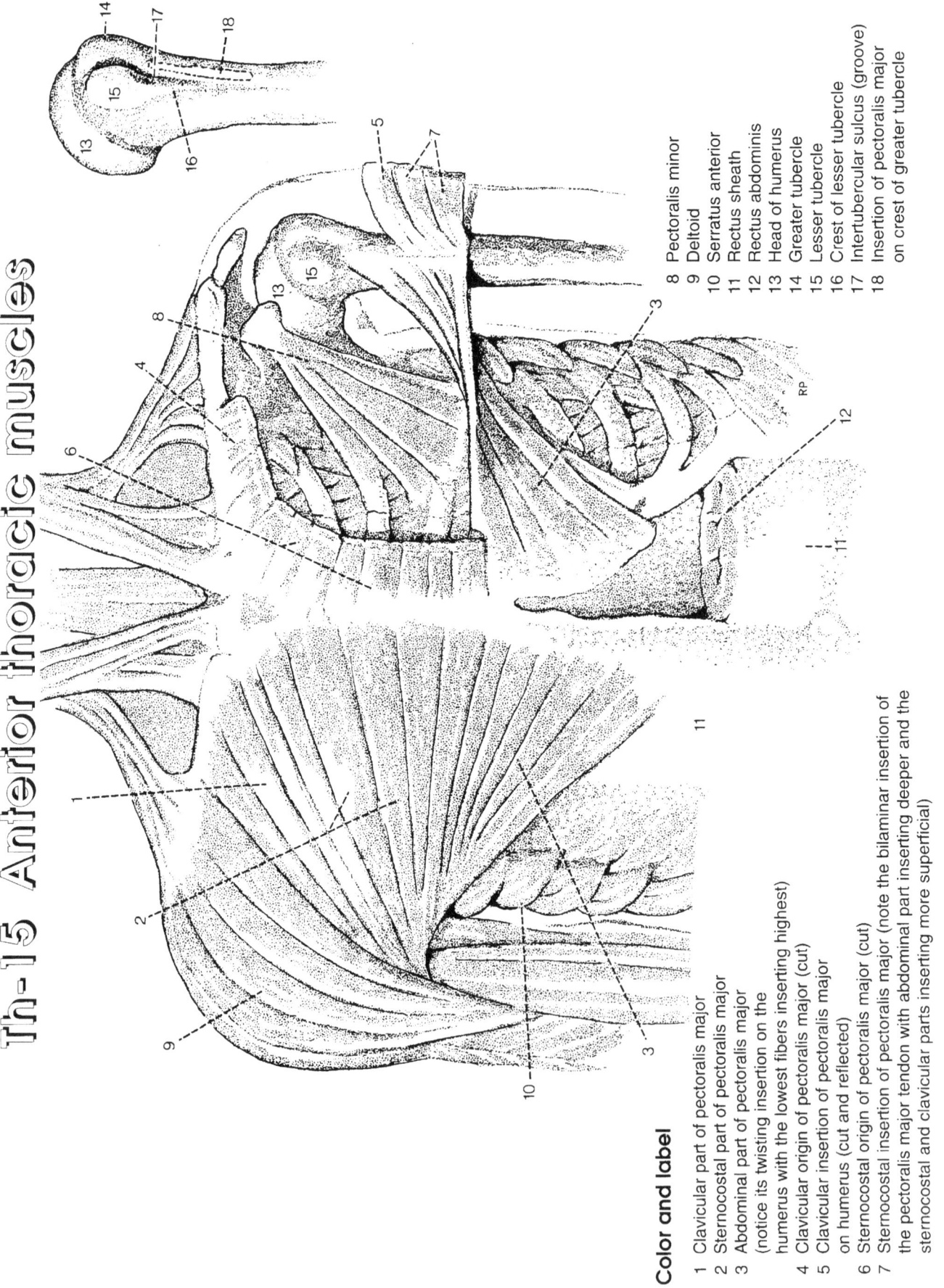

Color and label

1. Clavicular part of pectoralis major
2. Sternocostal part of pectoralis major
3. Abdominal part of pectoralis major (notice its twisting insertion on the humerus with the lowest fibers inserting highest)
4. Clavicular origin of pectoralis major (cut)
5. Clavicular insertion of pectoralis major on humerus (cut and reflected)
6. Sternocostal origin of pectoralis major (cut)
7. Sternocostal insertion of pectoralis major (note the bilaminar insertion of the pectoralis major tendon with abdominal part inserting deeper and the sternocostal and clavicular parts inserting more superficial)
8. Pectoralis minor
9. Deltoid
10. Serratus anterior
11. Rectus sheath
12. Rectus abdominis
13. Head of humerus
14. Greater tubercle
15. Lesser tubercle
16. Crest of lesser tubercle
17. Intertubercular sulcus (groove)
18. Insertion of pectoralis major on crest of greater tubercle

Th-15 Anterior thoracic muscles
(opposite page)

1. ___
2. ___
3. ___
4. ___
5. ___
6. ___
7. ___
8. ___
9. ___
10. ___
11. ___
12. ___
13. ___
14. ___
15. ___
16. ___
17. ___
18. ___

Th-16 Muscle attachments of the anterior thorax

Color and label the muscle origins (O) red and insertions (I) blue

1. Scalenus medius (I)
2. Scalenus anterior (I)
3. Subclavius (O)
4. Sternohyoid (O)
5. Sternocleidomastoid (clavicular head) (O)
6. Sternocleidomastoid (sternal head) (O)
7. Pectoralis major (clavicular head) (O)
8. Pectoralis major (sternocostal head) (O)
9. Rectus abdominis (I)
10. Pectoralis minor (I)
11. Pectoralis minor (O)
12. Omohyoid (I)
13. Deltoid (O)
14. Trapezius (I)
15. Common origin of biceps brachii and coracobrachialis (O)
16. Triceps brachii long head (O)
17. Subscapularis (I)
18. Supraspinatus (I)
19. Pectoralis major (I)
20. Latissimus dorsi (I)
21. Teres major (I)
22. Deltoid (I)
23. Coracobrachialis (I)
24. Serratus anterior (O)
25. External abdominal oblique (O)

Th-16 Muscle attachments of the anterior thorax
(opposite page)

1. ___
2. ___
3. ___
4. ___
5. ___
6. ___
7. ___
8. ___
9. ___
10. ___
11. ___
12. ___
13. ___
14. ___
15. ___
16. ___
17. ___
18. ___
19. ___
20. ___
21. ___
22. ___
23. ___
24. ___
25. ___

Th-17 Anterior thoracic wall seen from inside

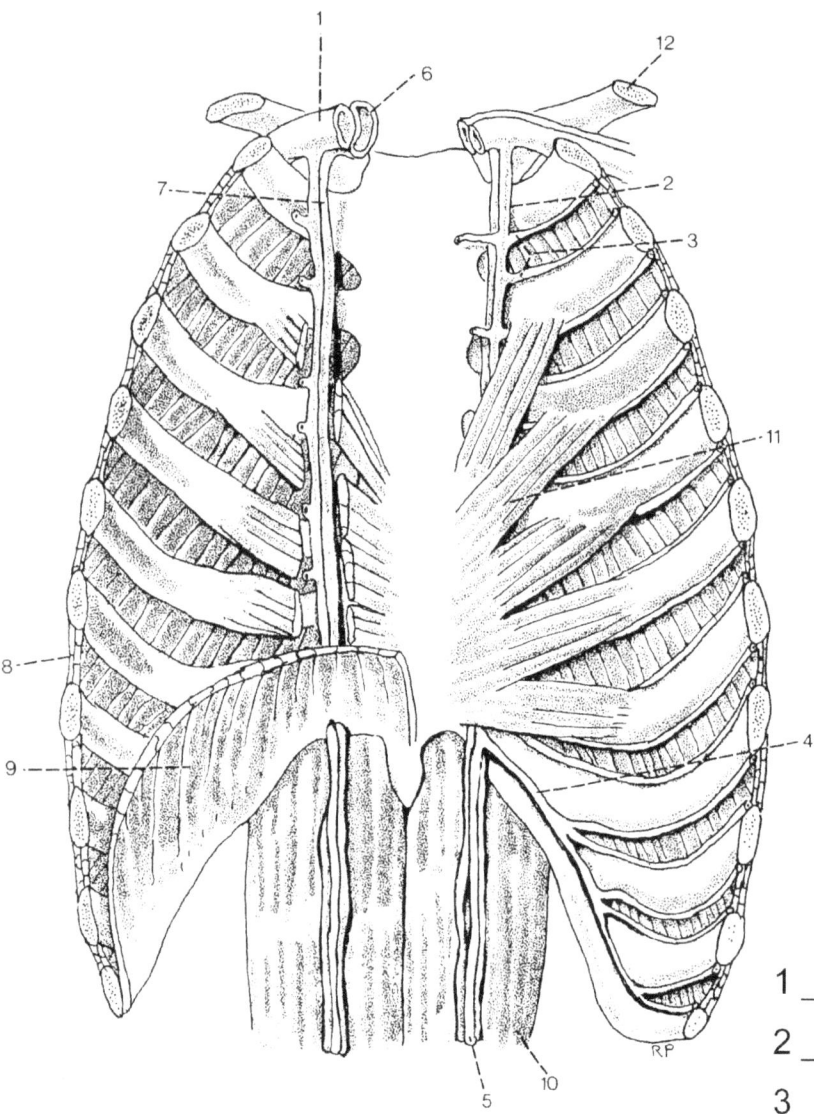

Color and label

1. Subclavian artery
2. Internal thoracic artery (old name, internal mammary artery)
3. Anterior intercostal arteries
4. Musculophrenic artery (phren refers to the diaphragm, which it helps supply)
5. Superior epigastric artery (the internal thoracic artery ends by dividing into the musculophrenic artery and the superior epigastric artery, which supplies the rectus abdominis muscle)
6. Subclavian vein
7. Internal thoracic vein (the internal thoracic vein is often doubled, resulting in two veins and one artery)
8. Intercostal muscles
9. Diaphragm
10. Rectus abdominis muscle
11. Transversus thoracis muscle
12. Clavicle (cut)

1 _____
2 _____
3 _____
4 _____
5 _____
6 _____
7 _____
8 _____
9 _____
10 _____
11 _____
12 _____

Th-18 Contents of thorax with anterior wall removed

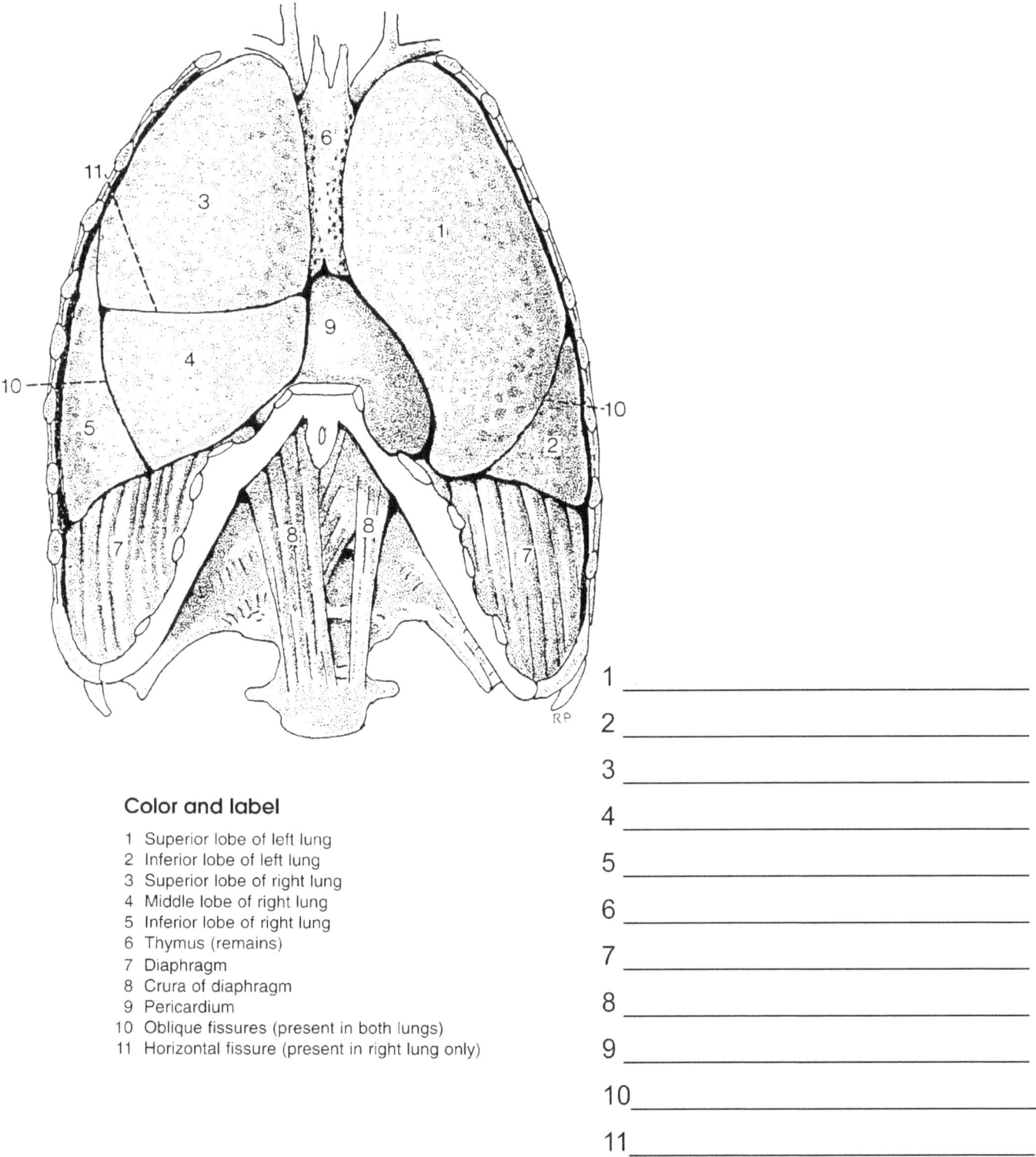

Color and label

1. Superior lobe of left lung
2. Inferior lobe of left lung
3. Superior lobe of right lung
4. Middle lobe of right lung
5. Inferior lobe of right lung
6. Thymus (remains)
7. Diaphragm
8. Crura of diaphragm
9. Pericardium
10. Oblique fissures (present in both lungs)
11. Horizontal fissure (present in right lung only)

1 _____
2 _____
3 _____
4 _____
5 _____
6 _____
7 _____
8 _____
9 _____
10 _____
11 _____

Note that the right lung has three lobes, whereas the left lung has only two. However, the fissures separating the lobes are not always present so that an isolated right lung with an obliterated horizontal fissure may appear to have only two lobes and be mistaken for the left lung.

Th-19 Intercostal muscles

The external intercostal muscles along with the parasternal (intercartilaginous) portions* of the internal intercostal muscles are active during inspiration. They raise the ribs, thus drawing air into the lungs. The remainder of the internal intercostal mucles depresses the ribs. In quiet breathing the elastic recoil of the costal cartilages and the elasticity of the lungs play the major role in depressing the ribs and pulling the thoracic wall inward. Both the external intercostal and internal intercostal muscles acting together strenghten the thoracic wall against strong internal and external pressure as occurs in singing, shouting, and breathing deeply.

*Note that the incline of the parasternal portions of the internal intercostal muscles bears the same geometric relation to the costal cartilages as that of the external intercostal muscles to the ribs. Their contraction will raise the costal cartilages.

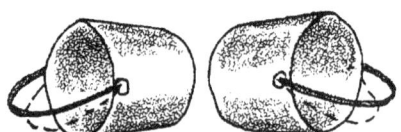

The movement of ribs in respiration may be likened to that of the handle on a pail or bucket. Just as the semicircular handle swings away from the rim of the pail, the ribs swing away from the midline when they are raised, thus increasing the transverse diameter of the thorax.

A simple two-dimensional model made from stiff cardboard or popsicle sticks and thumb tacks illustrates how the external intercostal muscle by raising the ribs increases the thoracic volume. The dimensions here apply only to the model and not necessarily to the human body.

During **expiration:** the external intercostal muscles are relaxed; the incline (slant) of ribs from back to front and from the midline to each side is greater; the spaces between the ribs are smaller.

During **inspiration:** the external intercostal muscles contract; the ribs are raised; the spaces between the ribs increase; the anterior-posterior diameter and the transverse diameter both increase, thus enlarging the thoracic (and pulmonary) volume, resulting in air being drawn into the lungs.

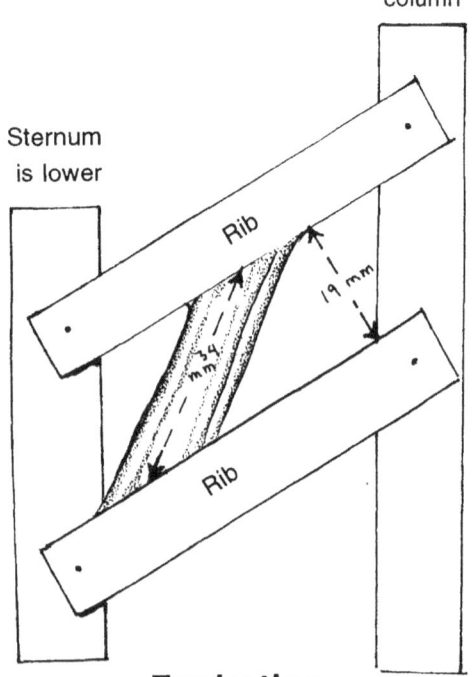

Expiration

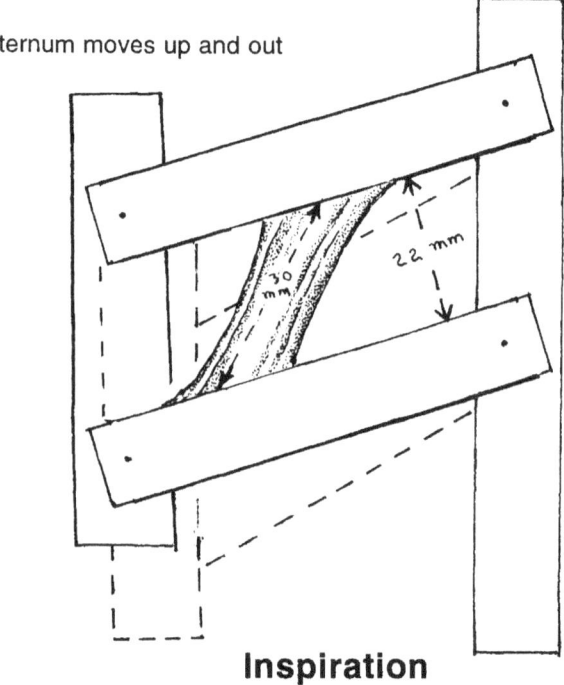

Inspiration

Th-20 Intercostal muscles

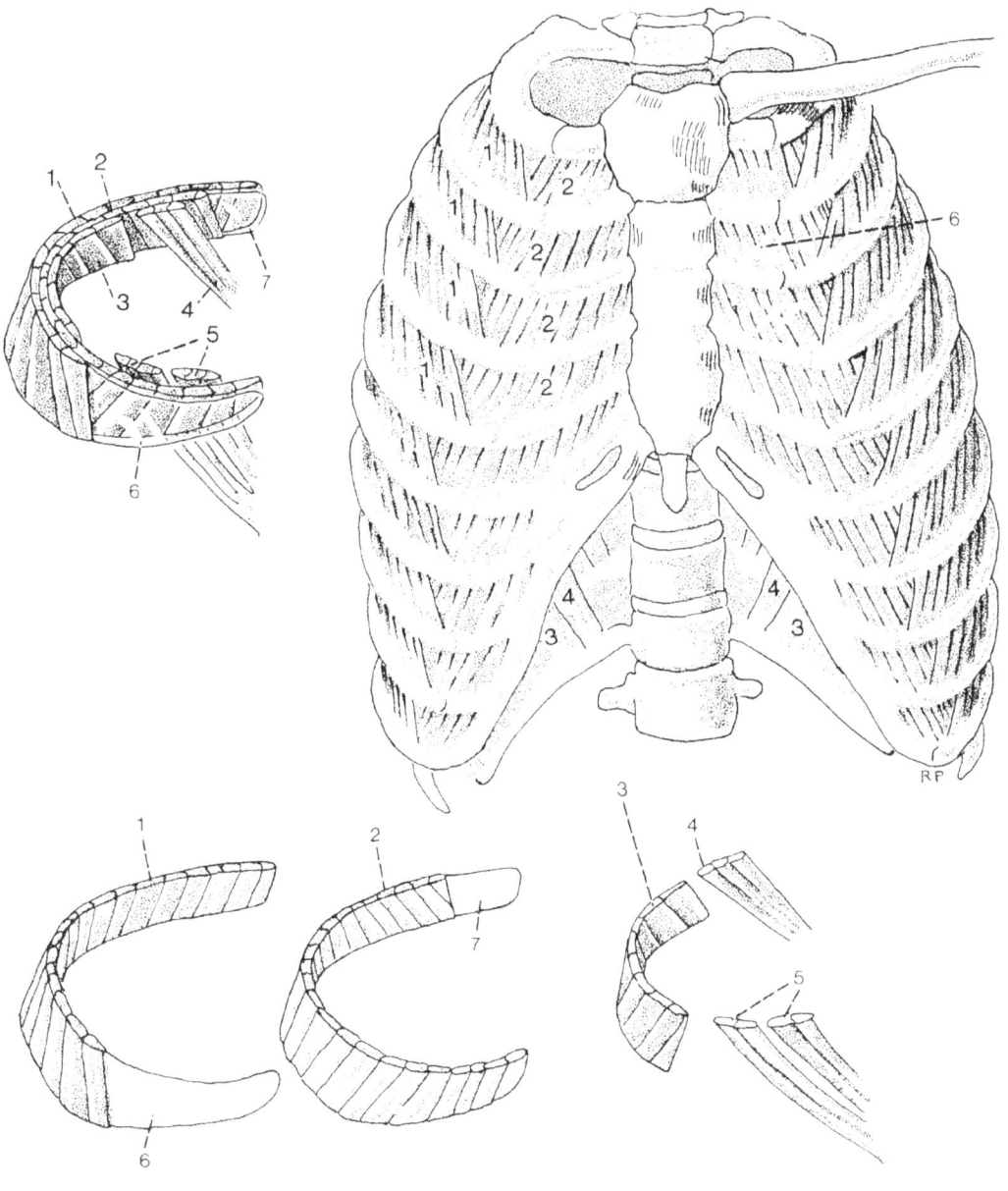

Color and label
1. External intercostal
2. Internal intercostal
3. Innermost intercostal
4. Subcostal
5. Transversus thoracis
6. External intercostal membrane
7. Internal intercostal membrane

Notice the direction of fibers in each layer. Also notice that neither the external intercostal nor the internal intercostal muscles completely fill in the intercostal spaces; rather each has a membranous portion that fills in its missing muscular portion. The parasternal (intercartilaginous) portions of the internal intercostal muscles (2) are visible beneath the membranes of the external intercostal muscles (6).

1 _____
2 _____
3 _____
4 _____
5 _____
6 _____
7 _____

Th-21 Cross section of thoracic wall with intercostal arteries

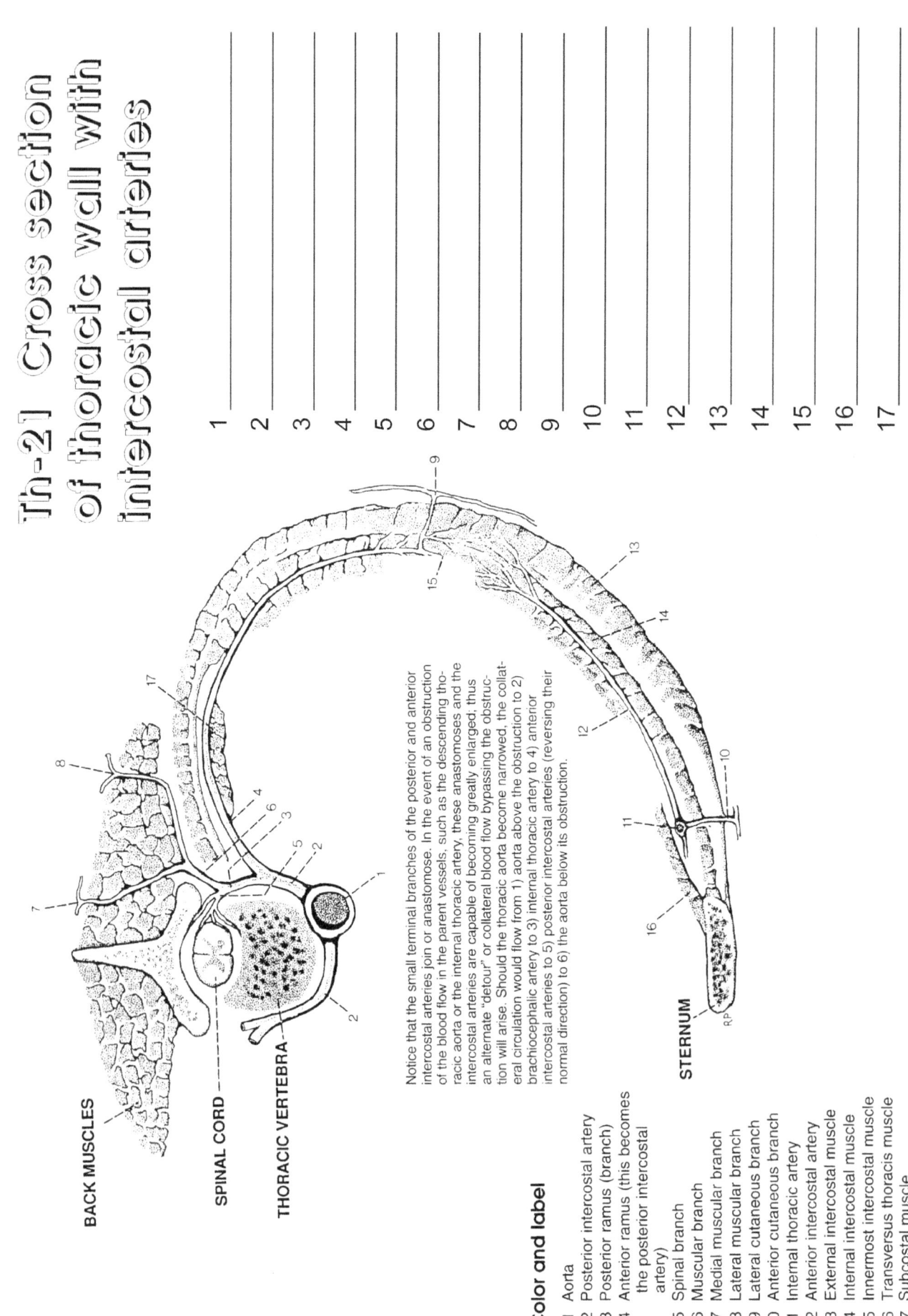

Notice that the small terminal branches of the posterior and anterior intercostal arteries join or anastomose. In the event of an obstruction of the blood flow in the parent vessels, such as the descending thoracic aorta or the internal thoracic artery, these anastomoses and the intercostal arteries are capable of becoming greatly enlarged, thus an alternate "detour" or collateral blood flow bypassing the obstruction will arise. Should the thoracic aorta become narrowed, the collateral circulation would flow from 1) aorta above the obstruction to 2) brachiocephalic artery to 3) internal thoracic artery to 4) anterior intercostal arteries to 5) posterior intercostal arteries (reversing their normal direction) to 6) the aorta below its obstruction.

Color and label

1. Aorta
2. Posterior intercostal artery
3. Posterior ramus (branch)
4. Anterior ramus (this becomes the posterior intercostal artery)
5. Spinal branch
6. Muscular branch
7. Medial muscular branch
8. Lateral muscular branch
9. Lateral cutaneous branch
10. Anterior cutaneous branch
11. Internal thoracic artery
12. Anterior intercostal artery
13. External intercostal muscle
14. Internal intercostal muscle
15. Innermost intercostal muscle
16. Transversus thoracis muscle
17. Subcostal muscle

Th-22 Section of thoracic wall with intercostal arteries

Color and label

1. Aorta
2. Posterior intercostal arteries
3. Collateral branch
4. Internal thoracic artery
5. Anterior intercostal arteries
6. Thoracic vertebra
7. Sternum
8. Internal intercostal muscle
9. Innermost intercostal muscle

Color and label

1. Intercostal vein
2. Intercostal artery
3. Intercostal nerve
4. Collateral intercostal artery and vein
5. Collateral branch of intercostal nerve
6. External intercostal muscle
7. Internal intercostal muscle
8. Innermost intercostal muscle
9. Parietal pleura (lines inner surface of thoracic wall)
10. Pleural cavity (potential space between parietal pleura and pulmonary [visceral] pleura)
11. Pulmonary pleura (covers the lungs)
12. Ribs
13. Lung

Th-23 Arteries of the thorax and upper arm

(opposite page)

Color and label

1. Arch of aorta (behind manubrium)
2. Brachiocephalic artery
3. Right subclavian artery
4. Right common carotid artery
5. Thyrocervical trunk
6. Axillary artery (continuation of subclavian artery)
7. Brachial artery (continuation of axillary artery)
8. Ulnar artery
9. Radial artery
10. Common interosseous artery
11. Posterior interosseous artery
12. Inferior thyroid artery
13. Vertebral artery
14. Ascending branch of superficial branch of transverse cervical artery
15. Deep branch of transverse cervical artery
16. Suprascapular artery
17. Supreme thoracic artery
18. Thoracoacromial trunk
19. Acromial branch of thoracoacromial trunk
20. Clavicular branch
21. Deltoid branch
22. Superficial branch of transverse cervical artery
23. Transverse cervical artery
24. Pectoral branch of thoracoacromial trunk
25. Lateral thoracic artery
26. Anterior humeral circumflex artery
27. Posterior humeral circumflex artery
28. Subscapular artery
29. Circumflex scapular artery
30. Thoracodorsal artery
31. Radial collateral artery of deep brachial artery
32. Superior ulnar collateral artery
33. Inferior ulnar collateral artery
34. Radial recurrent artery
35. Anterior ulnar recurrent artery
36. Posterior ulnar recurrent artery
37. Recurrent interosseous artery
38. Anterior interosseous artery
39. Internal thoracic artery
40. Descending branch of superficial branch of tranverse cervical artery
41. Perforating branches of internal thoracic artery
42. Anterior intercostal arteries
43. Superior epigastric artery
44. Musculophrenic artery
45. Xiphoid process
46. Deep (profunda) brachial artery (behind humerus)

1_____
2_____
3_____
4_____
5_____
6_____
7_____
8_____
9_____
10_____
11_____
12_____
13_____
14_____
15_____
16_____
17_____
18_____
19_____
20_____
21_____
22_____
23_____
24_____
25_____
26_____

Th-23 Arteries of the thorax and upper arm

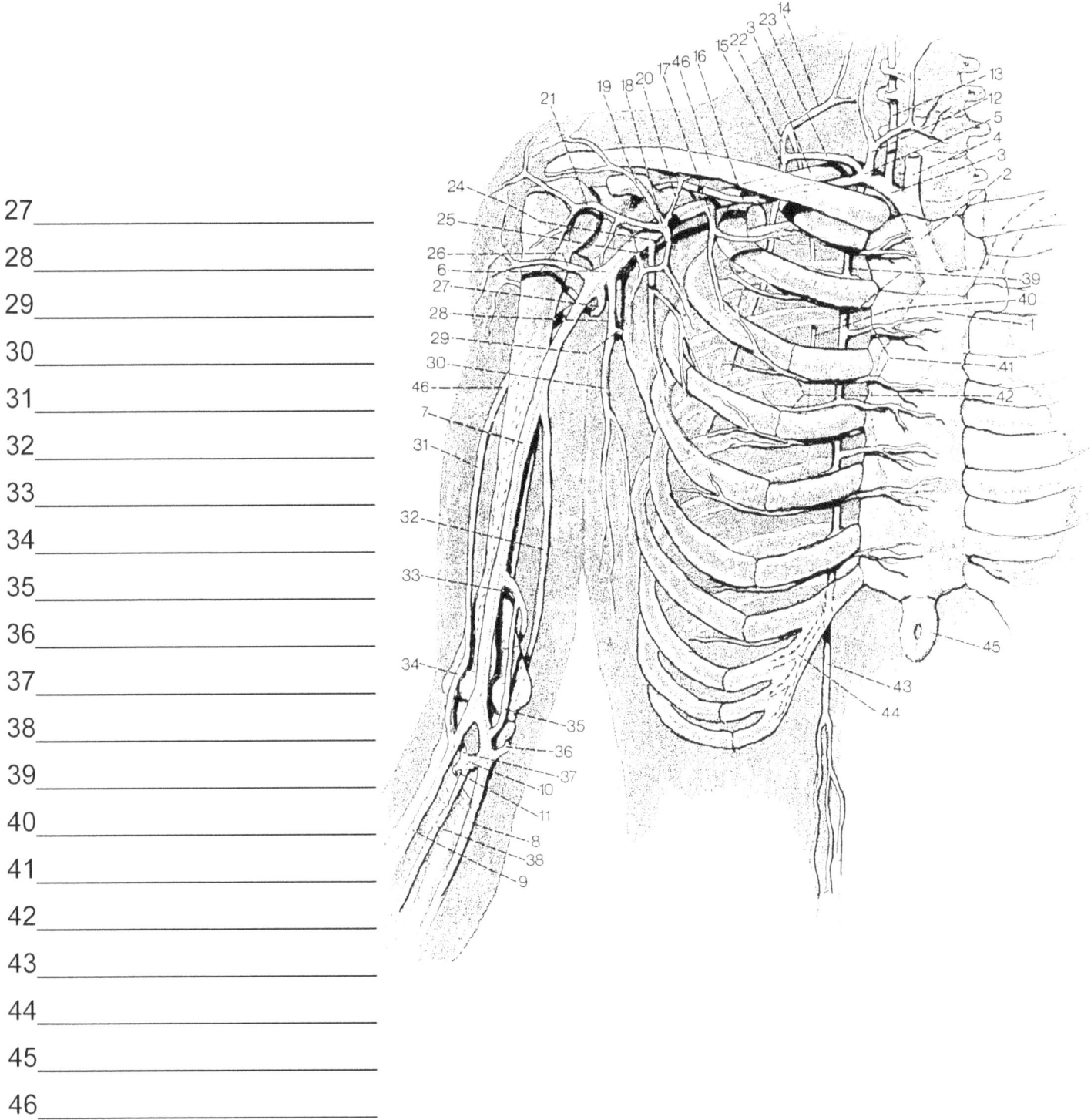

27 _____
28 _____
29 _____
30 _____
31 _____
32 _____
33 _____
34 _____
35 _____
36 _____
37 _____
38 _____
39 _____
40 _____
41 _____
42 _____
43 _____
44 _____
45 _____
46 _____

Th-24 Thoracic spinal nerve

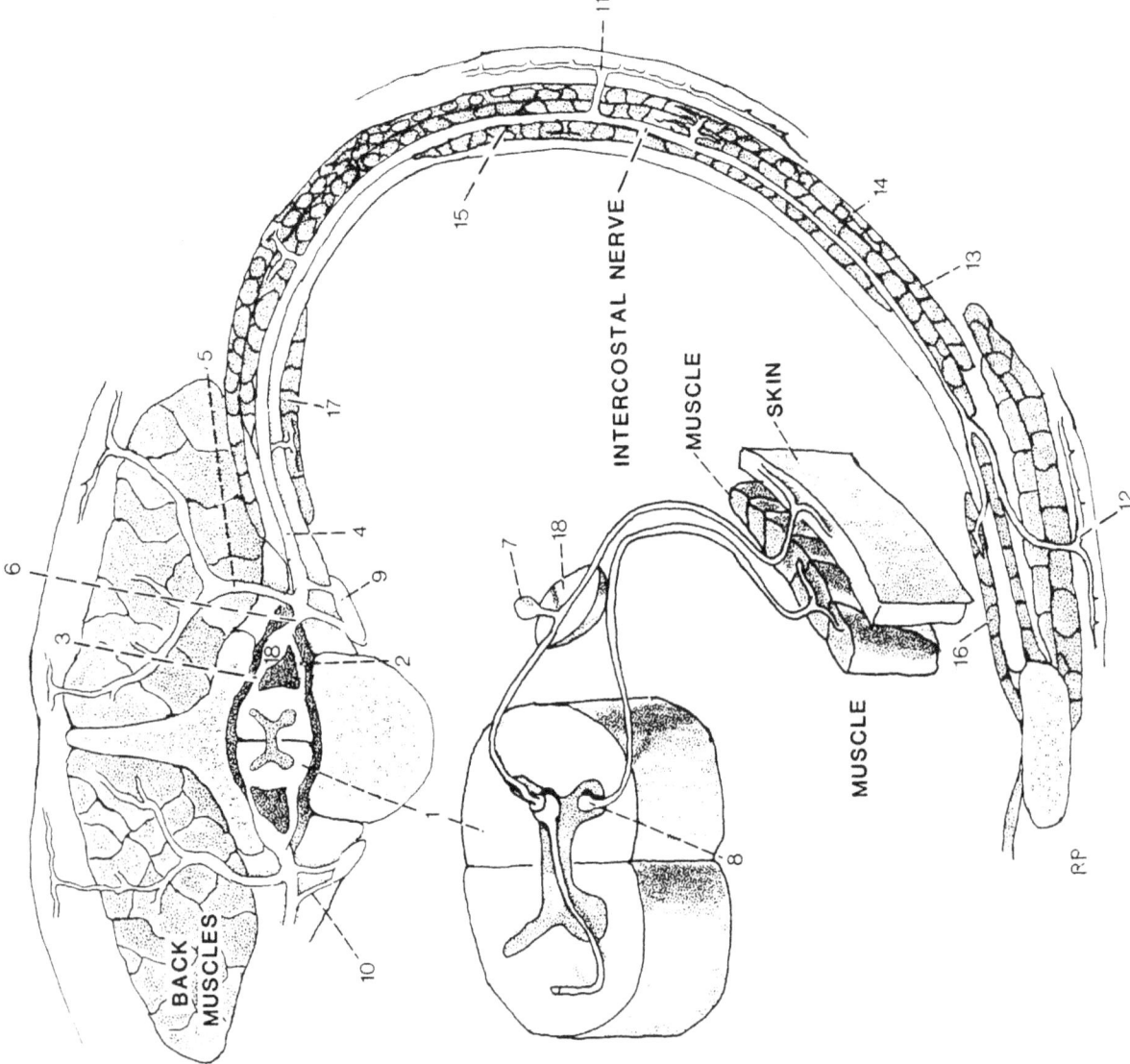

Color and label

1 Spinal cord
2 Ventral root of spinal nerve; contains out-going (efferent**) motor fibers; a nerve fiber is an axon.
3 Dorsal root of spinal nerve; contains in-coming (afferent**) sensory fibers.
4 Ventral ramus; the ventral and dorsal rami contain both motor fibers and sensory fibers.
5 Dorsal ramus
6 Spinal nerve; note that each spinal nerve arises from two roots, a ventral root and a dorsal root; it then divides into two rami, a ventral ramus and a dorsal ramus; the ventral ramus becomes the intercostal nerve; in fact all the nerves in our arms and legs are continuations of ventral rami; the dorsal rami innervate the large back muscles and supply sensation to the skin in the middle of the back.
7 Cell body of sensory neuron; all the sensory spinal nerve fibers have their cell bodies in the dorsal root ganglia.
8 Motor neuron cell body; these large alpha motor neurons innervate striated muscle, such as the intercostals.
9 Sympathetic ganglion*; these neurons give rise to fibers that supply blood vessels, sweat glands, and arrector pili (hair erector) muscles in hair follicles.
10 Communicating rami
11 Lateral cutaneous branch
12 Anterior cutaneous branch
13 External intercostal muscle
14 Internal intercostal muscle
15 Innermost intercostal muscle
16 Transversus thoracis muscle
17 Subcostal muscle; note that the intercostal nerve courses between the innermost intercostal muscle and the internal intercostal muscle.
18 Dorsal root ganglion* (or spinal ganglion)

* A ganglion is a collection of nerve cell bodies outside the brain and spinal cord. The brain and spinal cord comprise the central nervous system (CNS).
**Efferent and afferent simply mean "going away from" and "coming toward", respectively.

Th-24 Thoracic spinal nerve
(opposite page)

1.
2.
3.
4.
5.
6.
7.
8.
9.
10.
11.
12.
13.
14.
15.
16.
17.
18.

Th-25 The pericardium
(opposite page)

The pericardium, or pericardial sac, is a tough fibrous membrane that surrounds the heart. It consists of two fused membranes: a strong outer fibrous membrane, the fibrous pericardium, and an inner thin serous membrane, the serous pericardium. The inner serous pericardium both lines the inside of the pericardial sac (parietal part) and is reflected over the proximal parts of the eight great vessels and onto the heart where it forms the outer layer of the heart, the epicardium (visceral part of the pericardium). The pericardial sac is strong and not capable of expansion, so that if blood leaks into the pericardial space, the heart may be compressed to the degree that there is insufficient atrial capacity for blood to return and hence insufficient arterial outflow. This condition is called **tamponade** and can be life-threatening.

The relationship between the heart and the surrounding serous pericardium may be likened to a fist (the heart) being pushed into a soft balloon (the serous pericardium; top figures A and B). The part of the balloon that covers the fist corresponds to the visceral serous pericardium or epicardium, whereas the remainder of the balloon corresponds to the parietal serous pericardium that lines the inside of the pericardial sac, but without the surrounding fibrous pericardium. However, unlike the diagram of the balloon, which shows a considerable amount of space inside the indented balloon, the space between the pericardial sac and the heart is actually a potential space and contains only a small amount of slippery serous fluid secreted by the serous pericardium.

Th-25 The pericardium

Label the cut edge of the balloon
1 "Parietal" layer
2 "Visceral" layer

1 _____
2 _____

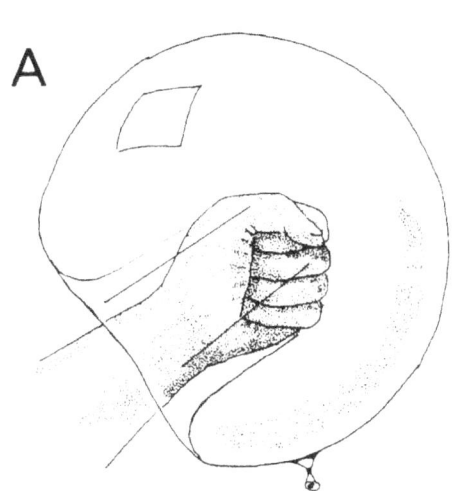

A

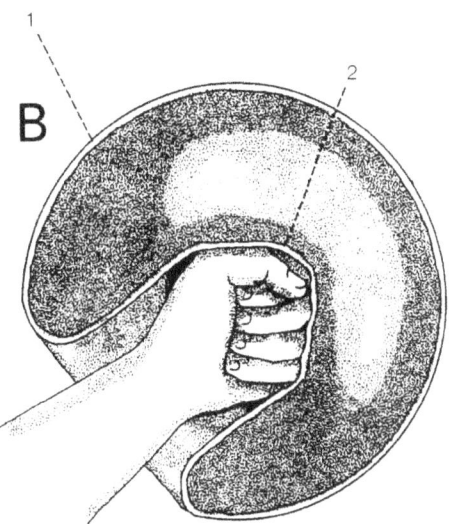

B

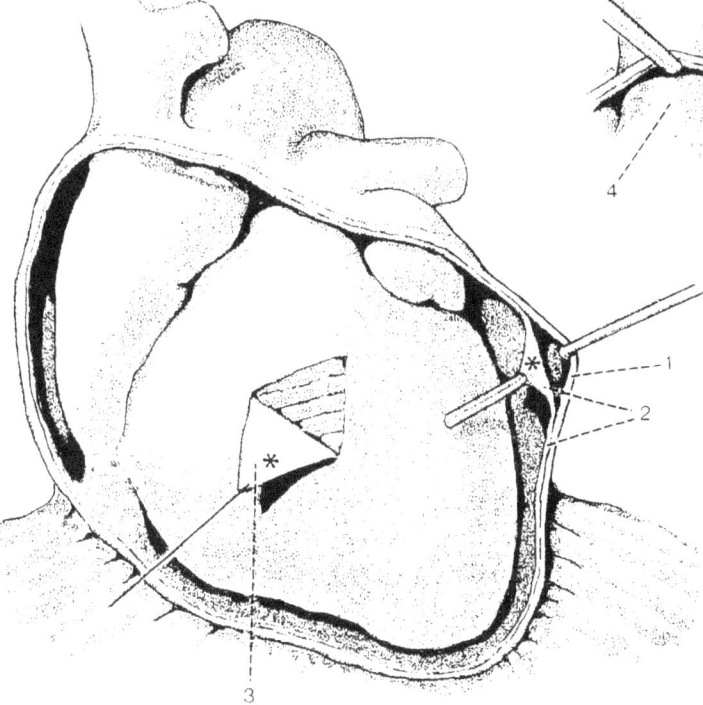

Color and label

1 Fibrous pericardium (forms the outer strong layer)
2 Parietal part of serous pericardium* (thin and delicate layer; lines inside of fibrous pericardium)
3 Visceral part of serous pericardium* (covers outside of heart; also called epicardium)
4 Great vessels such as the aorta penetrate pericardial sac and are covered by the serous pericardium inside the pericardial sac.

*Serous pericardium peeled off at asterisk

1 _____
2 _____
3 _____
4 _____

Th-26 The interior of the posterior pericardial sac with the heart removed and the great vessels cut
(opposite page)

1. _____
2. _____
3. _____
4. _____
5. _____
6. _____
7. _____
8. _____
9. _____
10. _____
11. _____
12. _____
13. _____
14. _____
15. _____
16. _____
17. _____
18. _____
19. _____
20. _____
21. _____

Th-26 The interior of the posterior pericardial sac with the heart removed and the great vessels cut

Viewed from the front

The serous pericardium forms two infolding covers of the great vessels which divide the area in back of the heart into the two pericardial sinuses, the straight sinus and the oblique sinus. One infolding of serous pericardium surrounds the intrapericardial parts of the aorta (5) and the pulmonary trunk (6); the other "tube" surrounds the intrapericardial portions of the remaining six great vessels.

Color and label

1. Oblique pericardial sinus (occupied by back of left atrium)
2. Transverse pericardial sinus (between arrowheads; immediately in front of right pulmonary artery)
3. Inferior vena cava
4. Superior vena cava
5. Aorta
6. Pulmonary trunk
7. Arch of aorta
8. Fibrous pericardium (its thickness somewhat exaggerated)
9. Serous pericardium (parietal layer; lines inside of fibrous pericardium)
10. Serous pericardium covering intrapericardial parts of great vessels
11. Right pulmonary artery
12. Bare area of fibrous pericardium (not lined with serous pericardium)
13. Left pulmonary artery
14. Left pulmonary veins
15. Right pulmonary veins
16. Right brachiocephalic vein
17. Left brachiocephalic vein
18. Brachiocephalic artery
19. Left common carotid artery
20. Left subclavian artery
21. Base of pericardium (fused inferiorly to central tendon of diaphragm)

Th-27 Exterior of the heart

(opposite page)

Label and color these veins blue
1. Right brachiocephalic vein
2. Left brachiocephalic vein
3. Superior vena cava
4. Inferior vena cava
5. Right internal thoracic vein
6. Left internal thoracic vein
7. Right pericardiacophrenic vein
8. Left pericardiacophrenic vein
9. Anterior cardiac veins (these drain directly into the right atrium)
10. Great cardiac vein* (this becomes the coronary sinus on inferior surface of heart)
11. Pulmonary trunk (color blue because it carries deoxygenated blood; remember, its name is trunk, not artery)
12. Small (or lesser) cardiac vein

Label and color these arteries red
13. Brachiocephalic artery
14. Right internal thoracic artery
15. Right pericardiacophrenic artery
16. Left common carotid artery
17. Left subclavian artery
18. Left internal thoracic artery
19. Left pericardiacophrenic artery
20. Right coronary artery*
21. Right marginal branch
22. Anterior interventricular artery* (branch of left coronary artery; also called left anterior descending)
23. Ascending aorta

Label the serous membranes
24. Cut edge of parietal pleura
25. Cut edge of pericardium; the phrenic nerve and the pericardiacophrenic artery and vein are "sandwiched" between these two membranes

Label and color these nerves yellow
26. Left phrenic nerve
27. Left vagus nerve (cranial nerve X; supplies parasympathetic fibers to the heart)
28. Recurrent laryngeal nerve (innervates the laryngeal muscles)
29. Right phrenic nerve (the two phrenic nerves arises from cervical nerves C3,C4,C5 and innervate the diaphragm)

Label
30. Right auricle (outpouching of right atrium; *auricula*, Latin for little ear)
31. Left auricle (outpouching of left atrium)
32. Root of left lung
33. Ligamentum arteriosum (remnant of fetal ductus arteriosus which diverted oxygenated blood headed for the nonfunctional lungs to be shunted from the pulmonary trunk directly to the aorta)

1_____
2_____
3_____
4_____
5_____
6_____
7_____
8_____
9_____
10_____
11_____
12_____
13_____
14_____
15_____
16_____
17_____
18_____
19_____
20_____
21_____
22_____
23_____
24_____
25_____

*Coronary vessels lie under fat which must be removed for the vessels to be seen.

Th-27 Exterior of the heart

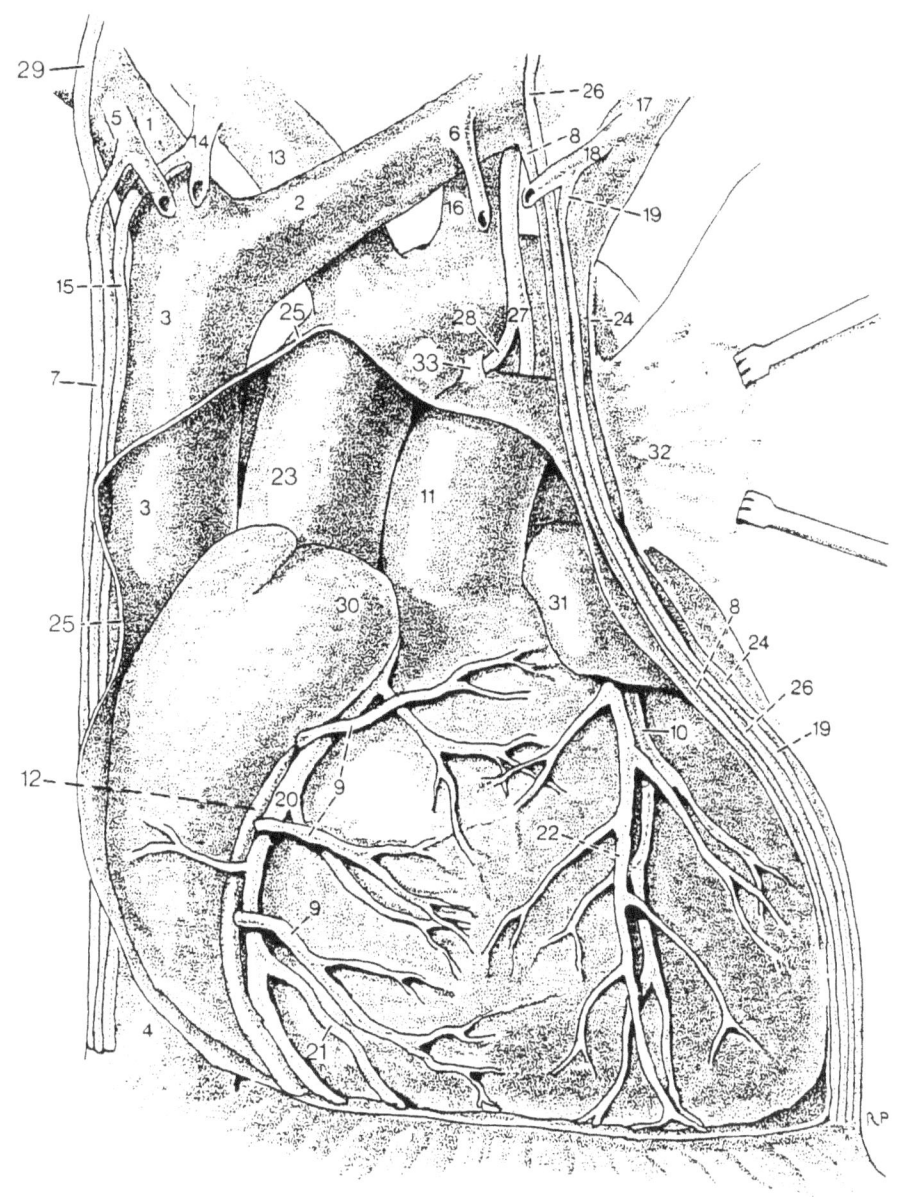

26 _____
27 _____
28 _____
29 _____
30 _____
31 _____
32 _____
33 _____

45

Th-28 Interior of the heart somewhat schematic
(opposite page)

Label and color these veins blue
1. Right brachiocephalic vein
2. Left brachiocephalic vein
3. Superior vena cava
4. Azygos vein
5. Inferior vena cava

Label and color the interior of the right atrium blue
6. Ostium (opening) of superior vena cava
7. Ostium of inferior vena cava
8. Ostium of coronary sinus (returns blood from the heart wall)
9. Fossa ovalis (remains of the opening between left and right atria in the fetus)
10. Musculi pectinati (comb-like strands of heart muscle; *pecten*, Latin, comb)
11. Crista terminalis
12. Sinoatrial node (pacemaker; here somewhat dissected out)
13. Right auricle (ear-like outpouching of right atrium)

Label and color the interior of the right ventricle blue
14. Anterior cusp of tricuspid valve (leave white)
15. Chordae tendineae (leave white)
16. Anterior papillary muscle (pink)
17. Trabeculae carneae (pink)
18. Septomarginal trabecula (moderator band) (pink)
19. Conus arteriosus
20. Anterior valvule of pulmonary valve (no muscles in valves; leave white)
21. Myocardium (heart muscle; pink)
22. Endocardium (leave white)
23. Epicardium (leave white)
24. Interventricular septum (muscular part; pink)
25. Pulmonary trunk (carries deoxygenated blood to lungs)
26. Right pulmonary artery
27. Left pulmonary artery
28. Superior branch of right pulmonary artery
29. Inferior branch of right pulmonary artery

Label and color the left atrium red
30. Ostia (openings of right pulmonary veins; these carry oxygenated blood from right lung back to heart)
31. Left pulmonary veins (carry oxygenated blood from left lung back to heart)

Label and color the left ventricle
32. Anterior cusp of mitral valve (leave white)
33. Posterior cusp of mitral valve (leave white)
34. Chordae tendineae (leave white)
35. Anterior papillary muscle (pink)
36. Left valvule of aortic valve (leave white)
37. Ostium of left coronary artery (coronary arteries supplies blood to the heart)
38. Aortic arch (aorta carries oxygenated blood to the whole body)
39. Brachiocephalic artery carries blood to right arm and right side of neck and head
40. Left common carotid artery (carries blood to left side of neck and head)
41. Left subclavian artery (carries blood to left arm)

1 _____
2 _____
3 _____
4 _____
5 _____
6 _____
7 _____
8 _____
9 _____
10 _____
11 _____
12 _____
13 _____
14 _____
15 _____
16 _____
17 _____
18 _____
19 _____
20 _____
21 _____
22 _____
23 _____
24 _____
25 _____
26 _____
27 _____
(use abbrevs.)

Th-28 Interior of the heart

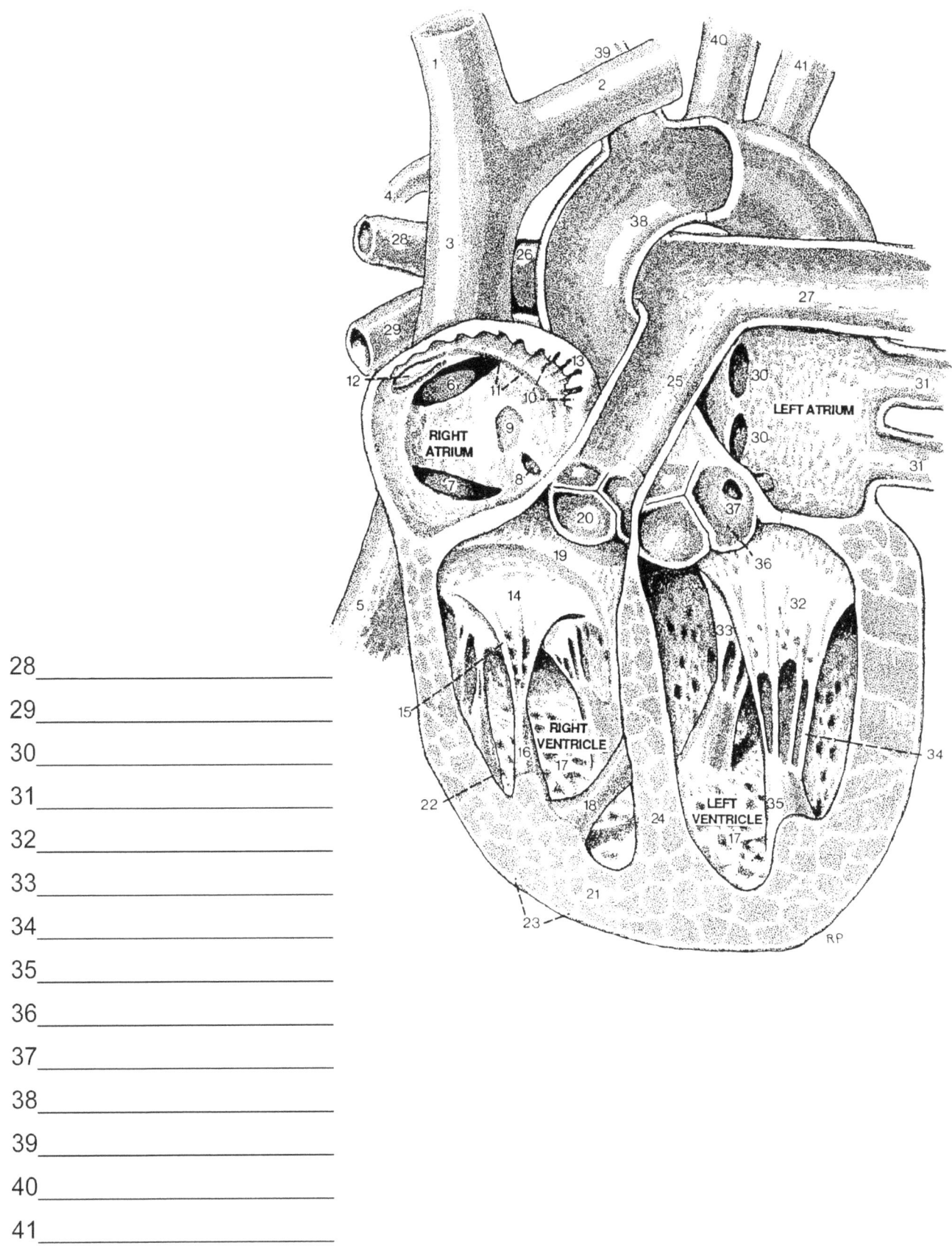

28 _____
29 _____
30 _____
31 _____
32 _____
33 _____
34 _____
35 _____
36 _____
37 _____
38 _____
39 _____
40 _____
41 _____

Th-29 Trace the course of blood through the heart

(opposite page)

Deoxygenated blood returns to the right atrium (R At) of the heart from the head, arms, and thorax by way of the superior vena cava **(1)**. Blood from the legs and abdomen reaches the right atrium by way of the inferior vena **(2)**. Blood from the heart wall returns mainly by way of the coronary sinus **(3)**, which also empties into the right atrium. Blood from the thoracic wall drains into the superior vena cava by way of the azygos vein. Blood leaves the right atrium through the right atrioventricular orifice and enters the right ventricle (RV) **(4)**. The tricuspid valve (TCV) allows blood to flow only from atrium to ventricle, thus preventing any backflow of blood from ventricle to atrium. Ventricular contraction closes the tricuspid valve and forces the blood through the pulmonary valve (PV) into the pulmonary trunk **(5)**, which divides into the left pulmonary artery **(6)** and the right pulmonary artery **(7)**. Oxygenated blood from the lungs is carried back to the the left atrium (L At) of the heart by way of four pulmonary veins **(8)**. The blood then passes through the bicuspid or mitral valve (MV), which guards the left atrioventricular orifice, and enters the left ventricle (LV) **(9)**. Ventricular contraction (the two ventricles contract simultaneously) closes the mitral valve and forces the blood through the aortic valve (AV) into the aorta **(10)**.

Although the systolic pressure in the left ventricle is six times greater than that in the right ventricle, the amount of blood pumped by the right ventricle to the lungs is approximately equal to the amount pumped by the left ventricle into the aorta.

Color arrows **1- 6** (deoxygenated blood) **blue** and arrows **6-10** (oxygenated blood) **red**

SVC	Superior vena cava	Pul Tr	Pulmonary trunk (note, *trunk*; not artery)
R At	Right atrium	L At	Left atrium
TCV	Tricuspid valve	MV	Mitral valve
RV	Right ventricle	LV	Left ventricle
PV	Pulmonary valve	AV	Aortic valve
LA	Ligamentum arteriosum		

SVC _____

RAt _____

TCV _____

RV _____

PV _____

LA _____

Pul Tr _____

L At _____

MV _____

LV AV _____

Th-29 Trace the course of blood through the heart

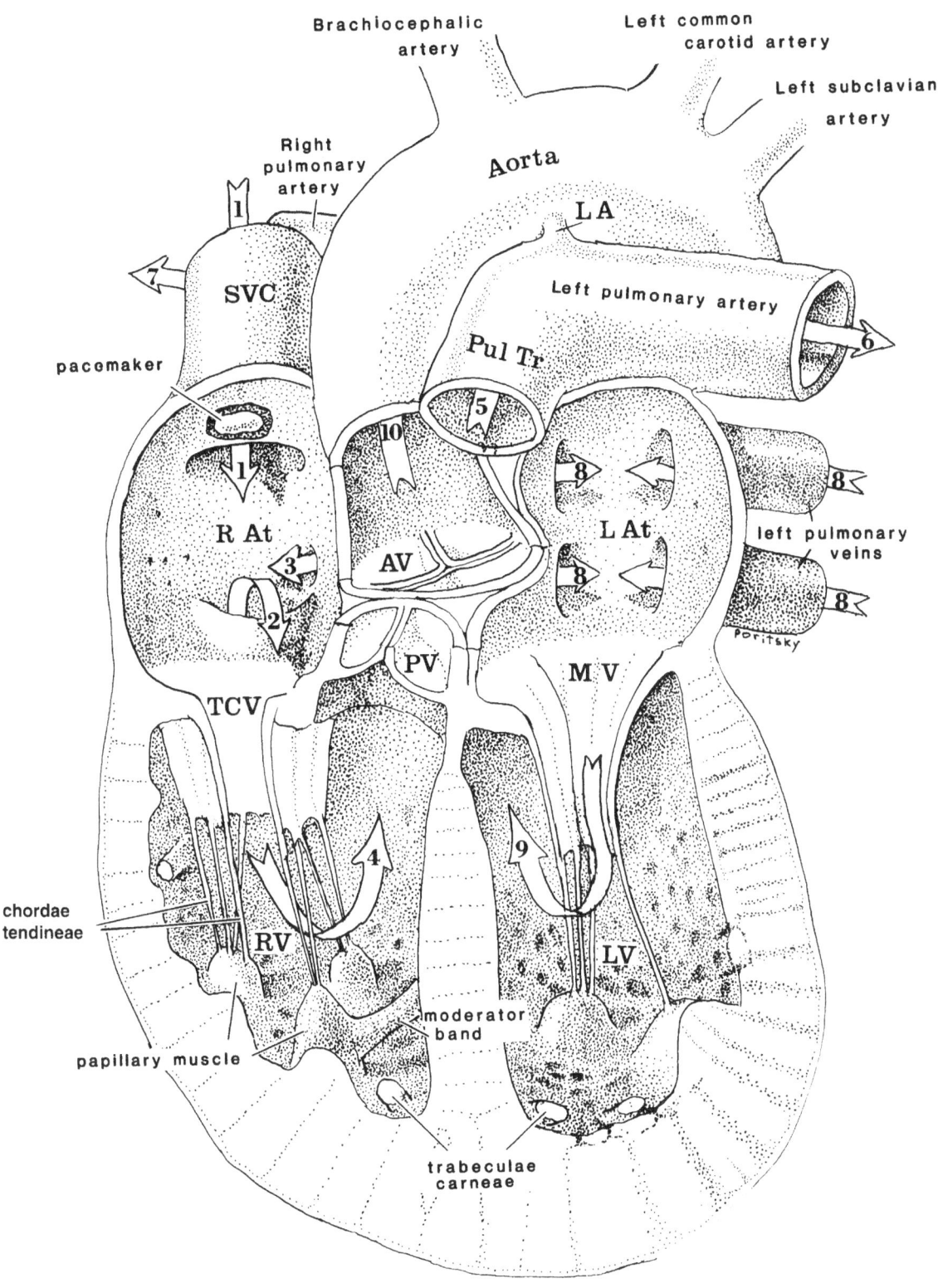

Th-30 The heart. Ventricles exposed

Much of the anterior wall has been removed to reveal the interior of the ventricles

(Opposite Page)

1 _____
2 _____
3 _____
4 _____
5 _____
6 _____
7 _____
8 _____
9 _____
10 _____
11 _____
12 _____
13 _____
14 _____
15 _____
16 _____

17 _____
18 _____
19 _____
20 _____
21 _____
22 _____
23 _____
24 _____
25 _____
26 _____
27 _____
28 _____
29 _____
30 _____
31 _____

Th-30 The heart. Ventricles exposed

Much of the anterior wall has been removed to reveal the interior of the ventricles

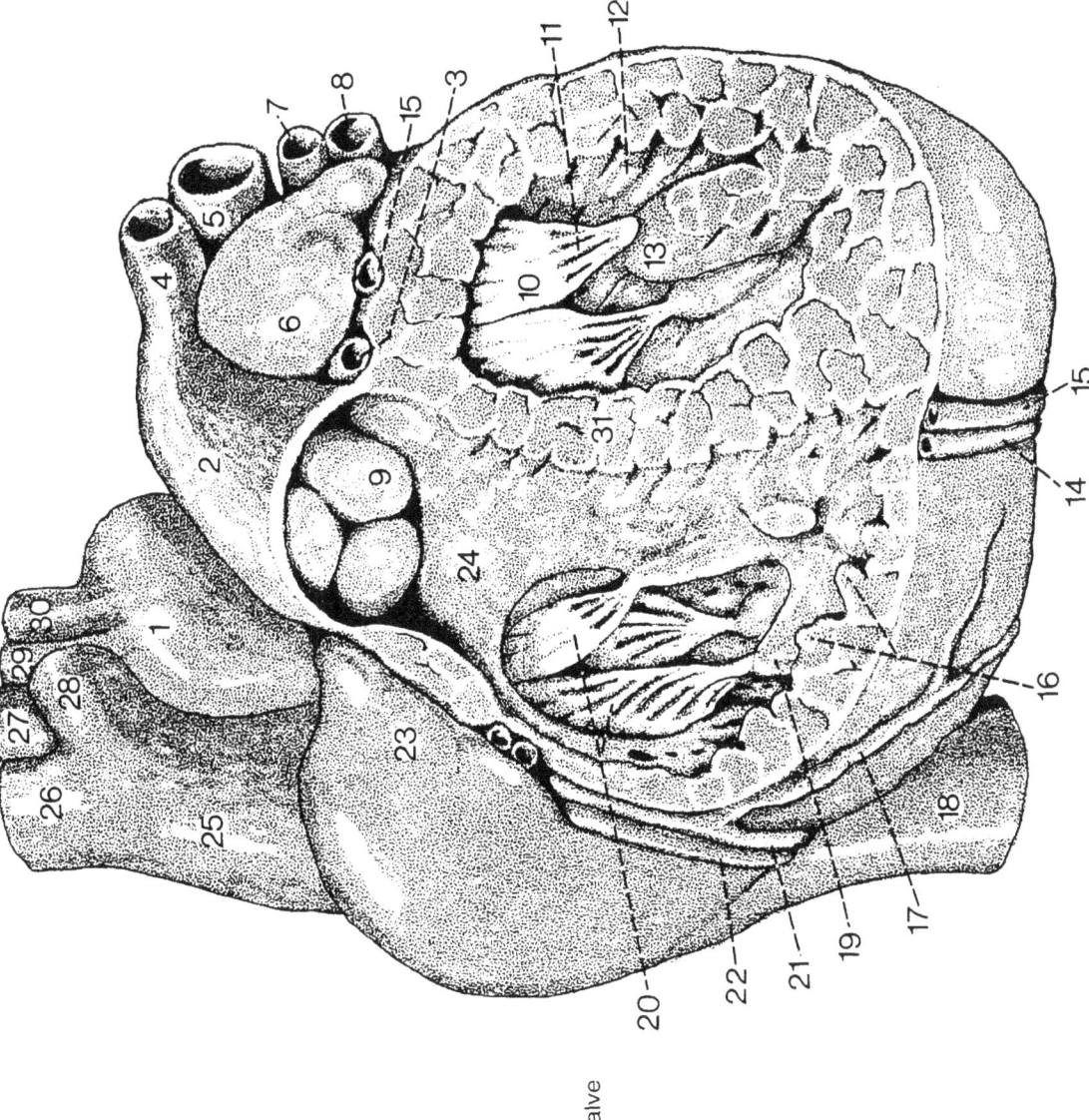

Color and label

1. Arch of aorta
2. Pulmonary trunk
3. Anterior interventricular artery
4. Superior branch of left pulmonary artery
5. Inferior branch of left pulmonary artery
6. Left auricle
7. Left superior pulmonary vein
8. Left inferior pulmonary vein
9. Pulmonary valve
10. Anterior cusp (leaflet) of mitral valve
11. Chordae tendineae
12. Trabeculae carneae in wall of left ventricle
13. Anterior papillary muscle in left ventricle
14. Anterior interventricular artery
15. Great cardiac vein
16. Trabeculae carneae in wall of right ventricle
17. Right marginal artery
18. Inferior vena cava
19. Papillary muscle
20. Chordae tendineae and septal leaflet of tricuspid valve
21. Right coronary artery
22. Small cardiac vein
23. Right auricle
24. Infundibulum (conus arteriosus) of right ventricle
25. Superior vena cava
26. Right brachiocephalic vein
27. Brachiocephalic artery ; notice that there are two brachiocephalic veins, but only a single brachiocephalic artery
28. Left brachiocephalic vein
29. Left common carotid artery
30. Left subclavian artery
31. Interventricular septum (largely removed)

51

Th-31 Base and diaphragmatic surface of heart

(opposite page)

Color and label

1. Left atrium (**base** or posterior surface of heart); it occupies the oblique pericardial sinus; it receives the oxygenated blood from the lungs via the 4 pulmonary veins.
2. Right atrium; it receives deoxygenated blood via the inferior and superior venae cavae.
3. Left ventricle (diaphragmatic or inferior surface of heart)
4. Right ventricle; the epicardium and epicardial fat have been stripped away.
5. Cusp of half valve at opening of inferior vena cava into right atrium
6. Superior vena cava
7. Arch of aorta; notice that the aortic arch curves posteriorly as well as to the left.
8. Beginning of descending aorta
9. Coronary sinus; largest intrinsic heart vein and main conduit of blood returning from the substance of the heart; opens into right atrium; note that the great cardiac vein becomes the coronary sinus.
10. Great cardiac vein; it becomes continuous with coronary sinus approximately 2.5 cm from the right atrium.
11. Circumflex artery (branch of left coronary artery)
12. Right coronary artery
13. Small (or lesser) cardiac vein; note that it empties into coronary sinus.
14. Ligamentum arteriosum (remains of the fetal ductus arteriosus)
15. Left subclavian artery
16. Left common carotid artery
17. Brachiocephalic artery; gives rise to the right subclavian artery and the right common carotid artery.
18. Opening (orifice) of azygos vein into the superior vena cava
19. Right pulmonary artery
20. Right superior pulmonary vein
21. Right inferior pulmonary vein
22. Posterior interventricular artery
23. Middle cardiac vein
24. **Apex** of heart
25. Left posterior ventricular branch of circumflex artery
26. Posterior vein of left ventricle
27. Superior left pulmonary vein
28. Left pulmonary artery
29. Inferior left pulmonary vein

1 _____
2 _____
3 _____
4 _____
5 _____
6 _____
7 _____
8 _____
9 _____
10 _____
11 _____
12 _____
13 _____
14 _____
15 _____
16 _____
17 _____
18 _____
19 _____
20 _____
21 _____
22 _____
23 _____
24 _____
25 _____
26 _____
27 _____
28 _____
29 _____

Th-31 Base and diaphragmatic surface of heart

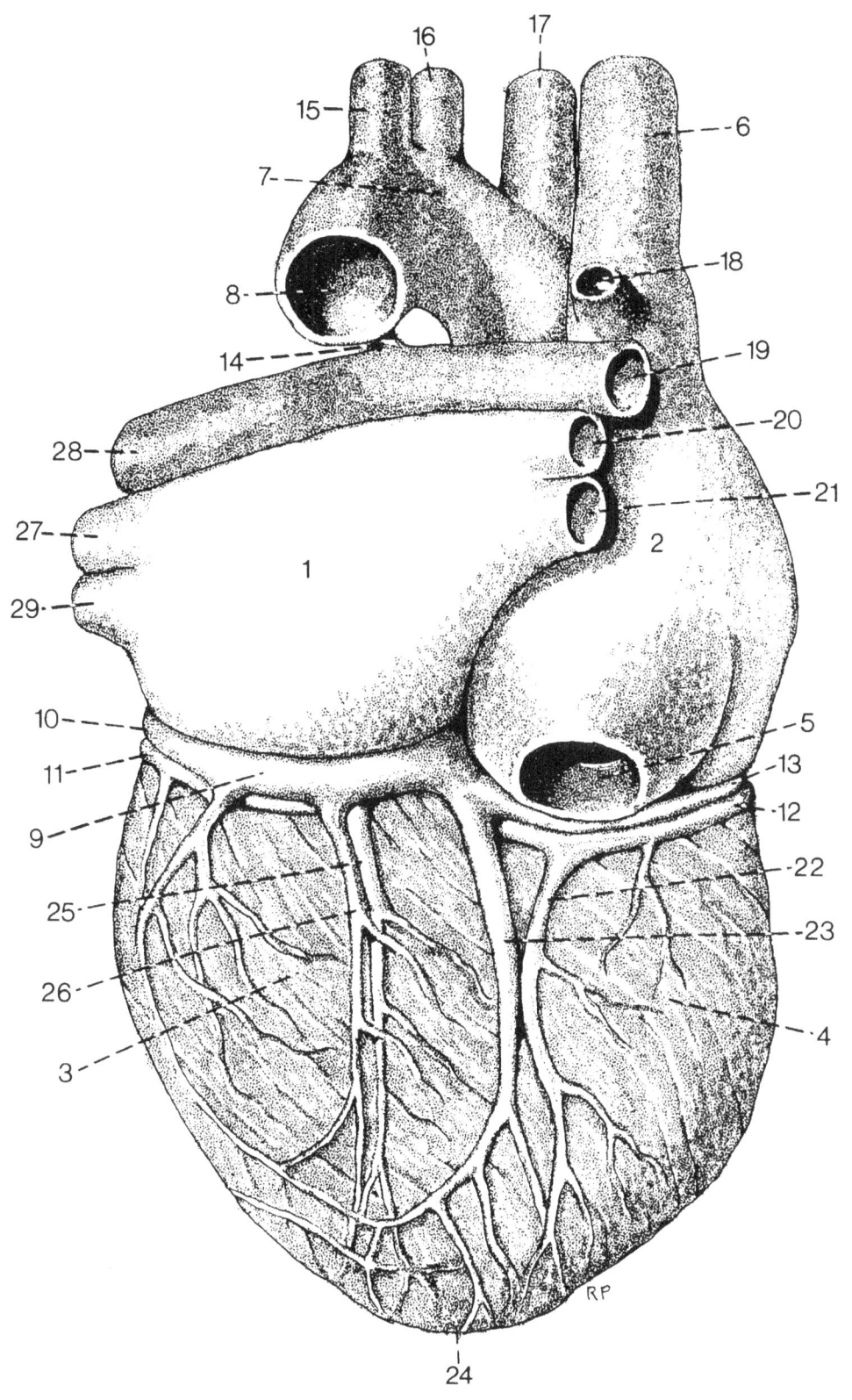

Th-32 Right atrium and right ventricle

(opposite page)

Color and label

1. Inferior vena cava
2. Superior vena cava
3. Azygos vein ending in superior vena cava
4. Right brachiocephalic vein
5. Left brachiocephalic vein
6. Ascending aorta
7. Pulmonary trunk
8. Left auricle (right auricle has been cut away)
9. Pectinate muscles (*musculi pectinati*, "comblike" muscles; *pecten*, Latin, comb) in right atrium
10. Right coronary artery
11. Pulmonary valve (closed in diastole; open in systole)
12. Anterior interventricular artery (branch of left coronary artery)
13. Great cardiac vein; continues as coronary sinus
14. Infundibulum of right ventricle (conus arteriosus)
15. Interventricular septum
16. Chordae tendineae of septal cusp (leaflet)
17. Trabeculae carneae (Latin, beams of flesh)
18. Moderator band (septomarginal trabecula)
19. Great cardiac vein
20. Anterior interventricular artery
21. Anterior papillary muscle
22. Chordae tendineae
23. Posterior papillary muscle
24. Anterior cusp of tricuspid valve (right atrioventricular valve)
25. Fibrous ring around right atrioventricular orifice (anchors the bases of tricuspid valve cusps or leaflets)
26. Right coronary artery
27. Small cardiac vein
28. Orifice (opening) of coronary sinus; returns most of the blood from the substance of the heart to the right atrium
29. Valve (half valve) of inferior vena cava
30. Crista terminalis (cut in two places)
31. Limbus (border) of fossa ovalis
32. Fossa ovalis (site of the fetal **foramen ovale** that fuctions as a one-way valve, directing oxygenated blood from the right atrium through the interatrial wall to the left atrium; closed after birth)
33. Sinuatrial node (pacemaker)
34. Septal cusp of tricuspid valve
35. Triangle of Koch (site of **atrioventricular node**); bounded by (1) base of septal leaflet of tricuspid valve, (2) anterior margin of orifice of coronary sinus, and (3) tendon of Todaro
36. Tendon of Todaro; rounded collagenous bundle that may be palpated extending from the valve of the inferior vena cava to the right fibrous trigone

1_____

2_____

3_____

4_____

5_____

6_____

7_____

8_____

9_____

10_____

11_____

12_____

13_____

14_____

15_____

16_____

17_____

18_____

19_____

20_____

21_____

22_____

23_____

24_____

25_____

26_____

27_____

28_____

29_____

30_____

31_____

32_____

33_____

34_____

35_____

36_____

Th-32 Right atrium and right ventricle

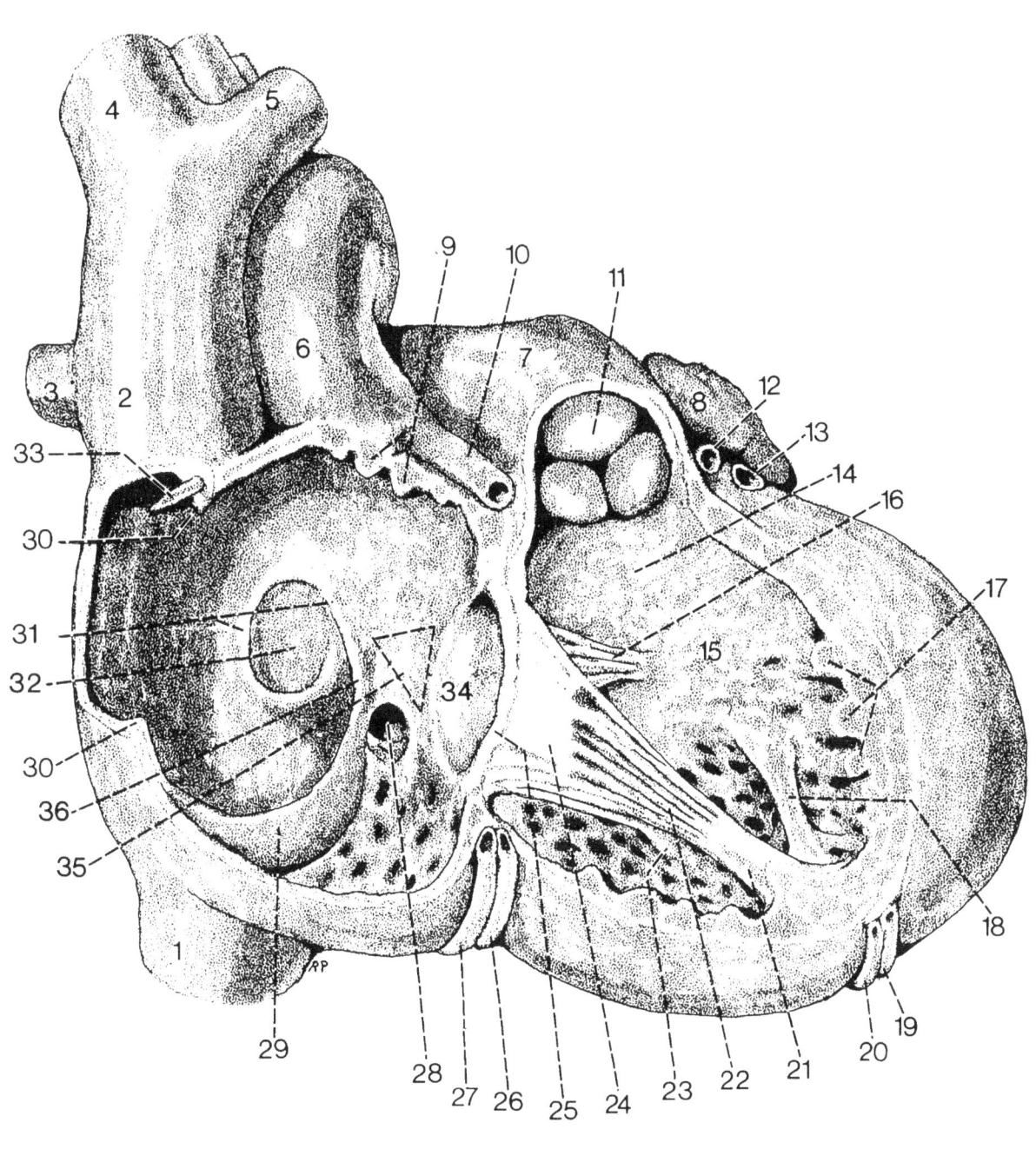

Right atrium   Right ventricle

Th-33 Left ventricle
(opposite page)

(use abbrevs.)

Color and label

1. Arch of aorta
2. Ligamentum arteriosum; remnant of embryonic ductus arteriosus which shunted blood from pulmonary artery to aorta; normally it closes and becomes ligamentous after birth.
3. Pulmonary trunk
4. Left inferior pulmonary artery
5. Left superior pulmonary artery
6. Left auricle; ear-like atrial appendage or outpouching of left atrium
7. Anterior interventricular artery
8. Great cardiac vein
9. Aortic valve (viewed from ventricular side)
10. Anterior cusp of mitral valve; this valve closes the left artrioventricular orifice during systole and prevents the reflux of blood into the left atrium.
11. Chordae tendineae; these tendinous chords extend from the valve cusps (or leaflets) to the papillary muscles and prevent the leaflets from being blown backwards into the atrium; the leaflets have no intrinsic muscles and close passively when ventricular contraction forces blood against their ventricular surfaces.
12. Apex of papillary muscle (cut)
13. Wall of left ventricle
14. Anterior papillary muscle; papillary muscles may have more than one apical nipple-like process, as shown here.
15. Apex of heart
16. Posterior papillary muscle; note that the chordae tendineae from both papillary muscles attach to both the anterior and posterior mitral valve cusps; thus the initial papillary muscle contraction causes apposition of the valve cusps.
17. Trabeculae carneae; muscular bundles on the inner walls of both ventricles; the two auricles contain the musculi pectinati.
18. Interventricular septum (largely removed)
19. Trabeculae carneae on interior wall of right ventricle
20. Posterior cusp and chordae tendineae of tricuspid valve; guards right atrioventricular orifice
21. Papillary muscle
22. Right marginal artery
23. Interior of right ventricle
24. Right atrium seen through right atrioventricular orifice
25. Wall of right ventricle
26. Anterior valve cusp and chordae tendineae of tricuspid valve
27. Lesser cardiac vein
28. Right coronary artery
29. Septal cusp and chordae tendinae of tricuspid valve
30. Conus arteriosus of right ventricle (infundibulum)
31. Pulmonary valve (viewed from ventricular aspect)
32. Superior vena cava
33. Ascending aorta
34. Right brachiocephalic vein
35. Brachiocephalic artery
36. Left brachiocephalic vein
37. Left common carotid artery
38. Left subclavian artery

1_____
2_____
3_____
4_____
5_____
6_____
7_____
8_____
9_____
10_____
11_____
12_____
13_____
14_____
15_____
16_____
17_____
18_____
19_____
20_____
21_____
22_____
23_____
24_____
25_____
26_____
27_____

Th-33 Left ventricle

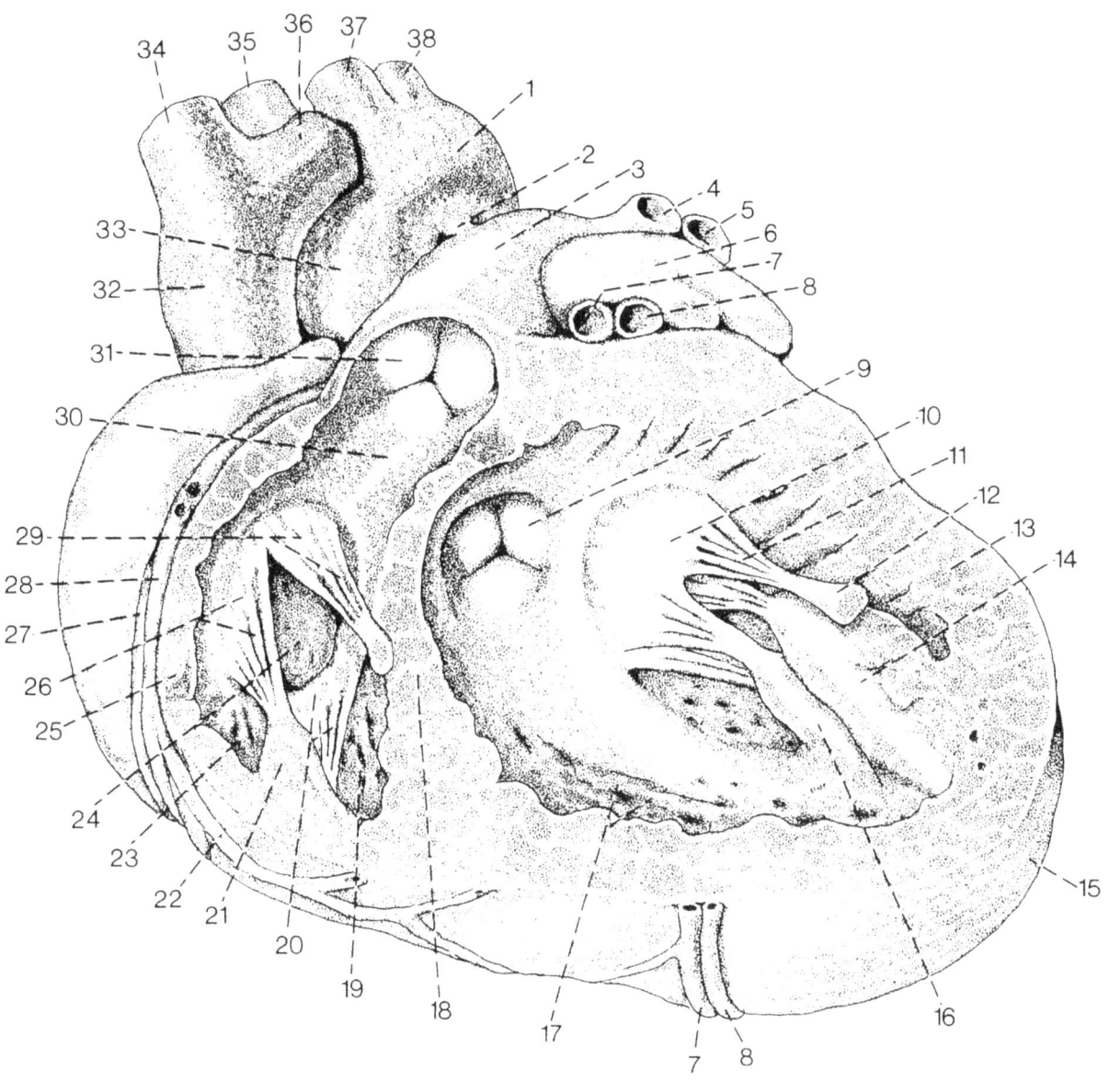

28 _____   34 _____
29 _____   35 _____
30 _____   36 _____
31 _____   37 _____
32 _____   38 _____
33 _____

Th-34 Heart valves and valve action
(opposite page)

Top figure shows the four heart valves viewed from the posterior aspect. Both the right and left atria have been removed (the atria lie **posterior** to the ventricles). The aorta and the pulmonary trunk have been cut just above their valves. Note that the two coronary arteries arise from the aorta; the right coronary artery (5) arises from the right aortic sinus (6) and the left coronary artery (7) arises from the left aortic sinus (8).

Color and label

1 Pulmonary valve
2 Aortic valve
3 Tricuspid valve
   (right atrioventricular valve)
4 Mitral valve (bicuspid or
   left atrioventricular valve)
5 Right coronary artery
6 Right aortic valvule and sinus and
   origin (orifice) of right coronary
   artery
7 Left coronary artery
8 Left aortic valvule and sinus and
   origin of left coronary artery
9 Anterior interventricular branch
   of left coronary artery
10 Circumflex branch of left coronary artery
11 Anterior cusp of tricuspid valve
   (right atrioventricular valve)
12 Posterior cusp of tricuspid valve
13 Septal cusp (not always present)
14 Anterior cusp of mitral valve
15 Posterior cusp of mitral valve

Bottom figure shows valve action in **diastole** and **systole**. Note that the heart valves consist of strong thin membranous leaflets or cusps (they are called valvules in the aortic and pulmonary valves) that have no muscle. They are shaped so that when the heart contracts, blood will flow in one direction only; from atria to ventricles, and from ventricles into the aorta and pulmonary trunk. They are closed by the blood being pushed **backwards** against the cusps.

Diastole. The heart muscle (myocardium) in the walls of both the atria and ventricles is **relaxed**. The **atrioventricular (AV) valves** (tricuspid and mitral) are both **open** (1 and 2) allowing blood to pass from the atria to the ventricles (arrows 1 and 2). The two **semilunar valves** (aortic 3 and pulmonary 4) are **closed** because the pressure in the aorta and pulmonary trunk is higher than that in the ventricles.

Systole. The atria and especially the **ventricles contract** forcing blood out of the heart and into the aorta and pulmonary trunk (arrows 3 and 4). The **mitral and tricuspid valves** are **closed** (5 and 6) and, once the pressure in the ventricles exceeds the pressure in the two great arteries, the **aortic and pulmonary valves** are forced **open** (7 and 8). The elastic walls of the aorta and pulmonary arteries bulge outward and absorb part of the systolic pressure wave and smooth out the pulse. Two-thirds of the time the heart is in distole and one-third it is in systole.

RA Right atrium
RV Right ventricule
LA Left atrium
PT Pulmonary trunk
A Aorta

RA_____

RV_____

LA_____

PT_____

A_____

Th-34 Heart valve action

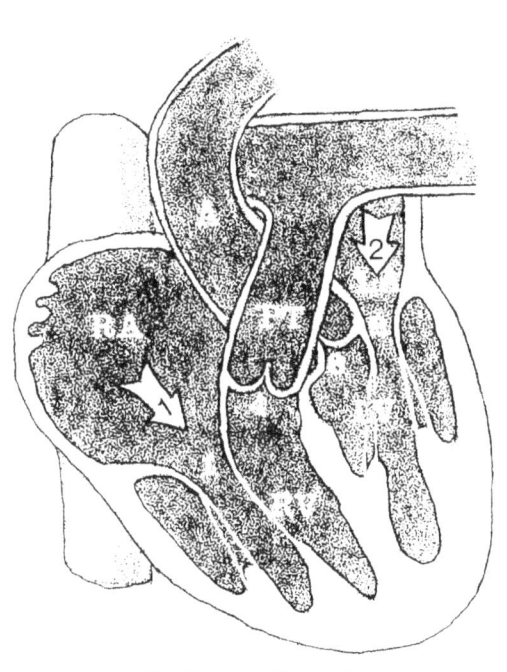

Diastole

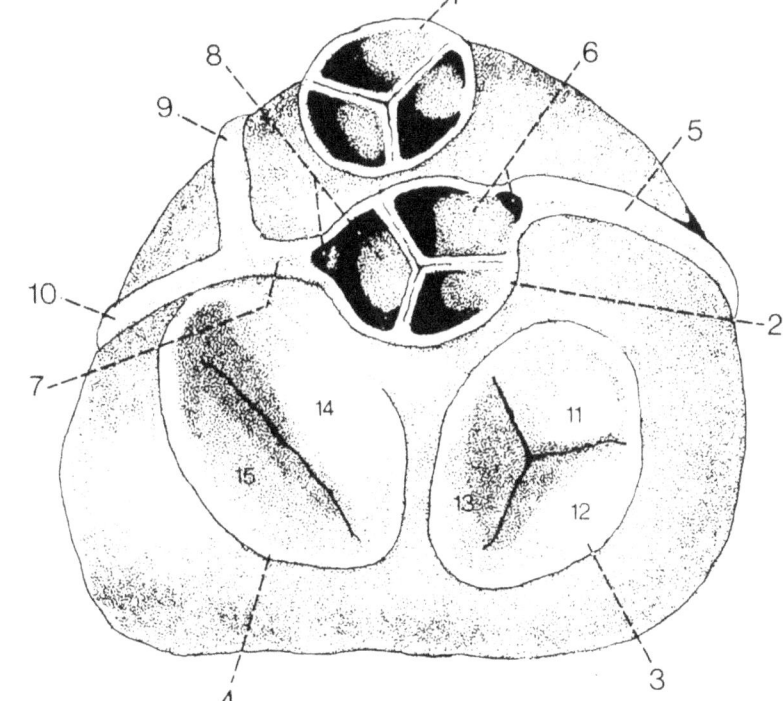

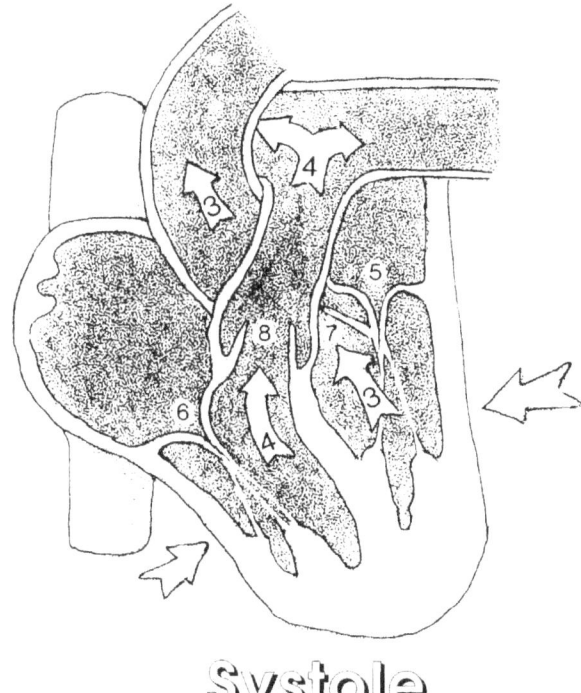

Systole

1 _____
2 _____
3 _____
4 _____
5 _____
6 _____
7 _____
8 _____
9 _____
10 _____
11 _____
12 _____
13 _____
14 _____
15 _____

Th-35 The four heart valves

Relation of the four valves of the heart to the sternum and ribs of the anterior thoracic wall and the best locations to listen to each (auscultation areas)

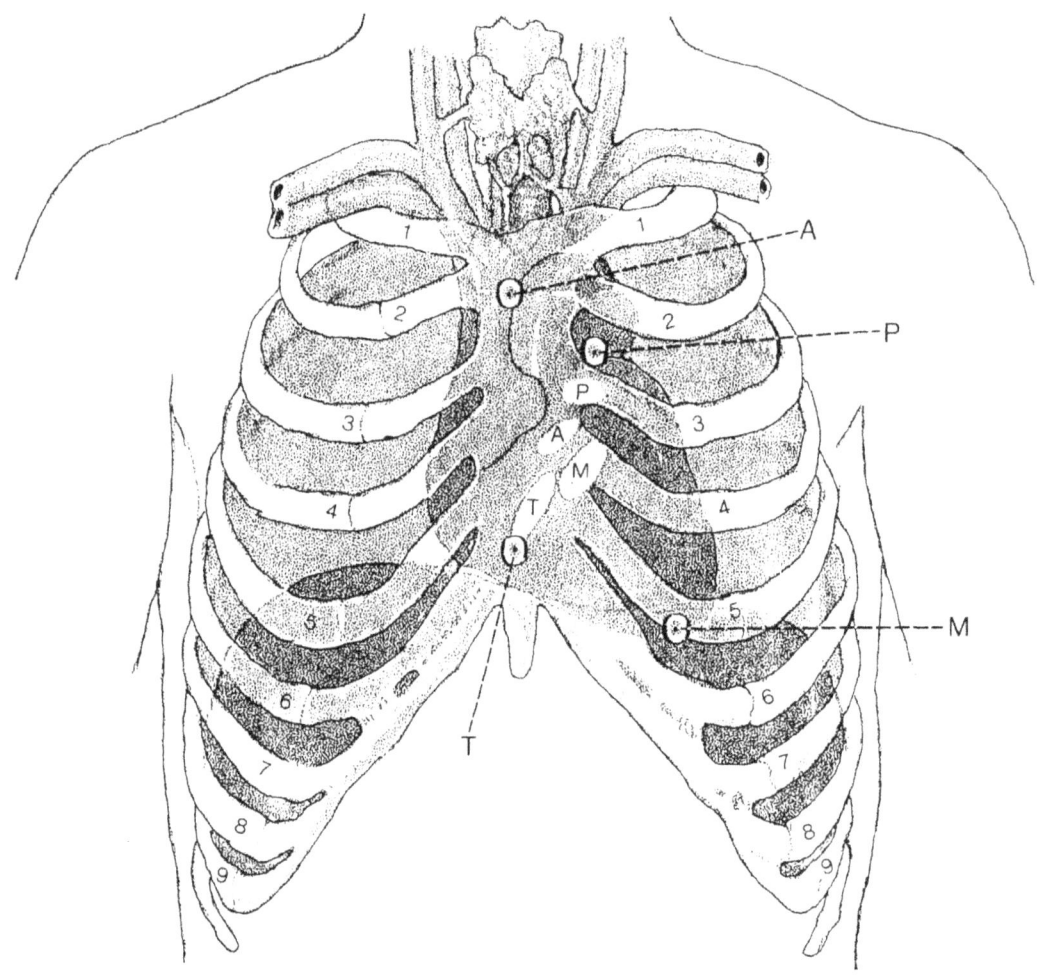

Color and label the position of the four heart valves (ellipses with letters T, P, M, A)

T   Tricuspid valve; color blue; guards the right atrioventricular orifice; prevents backflow of blood from right ventricle to right atrium.
P   Pulmonary valve; color blue; prevents backflow of blood from pulmonary trunk to right ventricle.
M   Mitral valve; color red; guards left atrioventridcular orifice; prevents backflow of blood from left ventricle to left atrium.
A   Aortic valve; color red; prevents backflow of blood from aorta to left ventricle.
White circles connected to letters indicate the best position to listen to each of the four heart valves (auscultation areas).

Label auscultation areas

T   Tricuspid valve auscultation area
P   Pulmonary valve auscultation area
M   Mitral valve auscultation area
A   Aortic valve auscultation area

T _____

M _____

P _____

A _____

Muscle: An etymological cartoon

To the ancient Greeks and Romans, contracted muscle looked like small mice running under the skin, so they named the fleshy red bundles of the body *musculi*, which means "little mice," *musculus* being the diminutive of *mus*, mouse.

A pedagogue, or teacher, orginally meant a leader of children and is derived from *pais*, a child, and *agogos*, to lead; hence, a leader of children.

Acropolis means a "high city," from *akron*, peak, and *polis*, city. The acromion is the lateral peak or extremity of the shoulder blade or scapula (*akron*, peak, and *omos*, shoulder). Acrophobia is the fear of heights. Akron, Ohio is built upon a hill.

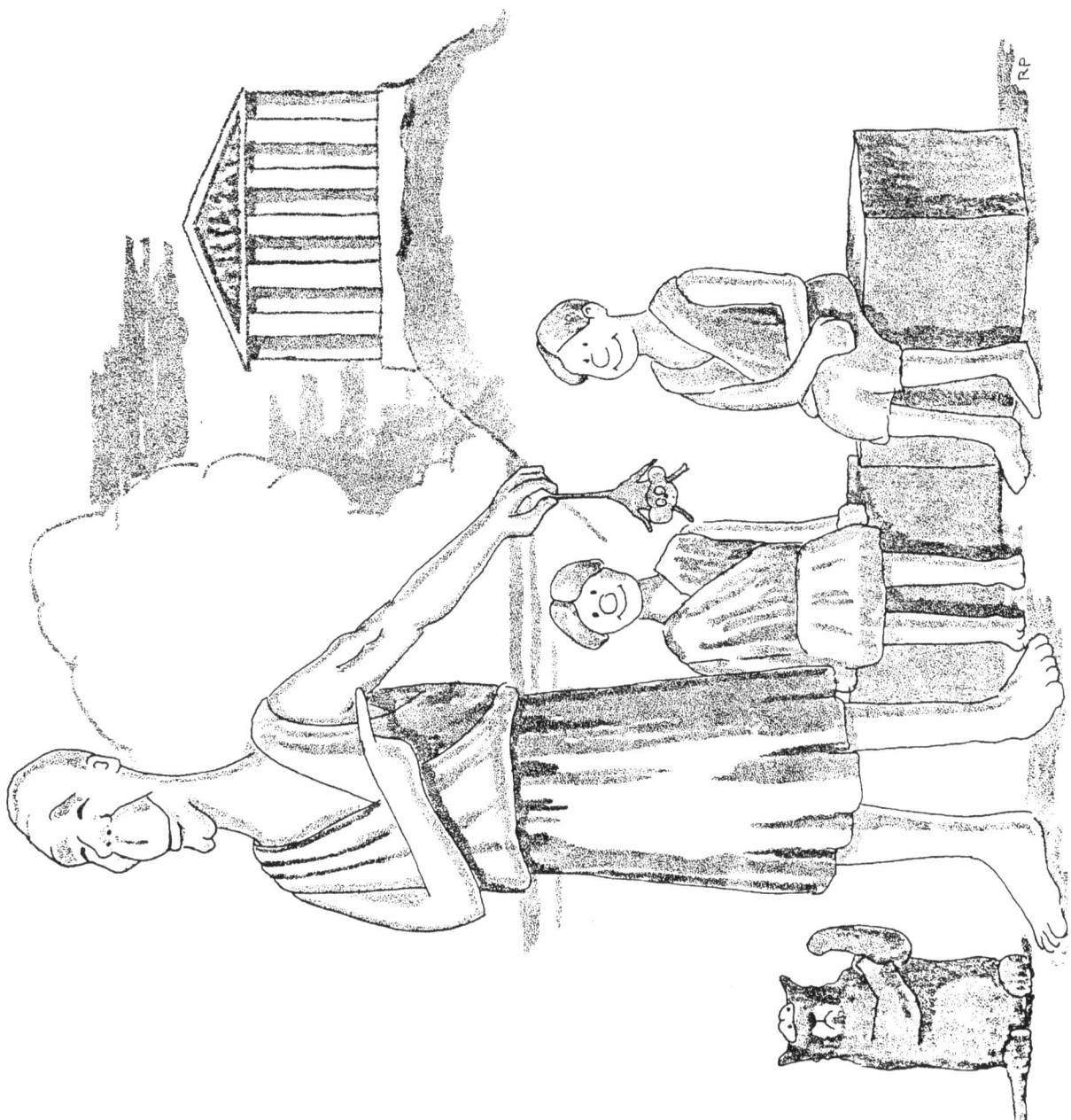

Th-36 Coronary arteries (most common pattern)

Anterior view of heart
Shaded vessels are on posterior surface

Color and label

1. Right coronary artery
2. Main atrial branch (usually called artery of sinuatrial node)
3. Sinuatrial nodal artery (arises from right coronary artery in 55% of hearts examined; from circumflex branch of left coronary artery in 45% of hearts)
4. Right conus artery
5. Right anterior ventricular rami
6. Right marginal artery (reaches apex of heart in 93% of hearts examined)
7. Right posterior ventricular rami
8. Posterior interventricular artery
9. Atrioventricular nodal artery (supplies AV node)
10. Anterior atrial rami
11. Left coronary artery
12. Circumflex artery
13. Anterior interventricular artery
14. Left conus artery
15. Left diagonal artery (present in 33-50% of hearts)
16. Left anterior ventricular arteries
17. Anterior septal rami (supplies anterior part of interventricular septum)
18. Posterior septal arteries
19. Left marginal artery (present in 90% of hearts)

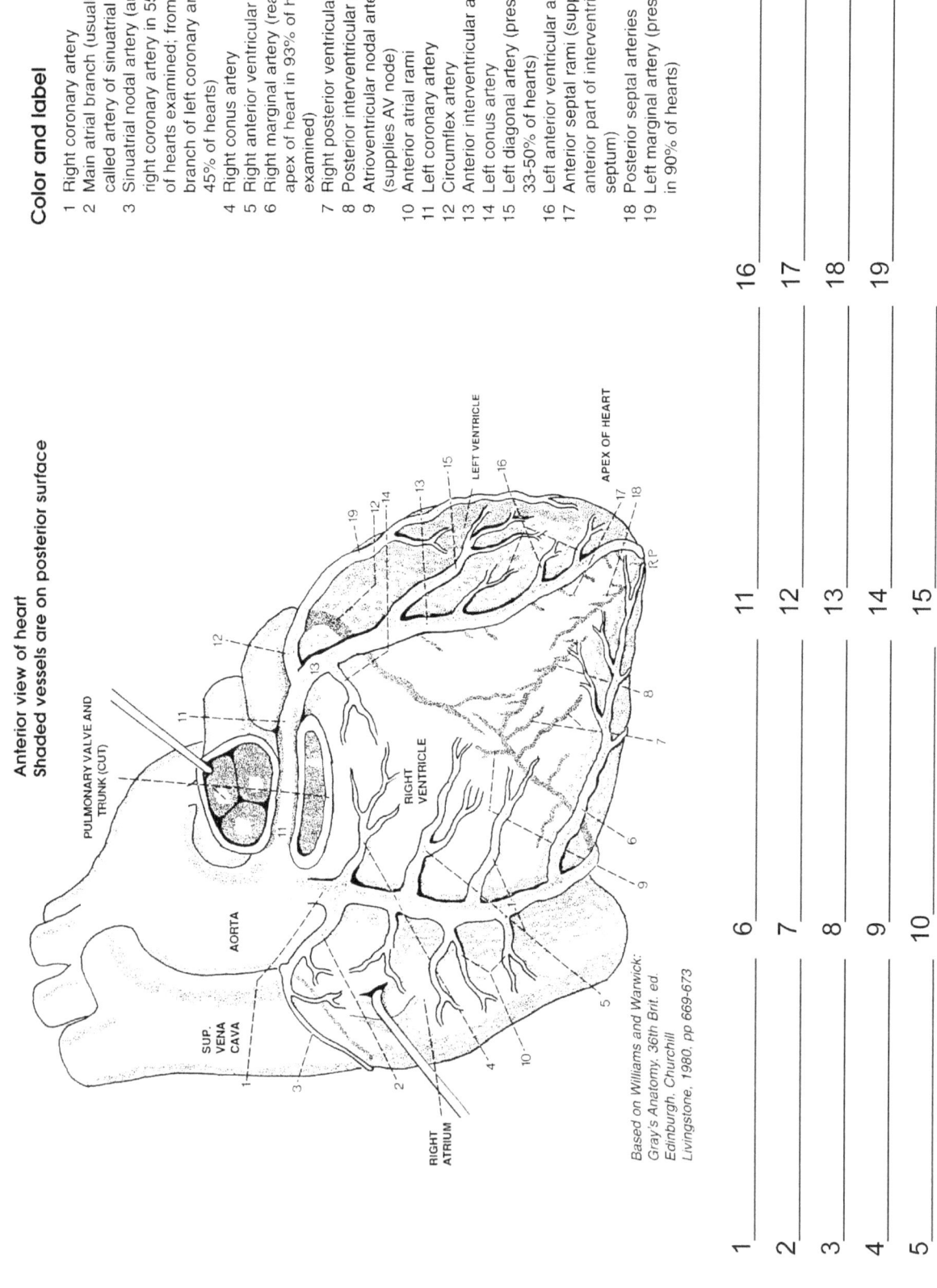

Based on Williams and Warwick:
Gray's Anatomy, 36th Brit. ed.
Edinburgh. Churchill
Livingstone, 1980, pp 669-673

1 _____ 6 _____ 11 _____ 16 _____
2 _____ 7 _____ 12 _____ 17 _____
3 _____ 8 _____ 13 _____ 18 _____
4 _____ 9 _____ 14 _____ 19 _____
5 _____ 10 _____ 15 _____

Th-37 Coronary veins

Venous drainage of the walls of the heart

Anterior view of heart
Shaded vessels are on posterior surface

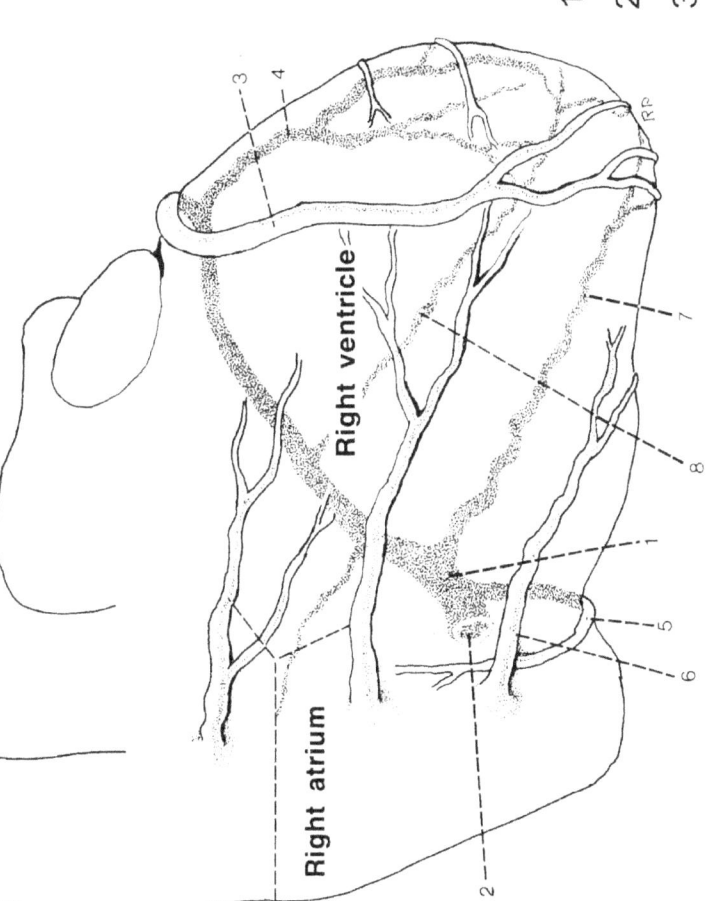

Color and label

1. Coronary sinus (on posterior surface of the heart); the coronary sinus is the main vein that drains blood from the substance (walls) of the heart.
2. Orifice (opening) of the coronary sinus into the right atrium
3. Great cardiac vein
4. Left marginal vein
5. Small cardiac vein
6. Right marginal vein; usually ends in right atrium as shown here; less frequently it drains into small cardiac vein, which then drains into coronary sinus.
7. Middle cardiac vein
8. Posterior vein of left ventricle
9. Anterior cardiac veins; notice these usually drain directly into the right atrium and not into the coronary sinus as do most of the cardiac veins.

The patterns of both veins and arteries vary considerably from one individual to another. Veins vary in their layout considerably more than arteries; the dissector should not expect to encounter arteries and veins especially the latter, exactly like those presented here.

Venae cordis minimae are small veins in the walls of the heart; they return blood from the walls of the heart directly into the chambers. Their openings, termed foramina venarum minimarum, are found in all four chambers, but chiefly in the atria.

1 _____
2 _____
3 _____
4 _____
5 _____
6 _____
7 _____
8 _____
9 _____

Th-38 Cardiac conducting system
(opposite page)

Color and label

1. Sinuatrial node (pacemaker); it initiates the cyclic wave of myocardial depolarization and contraction; its center is traversed by the sinoatrial nodal artery (nodal central artery); it receives a rich supply of sympathetic and parasympathetic nerves which can either speed up or slow down its rate of discharge.
2. Atrioventricular node; its discharge sets off a rapid-moving depolarization down the atrioventricular bundle.
3. Atrioventricular (common) bundle (of His); in membranous part of interventricular septum; notice that the atrioventricular bundle has penetrated the right fibrous trigone.
4. Right atrioventricular bundle branch
5. Left atrioventricular bundle branch
6. Subendocardial plexus of Purkinje cells in left ventricle; these form the terminal branches of left atrioventricular bundle.
7. Right bundle within moderator band (septomarginal trabecula); the papillary muscles contract immediately before ventricular wall contraction, thus pulling the atrioventricular valve leaflets closer together and allowing their concave surfaces to catch the initial force of systolic ventricular blood, which causes the leaflets to "balloon" backward into the closed position. In addition, during ventricular systole, tension on the chordae tendineae by the contracted papillary muscles prevents the valve leaflets from being blown backward into the atria and blood from being regurgitated into the atria.
8. Subendocardial plexus of Purkinje cells in right ventricle; as is the case in the left ventricle, these comprise the terminal branches of right atrioventricular bundle.
9. Pulmonary valve
10. Ascending aorta
11. Superior vena cava
12. Termination of the superior vena cava
13. Tendon of Todaro; a rounded subendocardial collagenous bundle extending from the right fibrous trigone (see figure 38) to the valve of the inferior vena cava; it forms part of the triangle of Koch, which marks the site of the atrioventricular node (see figure 31).
14. Orifice and valve of the coronary sinus
15. Termination and valve of the inferior vena cava
16. Base and posterior leaflet of tricuspid valve; both the septal leaflet and the anterior leaflet have been removed
17. Moderator band (septomarginal trabecula)
18. Posterior papillary muscle of left ventricle
19. Interventricular septum (muscular part)
20. Base and posterior leaflet of mitral valve
21. Right fibrous trigone (part of cardiac skeleton); the small opening in the right fibrous trigone through which the atrioventricular bundle passes affords the only connection between the atria and the ventricles; otherwise, the fibrous cardiac skeleton completely blocks atrial excitation from reaching the ventricles.

The existence and the exact role of "internodal tracts" connecting the sinuatrial node to the atrioventricular node have been intensely debated since the beginning of the 20th century. Early investigators identified what they believed to be three internodal tracts in the wall of the right atrium, an anterior, a middle, and a posterior. One investigator reported finding specialized cardiac cells in one tract that he felt supported the existence of a rapid-conducting pathway between the two nodes. However, current thinking dismisses the existence of any specialized tracts in the right atrium, and that the spread of atrial excitation, unlike that in the ventricles, travels from one myocardial cell to another across the atrial wall. Compact bundles of parallel myocardial cells in the atrial wall probably convey the excitatory impulse slightly faster than the excitatory wave that travels through the greater part of the wall.

Th-38 Cardiac conducting system

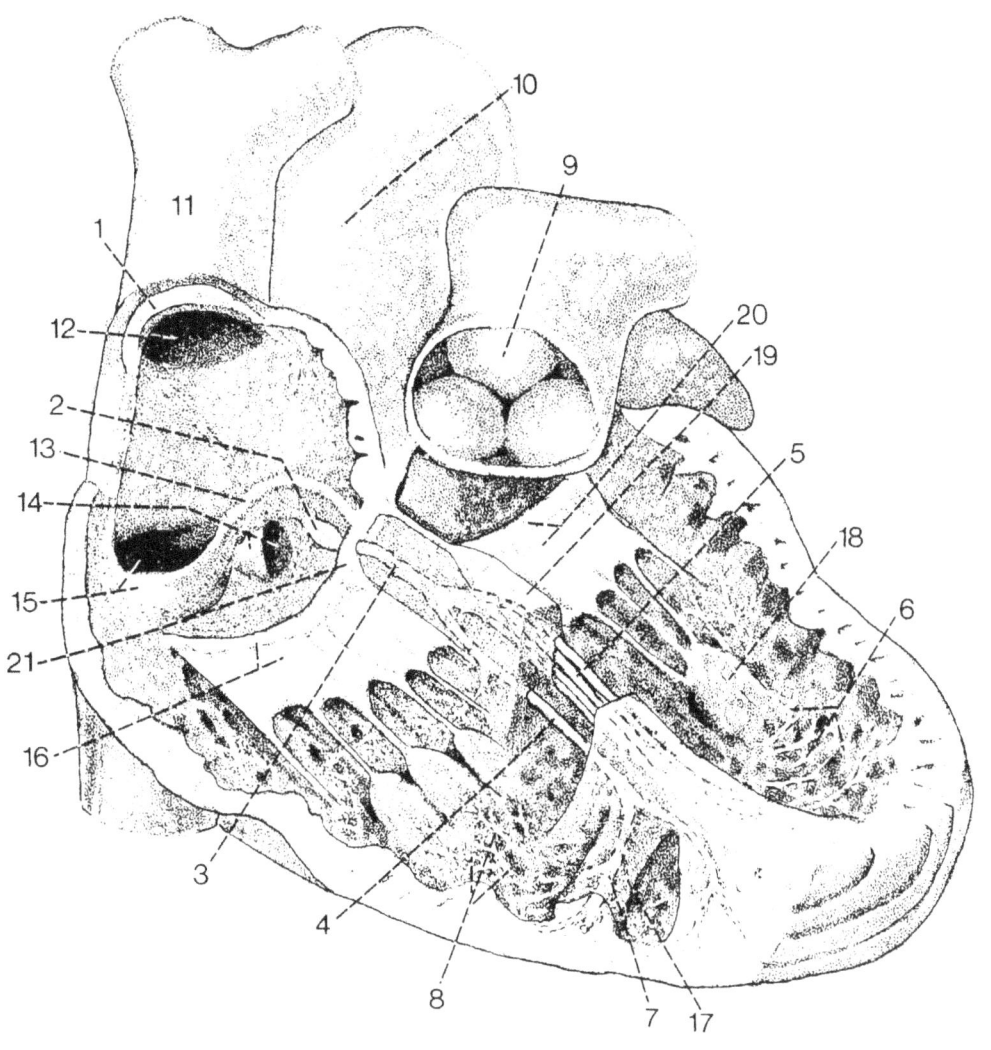

1_____
2_____
3_____
4_____
5_____
6_____
7_____
8_____
9_____
10_____
11_____

12_____
13_____
14_____
15_____
16_____
17_____
18_____
19_____
20_____
21_____

Th-39 Cardiac fibrous skeleton

(opposite page)

Label the indicated structures

Figure A. Posterior view (from atrial aspect) of four heart valves with their fibrous supporting skeleton. The atria have been removed.
1. Fibrous attachment of pulmonary valve cusps: **a**, anterior cusp; **r**, right cusp; **l**, left cusp (actually, left posterior)
2. Fibrous attachment for aortic valve cusps: **r**, right (actually, right-anterior) cusp; **p**, posterior cusp; **l**, left cusp;
3. Right fibrous trigone (central fibrous body; it appears trigone-shaped only when cut coplanar with the atrioventricular orifices; see figure B, below). Strongest part of fibrous skeleton.
4. Fibrous annulus of tricuspid valve leaflets: **a**, anterior leaflet; **p**, posterior leaflet; **s**, septal leaflet.
5. Fibrous annulus of mitral (bicuspid) valve: **p**, posterior leaflet; **a**, anterior leaflet.
6. Tendon of the infundibulum; extends from aortic valve skeleton to pulmonary valve skeleton
7. Site of passage of atrioventricular bundle through right fibrous trigone
8. Left fibrous trigone

Figure B. Fibrous cardiac skeleton viewed from the posterior right and slightly above. The two fibrous rings (tricuspid and mitral valve annuli) have been dissected free from the heart. The aortic and pulmonary valve fibrous supports are shown in the walls of the initial segments of the aorta and pulmonary trunk. The fibrous supports for both the aortic valve cusps and pulmonary valve cusps consist of three semicircular loops that anchor the semilunar cusps to the arterial walls (also described as triple scallops).
1. Aorta initial segment
2. Pulmonary trunk initial segment
3. Opening of left coronary artery
4. Opening of right coronary artery
5. Posterior semicircular support of the posterior aortic cusp. Note its continuity with the right fibrous trigone.
6. Right semicircular support of the right aortic cusp
7. Left semicircular support of the left aortic cusp. Note the fibrous skeleton of both semilunar valves are within the walls of the aorta and pulmonary trunk. The three fibrous semicircular loops are joined to each other at their free ends, which point away from the heart.
8. Pulmonary valve fibrous skeleton; it is similar in structure to that of the aortic valve.
9. Mitral valve fibrous ring (annulus fibrosus). It is not a complete ring but rather consists of two curved prongs (fila coronaria), one arising from the left fibrous trigone and the other arising from the right fibrous trigone. The incomplete part of the ring consists of small segments of fibrous connective tissue.
10. Tricuspid valve fibrous annulus; its structure is similar to the mitral valve fibrous ring. It consists mainly of two curved prongs with an incomplete part filled in by segments of fibrous tissue. It differs from that of the mitral valve in that both prongs are anchored to the right fibrous trigone.
11. Atrioventricular node
12. Membranous part of interventricular septum
13. Atrioventricular bundle (AV common bundle) traversing membranous part of interventricular septum
14. Right and left AV bundle branches (cut); the AV bundle divides into these two branches at the edge of the muscular interventricular septum (not shown).
15. Left fibrous trigone
16. Right fibrous trigone (central fibrous body)

After Williams et al., Gray's Anatomy, 38th British edition, 1995, with slight modification

Figure C. Front view of the heart with the anterior wall largely removed to show the position of the fibrous supporting elements: **T**, tricuspid valve; **M**, mitral valve; **A**, aortic valve; **P**, pulmonary valve. Note the three-loop configuration of both the aortic and pulmonary valve fibrous sleletons. As the ascending aorta leaves the heart, its valve is directed up, right, and slightly forward, whereas the pulmonary valve is directed slightly up, to the left and backward, so that the two valves are situated at right angles to one another.

Figure D. The initial segments of the ascending aorta (A) and the pulmonary trunk (P) viewed from the front. Note their 90-degree relation to each other.

Th-39 Cardiac fibrous skeleton

FIG A (use abbrevs.)

1 _____
2 _____
3 _____
4 _____
5 _____
6 _____
7 _____
8 _____

FIG B (use abbrevs.)

1 _____
2 _____
3 _____
4 _____
5 _____
6 _____
7 _____
8 _____
9 _____
10 _____
11 _____
12 _____
13 _____
14 _____
15 _____
16 _____

FIG C

T _____
M _____
A _____
P _____

FIG D

A _____
P _____

Th-40 Aortic valve and its fibrous support
(opposite page)

Color and label

Figure A. Initial segment of aorta cut open between right cusp and posterior cusp
1. Right aortic cusp
2. Left aortic cusp
3. Posterior (non-coronary) cusp. The three cusps and three aortic sinuses are named according to the origins of the coronary arteries. In the adult heart the **right cusp** (and sinus) are actually more anterior than right, the **left** is actually posterior, and the **posterior** tends to be more right than posterior (see figures C and D below). The cusps are folds of endocardium with a fibrous inner layer. The cusps, as is the case with mitral and tricuspid valve leaflets, have no muscle. Rather they are shaped so that higher pressure from the left ventricle (systolic ejection) will force them open. Whereas higher pressure in the aorta (ventricular diastolic relaxation) will force them to close (causing the "dupp" heart sound in "lubb-dupp, lubb-dupp". The "lubb" sound is the ventricular contraction and the closing of the AV valves. The pulmonary valve works in the same manner in relation to the right ventricle.
4. Right aortic sinus (the aortic sinuses were originally named the *sinuses of Valsalva*)
5. Left aortic sinus
6. Posterior aortic sinus; the aortic sinuses bulge outward giving the aortic root a tri-bulbous appearance.
7. Orifice of right coronary artery
8. Orifice of left coronary artery
9. Nodule (*of Arantius*); a small mass of fibrous tissue on the midpoint of the cusp free border
10. Lunule; thin translucent area of cusp on either side of the nodule
11. Triangular area of aortic wall between the cusp attachments. There are three of these.
12. Membranous part of interventricular septum
13. Left ventricle
14. Right ventricle
15. Muscular part of interventricular septum
16. Subaortic curtain (intervalvular septum); between left cusp and non-coronary cusp. It is continous with the anterior leaflet of the mitral valve.
17. Anterior leaflet of the mitral valve
18. Aortic wall (beginning of ascending aorta)

After Williams et al., Gray's Anatomy, 38th British edition, 1995.

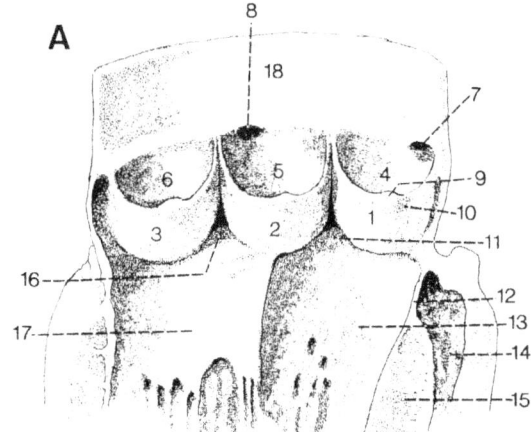

Figure B. Fibrous support for aortic valve cusps; dissected from aorta; viewed from right posterior aspect

1. Posterior cusp semicircular support; it arises from the right fibrous trigone
2. Right cusp semicircular support
3. Left cusp semicircular support; note all three semicircular supports are joined at their apices (10)
4. Right fibrous trigone
5. Left fibrous trigone
6. Anterior curved prong of tricuspid valve fibrous annulus (cut)
7. Posterior curved prong of tricuspid valve fibrous annulus (cut)
8. Posterior curved prong of mitral valve fibrous annulus (cut)
9. Anterior curved prong of mitral valve fibrous annulus (cut)
10. Joined apices of left and right semicircular fibrous loops (also described as three "triple scallops")

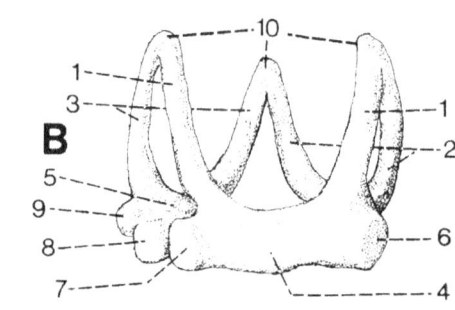

Figure C. Aorta valve **closed** viewed from above (aortic aspect); note apposed boundaries of the 3 cusps form a triradiate pattern.

1. Right cusp and sinus (each sinus is enclosed by the outer aortic wall and the inner ladle-shaped cusp).
2. Left cusp and sinus
3. Posterior cusp and sinus
4. Left coronary artery dividing into the anterior interventricular artery (5) and circumflex artery (6)
7. Right coronary artery

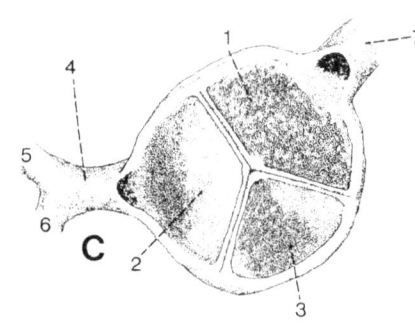

Figure D. Aortic valve in **open** position (ventricular systole). Aortic diameter increases during ventricular ejection. The free edges of the three cusps become taut and straight as the aortic wall expands, causing localized vortices of ejected blood in each sinus and insuring that the orifices of the coronary arteries remain open. All four heart valve fibrous supports are deformable and change shape considerably as the valves alternately open and close.

1. Right cusp
2. Left cusp
3. Posterior cusp
4. Left ventricle viewed through open aortic valve

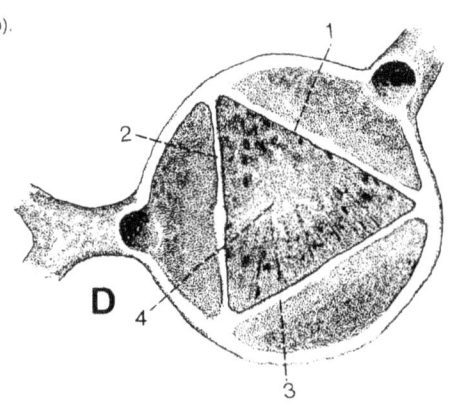

Th-40 Aortic valve and its fibrous support

FIG A

1 _____
2 _____
3 _____
4 _____
5 _____
6 _____
7 _____
8 _____
9 _____
10 _____
11 _____
12 _____
13 _____
14 _____
15 _____
16 _____
17 _____
18 _____

FIG B

1 _____
2 _____
3 _____
4 _____
5 _____
6 _____
7 _____
8 _____
9 _____
10 _____

FIG C

1 _____
2 _____
3 _____
4 _____
5 _____
6 _____
7 _____

FIG D

1 _____
2 _____
3 _____
4 _____

Th-41 Nerves to the heart
(opposite page)

Color and label

1. Heart (right ventricle)
2. Superior vena cava
3. Arch of aorta
4. Left vagus nerve (CN X, cranial nerve number ten; the cranial nerves are designated by Roman numerals; the two vagus nerves are the main outflow of the parasympathetic nervous system).
5. Right vagus nerve
6. Right phrenic nerve; the phrenic nerves innervate the diaphragm.
7. Left phrenic nerve
8. Right recurrent laryngeal nerve (branch of right vagus nerve; "recurrent" means "runs backward")
9. Left recurrent laryngeal nerve; note the different courses of the right and left recurrent laryngeal nerves.
10. Cardiac plexus*
11. Pulmonary trunk
12. Trachea
13. Left common carotid artery
14. Left subclavian artery
15. Right subclavian artery
16. Internal branch of superior laryngeal nerve (a branch of the vagus nerve)
17. Right common carotid artery
18. Left anterior scalene muscle
19. Thyroid gland (right lobe)
20. Cricoid cartilage
21. Thyroid cartilage
22. Superior larngeal branch of vagus nerve
23. Superior thyroid artery
24. External laryngeal branch of superior laryngeal branch of vagus nerve
25. Internal jugular vein
26. Hyoid cartilage

1 _____
2 _____
3 _____
4 _____
5 _____
6 _____
7 _____
8 _____
9 _____
10 _____
11 _____
12 _____
13 _____
14 _____
15 _____
16 _____
17 _____

*Cardiac plexus consists of both **sympathetic** and **parasympathetic nerve fibers**. The **preganglionic sympathetic** fibers originate bilaterally from nerve cell bodies in the **intermediolateral column** of the upper thoracic spinal cord gray matter. They leave the spinal cord with the ventral root of thoracic spinal nerves. Most of the fibers quickly exit the spinal nerve and enter the sympathetic trunk where most preganglionic fibers synapse upon postganglionic nerve cell bodies in the **sympathetic chain ganglia**. However, some preganglionic sympathetic fibers pass through the chain ganglia without synapsing and synapse instead upon sympathetic nerve cell bodies in the **cardiac plexus** (prevertebral ganglia). Postganglionic fibers from the ganglia then penetrate the heart and end mainly in the region of the SA node and AV node. They accelerate the heart beat and increase the force of systolic contraction. The preganglionic parasympathetic nerve fibers arise from **nuclei** in the brain stem **medulla** and travel within the vagus nerve and its cardiac branches, which supply the cardiac plexus with **parasympathetic fibers** that intermingle with sympathetc fibers. The parasympathetic fibers leave the cardiac plexus, penetrate the heart and synapse upon **postganglionic parasympathetic neurons** in the **walls of the right atrium** clustered mainly around the SA node and AV node. They have a slowing effect on the rate of the heart beat and an inhibitory effect on the force of the heart contraction. It is impossibe to distinguish sympathetic fibers from parasympathetic fibers by gross examination. The initiation of the cardiac cycle is myogenic; the physiologic demands of the body are conveyed to the heart by the parasympathetic and sympathetic nervous system, which modulate its rate and strength.

A **plexus** is a network of interlacing nerves or blood vessels.
A **nerve** is a collection of nerve cell fibers (axons) **outside** the central nervous system (brain and spinal cord; CNS). Larger nerves contain blood vessels and are enclosed by strong connective tissue sheaths.
A **ganglion** is a group of nerve cell bodies **outside** the central nervous system.
A neuroanatomical **nucleus** is a collection of nerve cell bodies within the central nervous system.
A **tract** is bundle of axons **within** the central nervous system.
A **synapse** is the **functional contact** between one nerve cell and another nerve cell or muscle fiber or gland. Most synapses occur at the junction between the tiny bulbous endings of axons of one neuron and the dendrites and cell body of another. It is the point where the nerve impulse is transmitted from one nerve cell to another.

Th-41 Nerves to the heart

18 _____
19 _____
20 _____
21 _____
22 _____
23 _____
24 _____
25 _____
26 _____

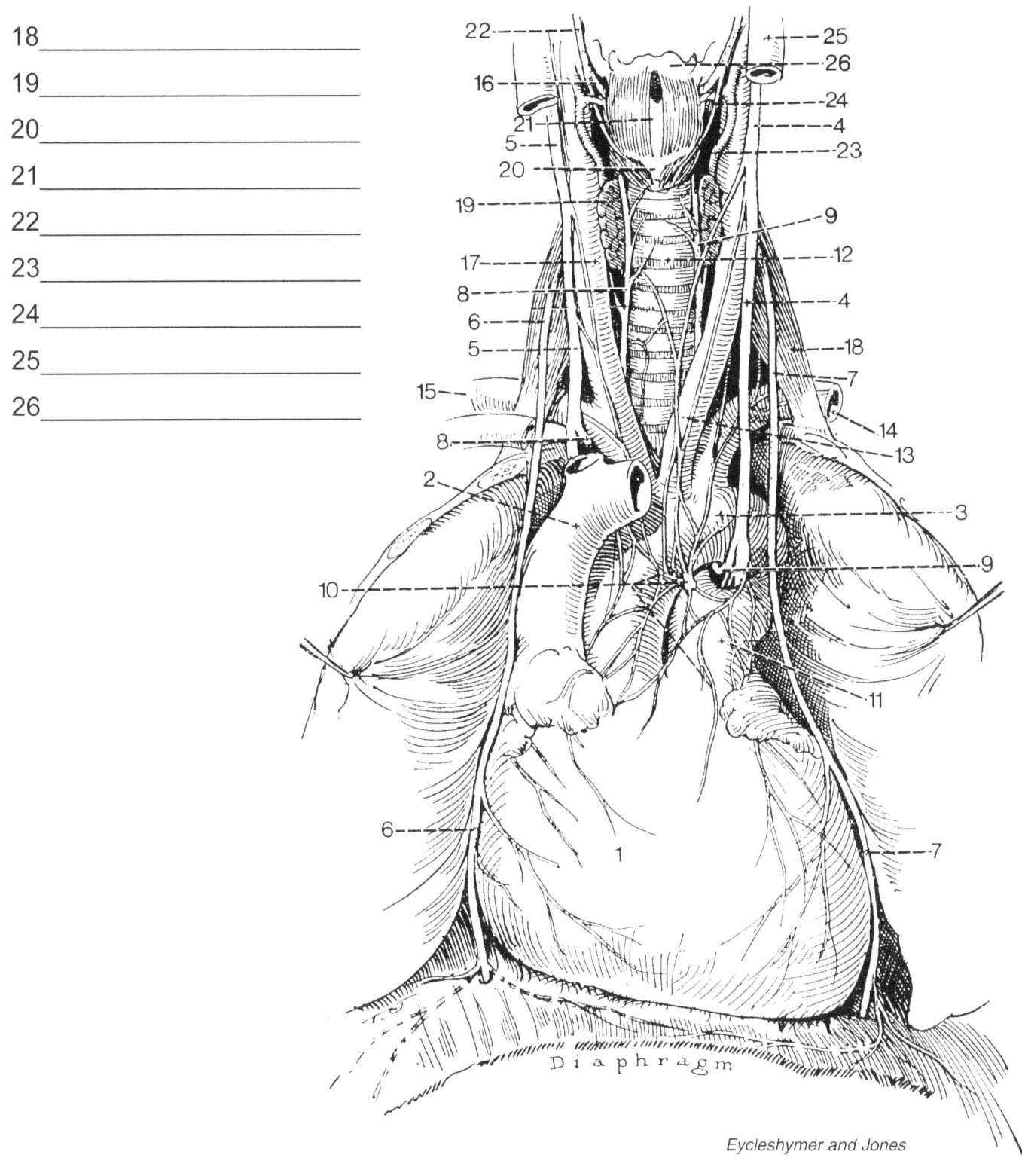

Eycleshymer and Jones

Th-42 Trachea, bronchi, and mediastinal surface of the lungs
(opposite page)

Figure A. The windpipe, or **trachea**, divides into two main or **principal bronchi**: the **right principal bronchus** supplying the right lung and the **left principal bronchus** supplying the left lung. Notice that the right principal bronchus is larger in diameter and more vertical than the left and more in line with the trachea, explaining why foreign objects usually become lodged in the right principal bronchus rather than in the left. The right principal bronchus divides into **three lobar bronchi** that each supply a lobe of the right lung: a **right superior lobar bronchus** to the superior lobe, a **right middle lobar bronchus** to the middle lobe, and a **right inferior lobar bronchus** to the inferior lobe. The **left principal bronchus** divides into a **superior lobar bronchus** which supplies the superior lobe of the left lung and an **inferior lobar bronchus** that supplies the inferior lobe. The left lung has only two lobes, a superior and an inferior, there being no middle lobe or horizontal fissure.

Color and label

1. Trachea
2. Right principal bronchus
3. Left principal bronchus
4. Right superior lobar bronchus
5. Right middle lobar bronchus
6. Right inferior lobar bronchus
7. Left superior lobar bronchus
8. Left inferior lobar bronchus

Notice the transverse rings of cartilage on the trachea* and bronchi. These rings are incomplete posteriorly, the void being filled by the nonstriated (smooth) tracheal muscle. Although these rings appear C-shaped when cut horizontally, they may bifurcate or fuse with the ring above or below. The cartilage rings, which give way to irregular plates of cartilage in the smaller branches of the bronchial tree, are essential in maintaining the patency of the air-conducting tubes and keeping them from collapsing as the air pressure inside them falls below the pressure exerted by the surrounding tissue during inspiration.

The lobar bronchi give off **segmental bronchi**, each of which supplies a **bronchopulmonary segment** of lung tissue. In the right lung the superior lobar bronchus gives off three segmental bronchi, the middle lobar bronchus gives off two segmental bronchi, and the inferior lobar bronchus gives off five segmental bronchi. In the left lung the superior lobar bronchus usually gives off four segmental bronchi and inferior lobar bronchus gives off five segmental bronchi. Each segmental bronchus has a designated number 1-10 plus B (for bronchus); for example, B1, B2, B3. Likewise each bronchopulmonary segment has the corresponding number 1-10 plus S (for segment); for example, S1, S2, S3 (figures 42 and 43). The bronchopulmonary segments are important in that they each contain a self-enclosed segment of lung tissue that is separated from its adjoining segments by connective tissue partitions (or septa) that allow single segments to be surgically removed—if diseased—leaving the rest of the lung intact.

*The word *trachea* comes from the Greek *tracheia,* which means "rough". Aristotle, who believed that the arteries contained air, named the trachea the "rough artery" as opposed to the arteries which he called the "smooth arteries". "Artery" was soon dropped from its name but *tracheia* persisted and became the accepted name for the windpipe.

Figures B and C. Medial surface of lungs

Color and label

1. Pleura surrounding hilum of both lungs
   The hilum is the point where structures enter and leave the lung
2. Principal bronchus
3. Pulmonary artery
4. Pulmonary veins
5. Pulmonary ligament
6. Oblique fissure
7. Horizontal fissure (right lung only)
8. Diaphragmatic (inferior) surface
9. Groove for azygos vein (right lung)
10. Groove for aorta (left lung)
11. Anterior sharp margin and anterior surface
12. Posterior surface and round margin

Th-42 Trachea, bronchi, and mediastinal surface of the lungs

1_____
2_____
3_____
4_____
5_____
6_____
7_____
8_____

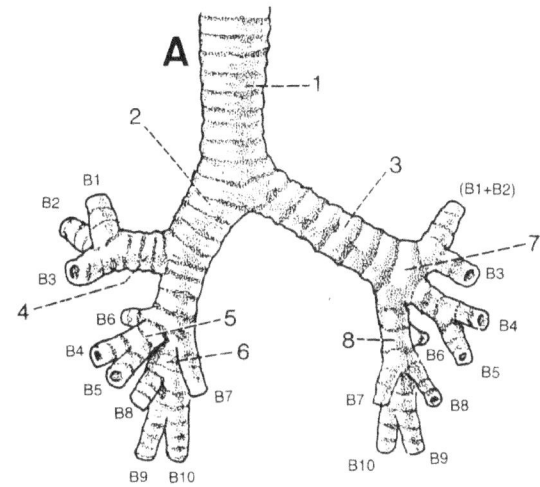

1_____
2_____
3_____
4_____
5_____
6_____
7_____
8_____
9_____
10_____
11_____
12_____

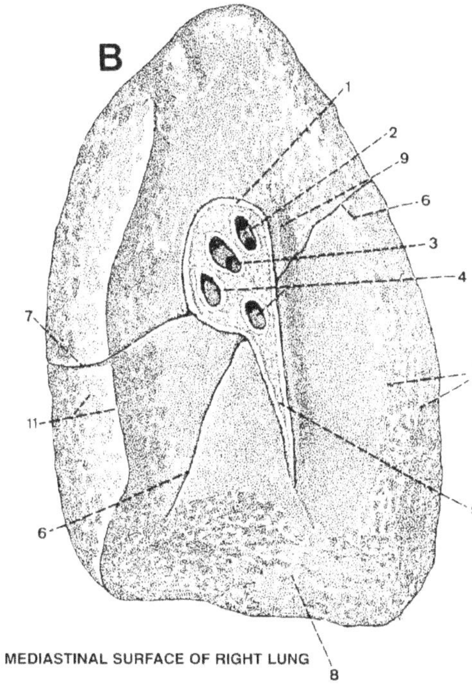

MEDIASTINAL SURFACE OF RIGHT LUNG

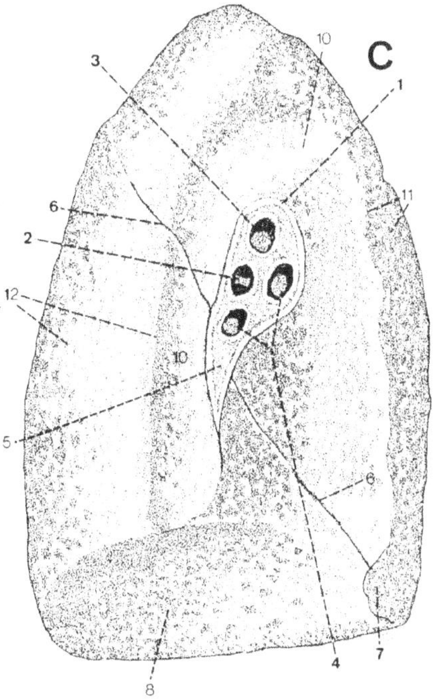

MEDIASTINAL SURFACE OF LEFT LUNG

Th-43 Bronchopulmonary segments Left Lung

(opposite page)

Each segmental bronchus and bronchopulmonary segment (bp) is designated by a letter and a number in addition to a name that indicates its position.

Segmental bronchi

Left superior lobar bronchus
B1+B2 Apicoposterior segmental bronchus

B3 Anterior segmental bronchus
B4 Superior lingual bronchus
B5 Inferior lingual bronchus

Left inferior lobar bronchus
B6 Superior segmental bronchus
B7 Medial basal segmental bronchus
B8 Anterior basal segmental bronchus
B9 Lateral basal segmental bronchus
B10 Posterior basal segmental bronchus

Bronchopulmonary (bp) segments

Superior lobe left lung
S1+S2 Apicoposterior bp segment
(segments S1 and S2 are often supplied by a single segmental bronchus)
S3 Anterior bp segment
S4 Superior lingual bp segment
S5 Inferior lingual bp segment

Inferior lobe left lung
S6 Superior bp segment
S7 Medial basal bp segment
S8 Anterior basal bp segment
S9 Lateral basal bp segment
S10 Posterior basal bp segment

B1 & 2 _____
B3 _____
B4 _____
B5 _____

S1 & 2 _____
S3 _____
S4 _____
S5 _____

B6 _____
B7 _____
B8 _____
B9 _____
B10 _____

S6 _____
S7 _____
S8 _____
S9 _____
S10 _____

Th-43 Bronchopulmonary segments Left Lung

Lateral surface

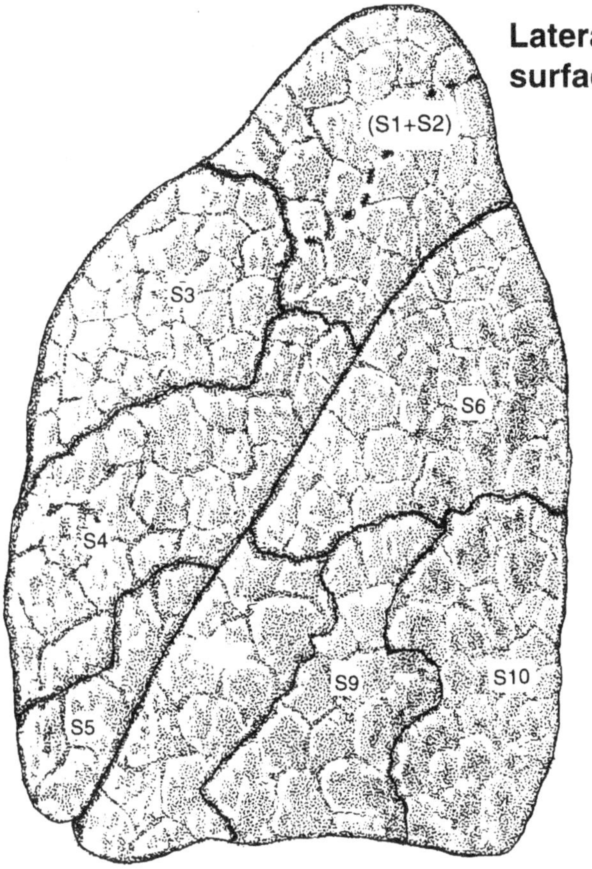

The left lung consists of only two lobes separated by the oblique fissure. Usually the upper lobe contains only four bronchopulmonary segments, as opposed to the right superior lobe which contains five. Segments S1 and S2 are supplied by a single segmental bronchus and, hence, function as a single segment. The lower lobe usually contains five segments, although bronchopulmonary segment S7 is missing in the lung pictured here.

After E. Pernkopf

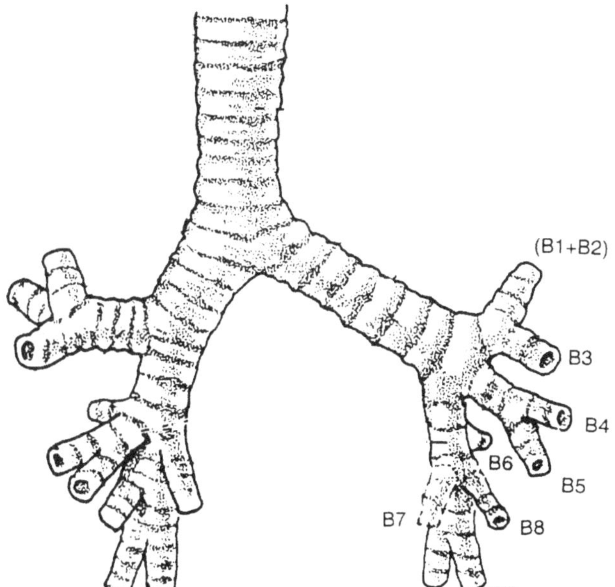

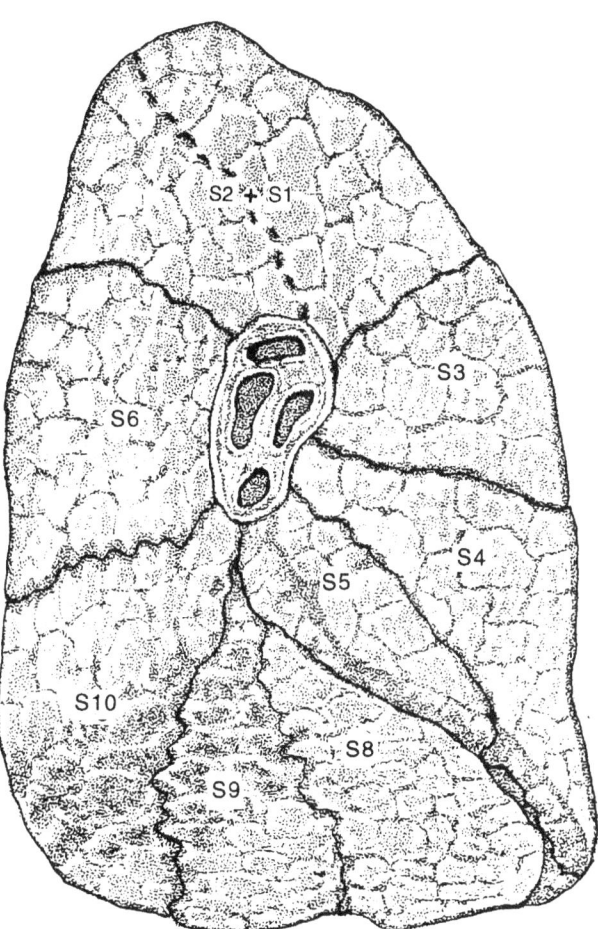

Medial and diaphragmatic surfaces

Color each segmental bronchus (B1-B10) the same color as the bronchopulmonary segment (S1-S10) that it supplies

Th-44 Bronchopulmonary segments Right Lung

(opposite page)

Segmental bronchi

Right superior lobar bronchus
- B1 Apicoposterior segmental bronchus
- B2 Posterior segmental bronchus
- B3 Anterior segmental bronchus

Right middle lobar bronchus
- B4 Lateral segmental brnchus
- B5 Medial segmental bronchus

Right inferior lobar bronchus
- B6 Superior segmental bronchus
- B7 Medial basal segmental bronchus
- B8 Anterior basal segmental bronchus
- B9 Lateral basal segmental bronchus
- B10 Posterior basal segmental bronchus

Bronchopulmonary (bp) segments

Superior lobe right lung
- S1 Apicoposterior bp segment
- S2 Posterior bp segment
- S3 Anterior bp segment

Middle lobe right lung
- S4 Lateral bp segment
- S5 Medial bp segment

Inferior lobe right lung
- S6 Superior bp segment
- S7 Medial basal bp segment
- S8 Anterior basal bp segment
- S9 Lateral basal bp segment
- S10 Posterior basal bp segment

B1 _____
B2 _____
B3 _____

B4 _____
B5 _____

B6 _____
B7 _____
B8 _____
B9 _____
B10 _____

S1 _____
S2 _____
S3 _____

S4 _____
S5 _____

S6 _____
S7 _____
S8 _____
S9 _____
S10 _____

Th-44 Bronchopulmonary segments Right Lung

Color each segmental bronchus (B1-B10) the same color as the bronchopulmonary segment (S1-S10) that it supplies

The right lung differs from the left lobe by having three lobes instead of two and a horizontal fissure (which may not always be present) in addition to an oblique fissure. The boundaries of the bronchopulmonary segments are not visible on the surface of the lung as pictured here. Each bronchopulmonary segment is a self-contained unit of respiratory tissue which, if diseased, may be surgically excised rather than having a whole lobe or the entire lung removed. The right upper lobe has three segments, the middle lobe has two segments, and the inferior lobe has five segments.

After E. Pernkopf

Lateral surface

Medial and diaphragmatic surfaces

Th-45A Bronchopulmonary segment

Air passages

The air passages in 9 to 10 bronchopulmonary segments in each lung are self-contained branching tubes that divide into smaller and smaller tubes; that is, they do not pass into adjacent segments, but rather remain entirely within the connective tissue septa that separate the segments from one another. In cases of disease or damage, a single diseased segment rather than a whole lobe may be surgically excised. Unfortunately, the exact positions of the septa are not evident on the exterior of the lungs. The dissector should, however, appreciate their importance and have an approximate idea of the position of each segment.

Color and label

1. Lobar broncus. Each lobar bronchus supplies air to a single lobe of the lungs; the 3 lobar bronchi supply the 3 lobes in the right lung, and 2 lobar bronchi supply the 2 lobes in the left lung.
2. Segmental bronchus. The lobar bronchi divide into segmental bronchi, each of which supplies a single bronchopulmonary segment.
3. Divisions (branches) of segmental bronchus. Note that the air passageways remain entirely within the bronchopulmonary segment and do not cross into adjacent segments. The arteries sometimes extend into adjacent segments, and the veins tend to lie intersegmentally between the segments as well as under the pulmonary pleura on the exterior surface of the lungs (see opposite page).
4. Intersegmental (between the segments) connective tissue septa (partitions)
5. Intrasegmental (within the segment) septa
6. Pulmonary pleura (being pulled off the exterior of the lung)

Air passage (segmental bronchus) in one bronchopulmonary segment

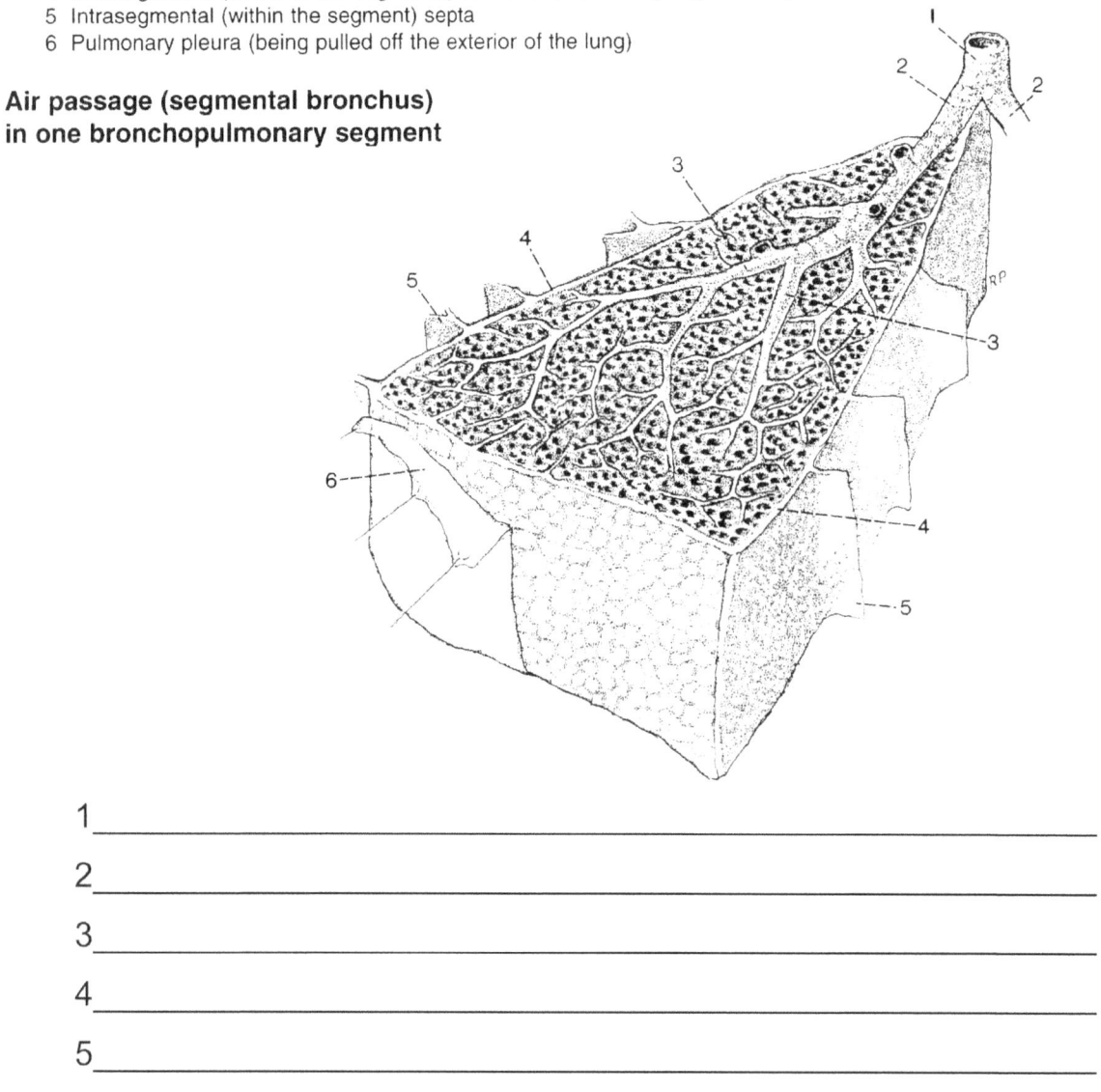

1. _____
2. _____
3. _____
4. _____
5. _____
6. _____

Th-45B Bronchopulmonary segment

Color and label

1. Lobar bronchus (branch of principal bronchus)
2. Segmental bronchus (branch of lobar bronchus)
3. Lobar artery (branch of pulmonary artery)
4. Segmental artery (branch of lobar artery)
5. Branch (tributary) of pulmonary vein
6. Intersegmental (between segments) vein
7. Venous plexus in connective tissue intersegmental septum (partition between bronchopulmonary segments)
8. Subpleural venous plexus
9. Arteries penetrating septum and entering adjacent segment
10. Connective tissue septum between segments
11. Pleura (reflected)
12. Septa extending into segment and into adjacent segments (not shown)

Air passage (segmental bronchus) and accompanying blood vessels in one bronchopulmonary segment

The right lung usually contains ten bronchopulmonary (BP) segments and the left lung usually has nine segments. Each BP segment has its own self-contained air supply consisting of a single segmental bronchus (2) and its progressively smaller branches. The segmental artery, which may be more than one (3), tends to accompany the segmental bronchus and its descendant divisions. Arteries occasionally become intersegmental and enter adjacent segments (9). The smaller veins are intrasegmental and drain peripherally into the larger intersegmental veins that course in the connective tissue septums (6,7). The veins also form venous plexuses beneath the pleura (11).

1. _____
2. _____
3. _____
4. _____
5. _____
6. _____
7. _____
8. _____
9. _____
10. _____
11. _____
12. _____

Th-46 Lungs and pleura
(opposite page)

The pleura is a serous membrane that invests the lungs and lines the inside of the rib cage. The **pulmonary** pleura covers the lungs and the **parietal** pleura lines the inside of the chest cavity. The parietal pleura is made up of: 1) the costal pleura, which lines the inside of the ribs; 2) the diaphragmatic pleura, which covers the upper surface of the diaphragm, and 3) the mediastinal pleura, which covers most of the pericardium. The pleura is actually two closed sacs that the lungs grow into just as the heart pushes into the pericardium. The actual space in the pleural sacs (pleural cavity) is a potential space that contains only a little serous fluid that allows the pulmonary pleura covering the lungs to slide against the parietal pleura.

Color and label

Figure A. Front view of lungs
1. Thymus gland (remnant)
2. Pulmonary (visceral) pleura (invests the lungs; reflected)
3. Superior lobe of left lung
4. Cardiac notch
5. Mediastinal pleura (fused to pericardium; part of the parietal pleura); note that the two pleural sacs are totally separate.
6. Oblique fissure
7. Inferior lobe of left lung
8. Reflection (folding) of diaphragmatic pleura with costal pleura forming the costodiaphragmatic recess
9. Pericardium
10. Diaphragm
11. Diaphragmatic pleura (fused to top of diaphragm)
12. Costodiaphragmatic recess of right lung. Note that the lung does not completely occupy the recess and that the pleura extends more caudally than does the lung. During normal breathing the lung will push partly into this recess and withdraw with every breath.
13. Inferior lobe of right lung
14. Oblique fissure
15. Middle lobe of right lung
16. Horizontal fissure
17. Parietal pleura (cut edge)
18. Superior lobe of right lung
19. Pulmonary pleura (reflected)

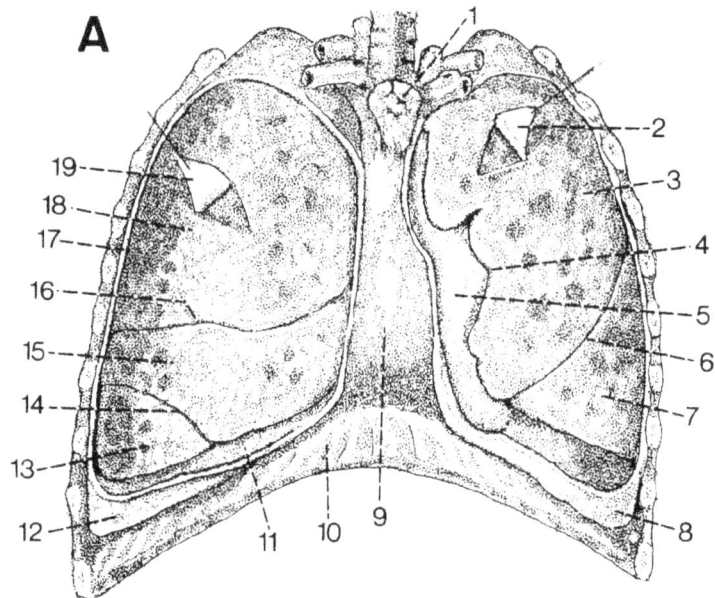

Figure B. Inferior view of lungs and heart
1. Heart
2. Inferior lobe of left lung
3. Oblique fissure
4. Pericardiacophrenic artery and vein ("sandwiched" between the pericardium and the mediastinal pleura)
5. Phrenic nerve (also "sandwiched")
6. Left lung (inferior surface of inferior lobe)
7. Aorta (giving rise to two posterior intercostal arteries)
8. Sympathetic trunk
9. Azygos vein receiving two posterior intercostal veins
10. Thoracic duct
11. Esophagus and esophageal plexus (on its exterior)
12. Inferior vena cava
13. Inferior lobe of right lung
14. Oblique fissure
15. Superior lobe of right lung
16. Phrenic nerve and accompanying pericardiacophrenic artery and vein

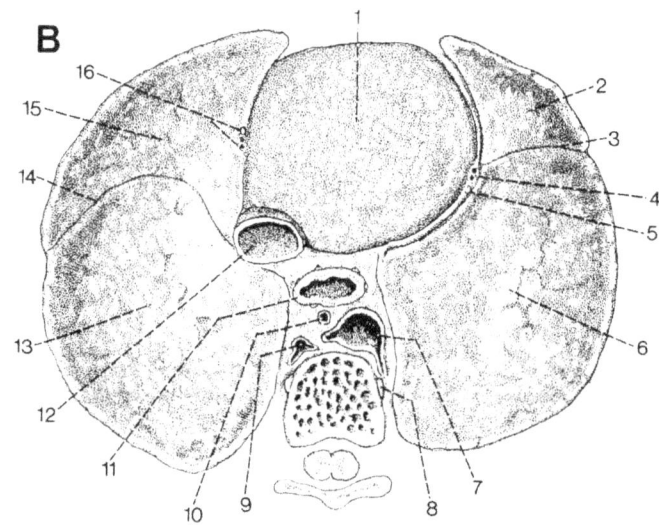

Figure C. Bifurcation of the trachea into right and left principal bronchi. Cut coronally. Viewed from behind
1. Trachea (wind pipe)
2. Right main bronchus; note it is larger and more vertical than the left main bronchus.
3. Left main bronchus; note it is more horizontal than the right main bronchus
4. Carina (keel-like projection at bifurcation); foreign objects often become lodged on the carina.

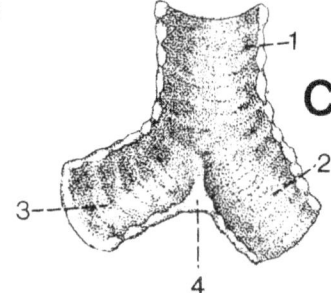

Th-46 Lungs and pleura

FIG A

1 _____
2 _____
3 _____
4 _____
5 _____
6 _____
7 _____
8 _____
9 _____
10 _____

11 _____
12 _____
13 _____
14 _____
15 _____
16 _____
17 _____
18 _____
19 _____

FIG B

1 _____
2 _____
3 _____
4 _____
5 _____
6 _____
7 _____
8 _____
9 _____

10 _____
11 _____
12 _____
13 _____
14 _____
15 _____
16 _____

FIG C

1 _____
2 _____
3 _____
4 _____

Th-47 The pleura and pleural recesses

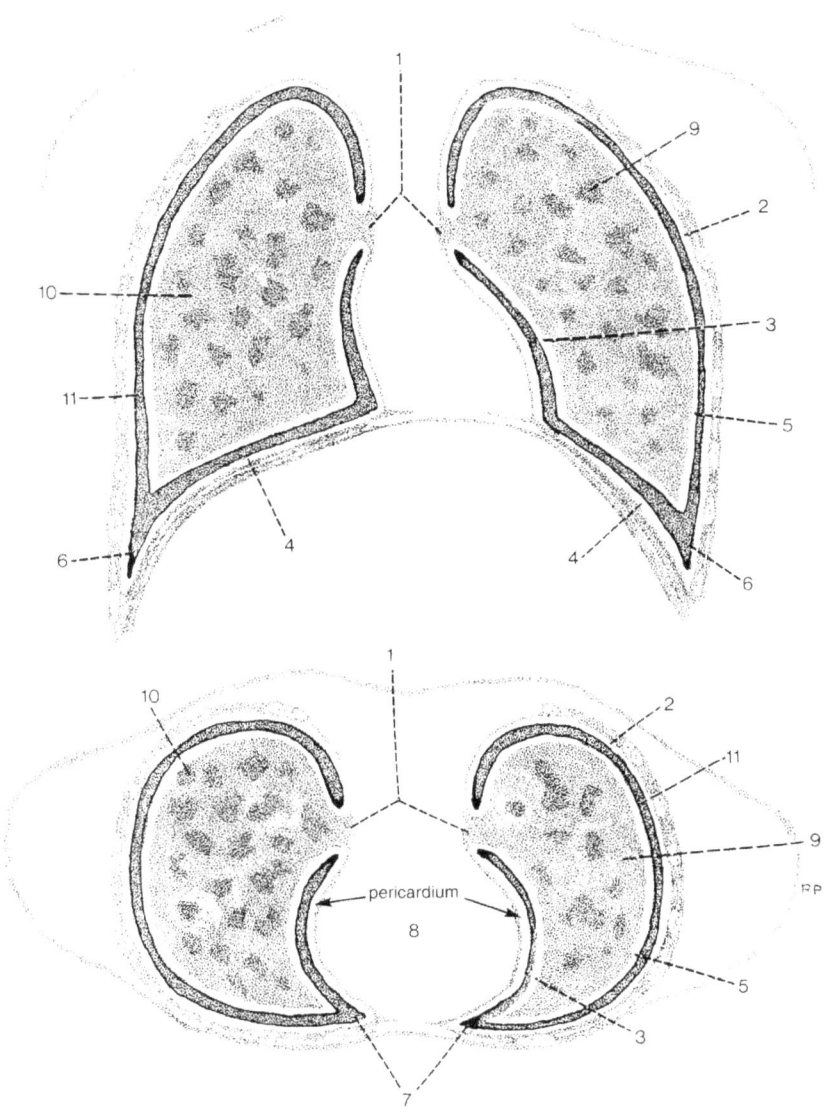

Color and label

1. Roots of lung; these contain the principal bronchi, arteries, veins, nerves, and lymphatics entering and leaving the lungs
2. Costal pleura
3. Mediastinal pleura (fused to pericardium)
4. Diaphragmatic pleura
5. Pulmonary (visceral) pleura
6. Costodiaphragmatic recess; normally only a slit. Note that it extends considerably further caudally than does the lung.
7. Costomediastinal recess; also only a slit. The recesses are important in that their accidental puncture may introduce infection into the pleural cavity
8. Heart
9. Left lung
10. Right lung
11. Pleural cavity (a potential space)

1 _____
2 _____
3 _____
4 _____
5 _____
6 _____
7 _____
8 _____
9 _____
10 _____
11 _____

Th-48 Trachea, esophagus and vagus nerve

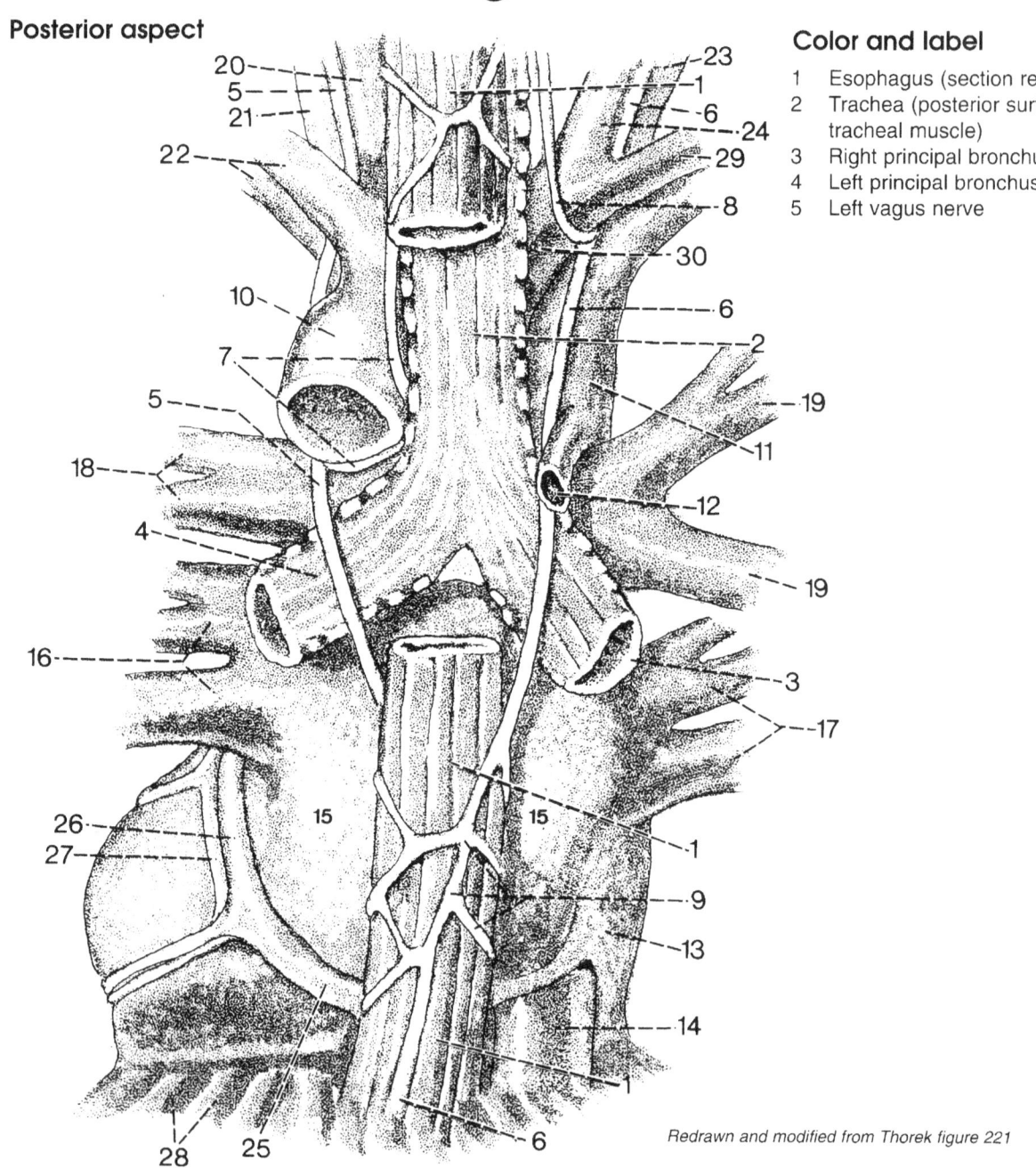

Posterior aspect

Color and label
1. Esophagus (section removed)
2. Trachea (posterior surface; tracheal muscle)
3. Right principal bronchus
4. Left principal bronchus
5. Left vagus nerve
6. Right vagus nerve
7. Left recurrent laryngeal nerve
8. Right recurrent laryngeal nerve
9. Esophageal plexus
10. Arch of aorta
11. Superior vena cava
12. Azygos vein
13. Right atrium
14. Inferior vena cava
15. Left atrium
16. Left pulmonary veins (red)
17. Right pulmonary veins (red)
18. Left pulmonary arteries (blue)
19. Right pulmonary arteries (blue)
20. Left common carotid artery
21. Internal jugular vein
22. Left subclavian artery and vein
23. Right jugular vein
24. Right common carotid artery
25. Coronary sinus
26. Great cardiac vein
27. Circumflex artery
28. Diaphragm
29. Right subclavian artery
30. Brachiocephalic artery

Redrawn and modified from Thorek figure 221

Th-48 Trachea, esophagus and vagus nerve

(opposite page)

1_____
2_____
3_____
4_____
5_____
6_____
7_____
8_____
9_____
10_____
11_____
12_____
13_____
14_____
15_____
16_____
17_____
18_____
19_____

20_____
21_____
22_____
23_____
24_____
25_____
26_____
27_____
28_____
29_____
30_____

Th-49 Right mediastinum

Right lung has been removed (opposite page)

Color and label

1. Right vagus nerve
2. Internal jugular vein
3. Internal thoracic artery; its origin is variable, but it usually arises from the first part of the subclavian artery
4. Subclavian vein
5. Cupula of pleura; covers apex of lung (the part above the first rib)
6. Internal thoracic vein; usually ends in the brachiocephalic vein
7. Manubrium
8. Vagus nerve
9. Anterior intercostal artery and vein (cut); each intercostal space has two pairs of these vessels: one pair below the rib above and one pair above the lower rib
10. Superior vena cava and remains of thymus gland
11. Ascending aorta
12. Lobar branches of right pulmonary artery
13. Internal thoracic artery and vein; note cut origins of anterior intercostal arteries and veins. The internal thoracic vessels also give off branches to the sternum and perforating branches to the muscle and to the breast pectoralis major
14. Phrenic nerve with pericardiacophrenic artery and vein (mediastinal pleura has been stripped away)
15. Pericardium and cut edge of parietal pleura
16. Sternum (body)
17. Pulmonary veins
18. Pulmonary ligament; visceral ligaments are made up of a double layer of serous membrane — here it is pleura — and connective tissue. In the abdomen visceral ligaments are a double layer of peritoneum.
19. Diaphragm
20. Greater splanchnic nerve (roots)
21. Intercostal nerve
22. Intercostal vein, artery, and nerve (**vein** is usually superior to the **artery**, which lies above the **nerve**; a useful mnemonic — from top to bottom — is VAN for vein, artery, and nerve).
23. Sympathetic ganglionated trunk
24. Right superior and inferior lobar bronchi
25. Azygos vein and azygos arch
26. Superior intercostal vein; note it is larger than the other intercostal veins
27. Trachea
28. Posterior intercostal vein, artery, and intercostal nerve
29. First rib
30. Right subclavian artery
31. Right common carotid artery

1 _____
2 _____
3 _____
4 _____
5 _____
6 _____
7 _____

8 _____
9 _____
10 _____
11 _____
12 _____
13 _____
14 _____
15 _____
16 _____
17 _____
18 _____
19 _____
20 _____
21 _____
22 _____
23 _____
24 _____
25 _____
26 _____
27 _____
28 _____
29 _____
30 _____
31 _____

Th-49 Right mediastinum

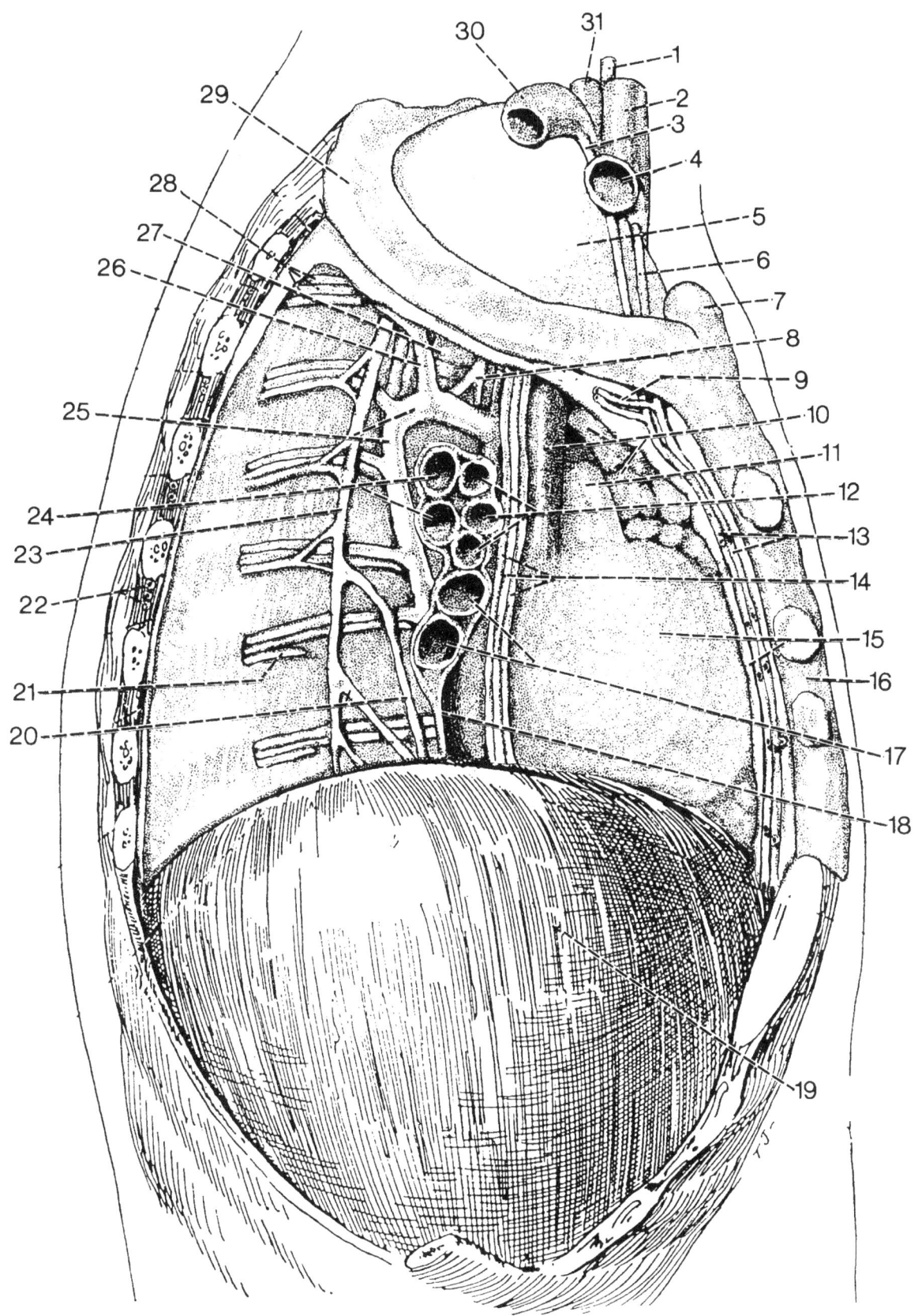

Eycleshymer and Jones with modification

Th-50 Left mediastinum

Left lung has been removed (opposite page)

Color and label

1. First rib
2. Arch of aorta
3. Sympathetic ganglion
4. Left vagus nerve
5. Posterior intercostal vein
6. Posterior intercostal artery
7. Intercostal nerve
8. Sympathetic trunk
9. Left principal bronchus
10. Thoracic aorta
11. Esophagus
12. Hemiazygos vein; highly variable; often absent.
13. Greater splanchnic nerve; consisting mainly of preganglionic sympathetic nerve fibers destined for the abdomen.
14. Esophageal plexus (vagus nerve)
15. Diaphragm
16. Pericardium and heart
17. Pulmonary ligament
18. Pulmonary veins
19. Pericardiacophrenic artery and vein
20. Remains of thymus gland
21. Phrenic nerve
22. Left pulmonary artery
23. Manubrium of sternum
24. Ligamentum arteriosum; remains of the fetal ductus arteriosum which shunted oxygenated blood from the left pulmonary artery to the aorta.
25. Subclavian vein
26. Left recurrent laryngeal nerve; a branch of the vagus nerve; it supplies all the intrinsic muscles of the larynx except one.
27. Internal thoracic artery
28. Subclavian artery
29. Cupula of the pleura

Th-50 Left mediastinum

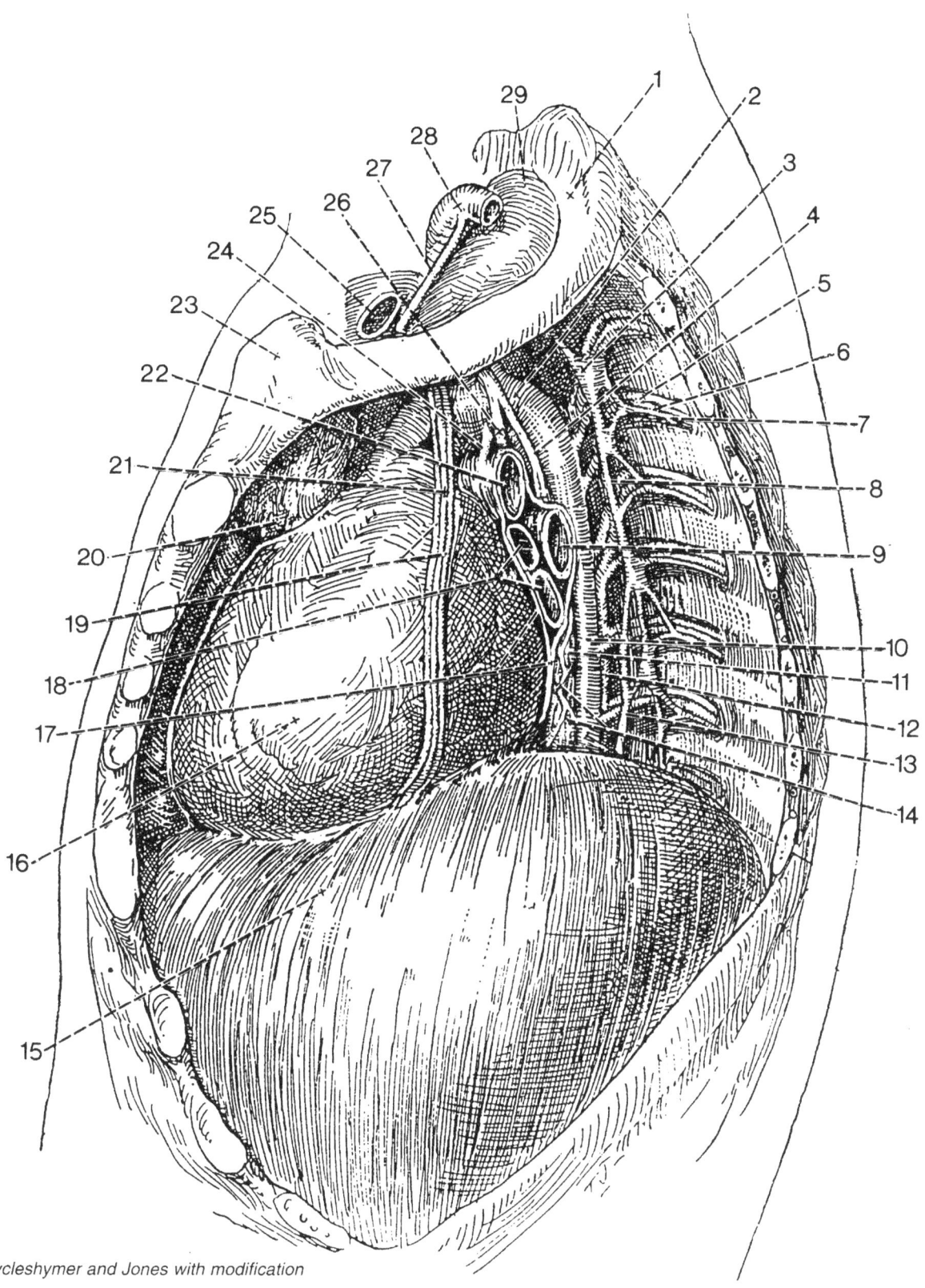

Eycleshymer and Jones with modification

89

Th-51 Diaphragm
Viewed from below
(opposite page)

1. _____
2. _____
3. _____
4. _____
5. _____
6. _____
7. _____
8. _____
9. _____
10. _____
11. _____
12. _____
13. _____
14. _____

Th-51 Diaphragm
Viewed from below

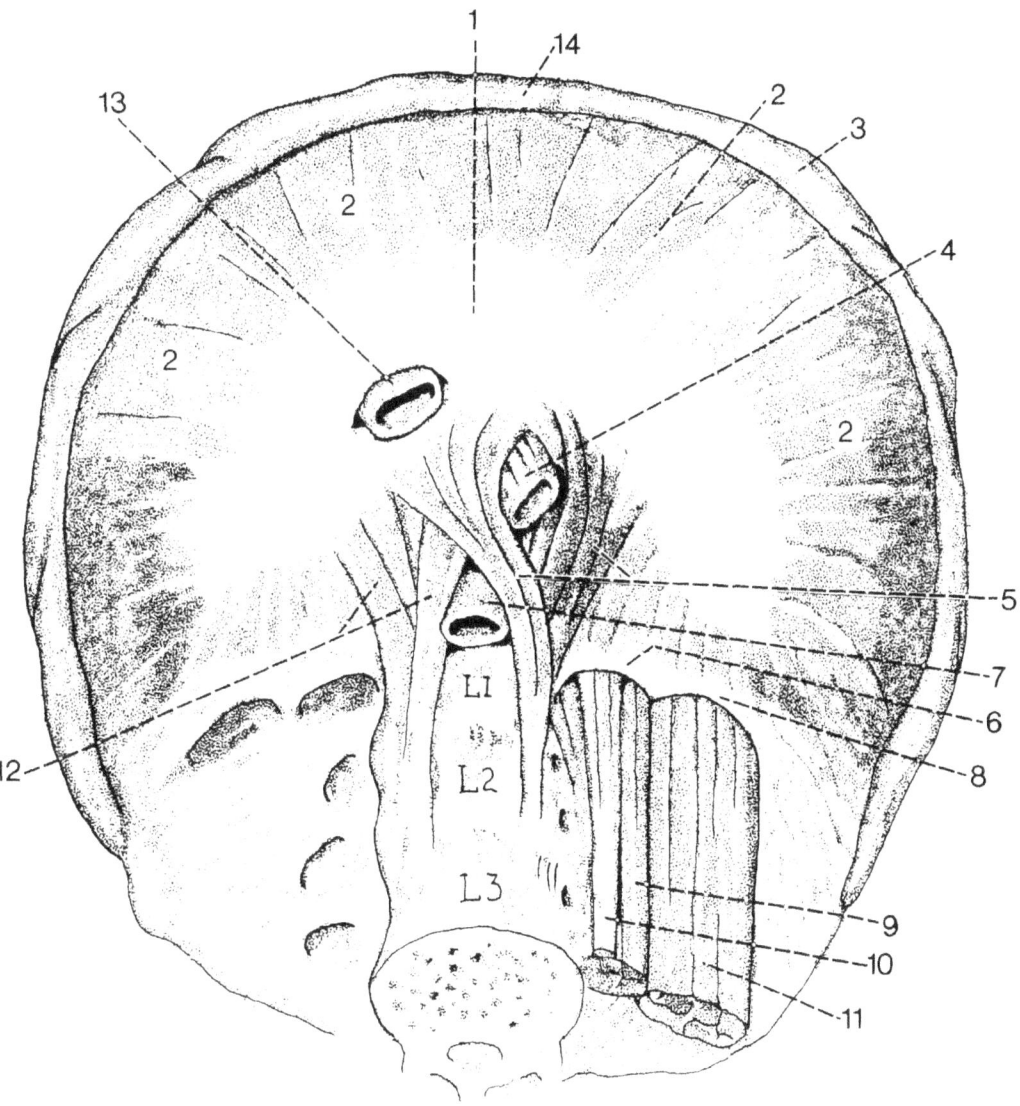

Color and label

1. Central tendon; a strong fibrous sheet into which the peripheral muscular diaphragm inserts. It forms the superior part of the dome-shaped diaphragm. It is pulled down with each inspiration (diaphragmatic contraction) and rises up with each expiration (diaphragmatic relaxation).
2. Muscular part of diaphragm. The diaphragm arises from the sternum (14), the lower border of the rib cage (3), the right (12) and left crura (5), and the medial (7) and lateral (8) arcuate ligaments.
3. Rib cage lower border
4. Esophagus. The right and left vagus nerves pass with the esophagus into the abdomen. A hiatal hernia is the protrusion of part of the stomach through the esophageal hiatus into the thorax.
5. Left crura of diaphragm
6. Medial arcuate ligament
7. Aorta; the thoracic duct and occasionally the azygos vein pass through the aortic opening. The aorta actually enters the abdomen **behind** the diaphragm and **not through** it.
8. Lateral arcuate ligament
9. Psoas major muscle
10. Psoas minor muscle (tendon)
11. Quadratus lumborum muscle
12. Right crura of the diaphragm
13. Inferior vena cava
14. Sternum (xiphoid process)

Th-52 Azygos vein and its tributaries
(opposite page)

Color and label

1. Azygos vein. Azygos means "not paired, without a twin or a mate" (Greek). The name probably arose because the hemiazygos and accessory hemiazygos veins, even when present, do not present a symmetrical mirror-image "twin".
2. Opening of azygos vein into the superior vena cava
3. Hemiazygos vein. The hemiazygos and accessory hemiazygos veins may both be absent. In this situation the azygos vein receives the posterior intercostal veins from the left side as well as the right side.
4. Accessory hemiazygos vein. The azygos system of veins is highly variable.
5. Horizontal connecting vein draining hemiazygos vein on the left into the azygos vein on the right
6. Left superior intercostal vein. The second, third, and sometimes the fourth intercostal veins unite to form the superior intercostal vein, which drains into the left brachiocephalic vein. The right superior intercostal vein joins the azygos vein where it begins its arch towards the superior vena cava.
7. Posterior intercostal vein
8. Left ascending lumbar vein
9. Right ascending lumbar vein. The azygos and hemiazygos veins begin at the junction of the ascending lumbar vein and the subcostal vein (not shown).
10. Left ascending lumbar vein connecting with left renal vein. The lumbar veins drain mainly into the superior vena cava by way of the azygos system.
11. Superior vena cava
12. Right brachiocephalic vein
13. Left brachiocephalic vein
14. Right renal vein
15. Inferior vena cava
16. Portion of inferior vena cava receiving hepatic veins. This portion is surrounded by the liver, which has been removed.
17. Lumbar vein
18. Aorta (cut)
19. Diaphragm
20. Esophagus (cut)
21. Pectoralis major muscle
22. Pectoralis minor muscle
23. Right kidney
24. Left kidney

1 _____
2 _____
3 _____
4 _____
5 _____
6 _____
7 _____
8 _____
9 _____
10 _____
11 _____
12 _____
13 _____
14 _____
15 _____
16 _____
17 _____
18 _____
19 _____
20 _____
21 _____
22 _____
23 _____
24 _____

Th-52 Azygos vein and its tributaries

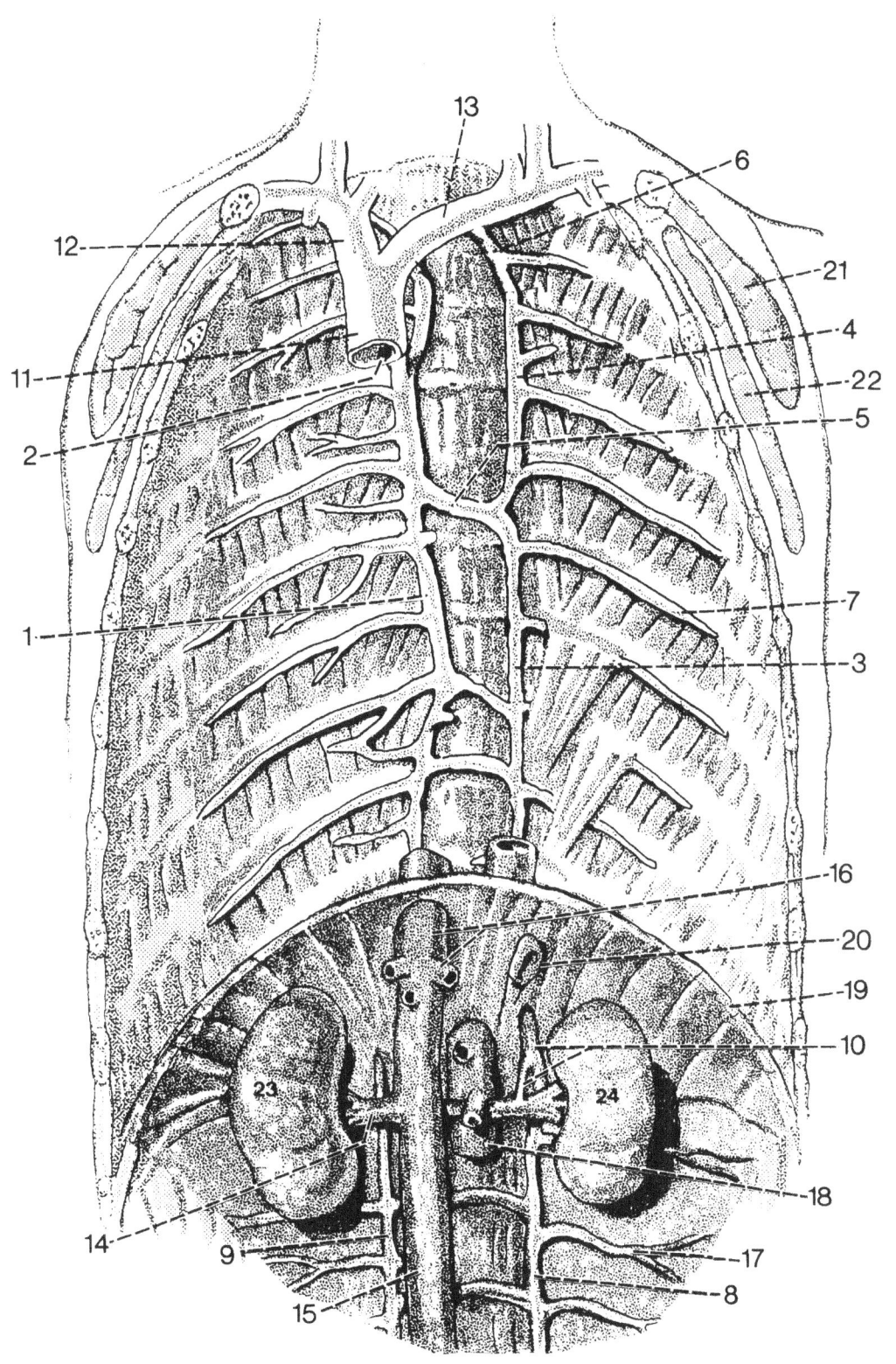

Th-53 Blood flow in the fetus
(opposite page)

Fetal blood gains its oxygen and gives off its carbon dioxide in the placenta (1). Oxygen-rich blood is carried from the placenta to the fetus by the umbilical vein (2). The umbilical vein enters the abdomen and ends in the liver where it attaches to the left branch of the portal vein. A short shunt within the liver, the ductus venosus (5), conveys the blood to the inferior vena cava (6) which empties the oxygen-rich blood — along with some oxygen-poor blood from the fetus's abdomen and legs — into the right atrium (7) of the heart. The superior vena cava also returns oxygen-poor blood from the arms, head, neck to the right atrium. As blood enters the right atrium, a considerable portion of the oxygen-rich blood passes through two holes in the interatrial septum (8) (see figure 54), into the left atrium (10), thus bypassing the right ventricle and the lungs. Most of the remaining oxygen-rich blood ejected by the right ventricle (9) will be shunted from the pulmonary trunk (12) to the aorta (13) by a connection between the pulmonary trunk and the aortic arch (14), the ductus arteriosus (13) (figure B); thus only a small portion of oxygenated blood will go to the lungs.

Color and label
Figure A
1. Placenta (blood oxygenated here)
2. Umbilical vein (within umbilical cord with two umbilical arteries)
3. Umbilicus
4. Umbilical vein (intra-abdominal); attaches to left branch of portal vein.
5. Ductus venosus; venous shunt in liver that connects end of umbilcal vein with inferior vena cava; closes after birth; its origin is encircled by a muscular sphincter.
6. Inferior vena cava
7. Right atrium
8. Foramen ovale (opening in fetal interatrial septum; closes after birth) (see figure 54)
9. Right ventricle)
10. Left atrium
11. Left ventricle
12. Pulmonary trunk
13. Ductus arteriosus; shunts oxygen-rich blood from pulmonary trunk to arch of aorta; the great vessels arising from the aortic arch will convey oxygenated blood to the head and neck; closes after birth.
14. Aorta
15. Internal iliac artery
16. Umbilical arteries. These close off and become ligamentous after birth except for the proximal portions that become parts of the superior vesical arteries.
17. Liver
18. Portal vein

Figure B Fetal heart showing the ductus arteriosus diverting oxygen-rich blood from the pulmonary trunk to the aortic arch

1_____
2_____
3_____
4_____
5_____
6_____
7_____
8_____
9_____
10_____
11_____
12_____
13_____
14_____
15_____
16_____
17_____
18_____

Th-53 Blood flow in the fetus

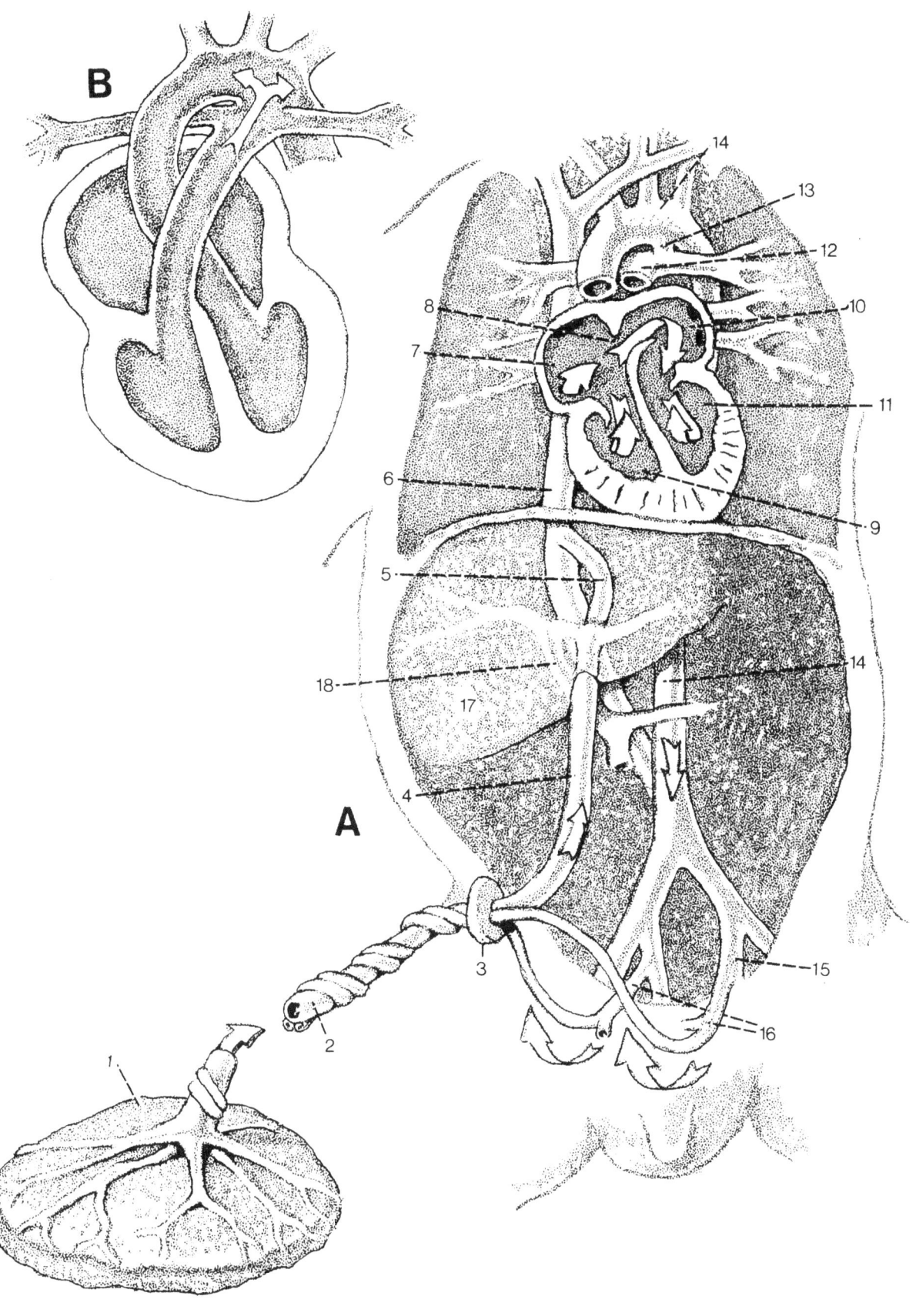

Th-54 Fetal heart in late development

A
1. _____
2. _____
3. _____
4. _____
5. _____
6. _____
7. _____
8. _____
9. _____
10. _____
11. _____
12. _____
13. _____
14. _____
15. _____
16. _____
17. _____
18. _____
19. _____
20. _____

B
1. _____
2. _____
3. _____
4. _____
5. _____

Th-54 Fetal heart in late development

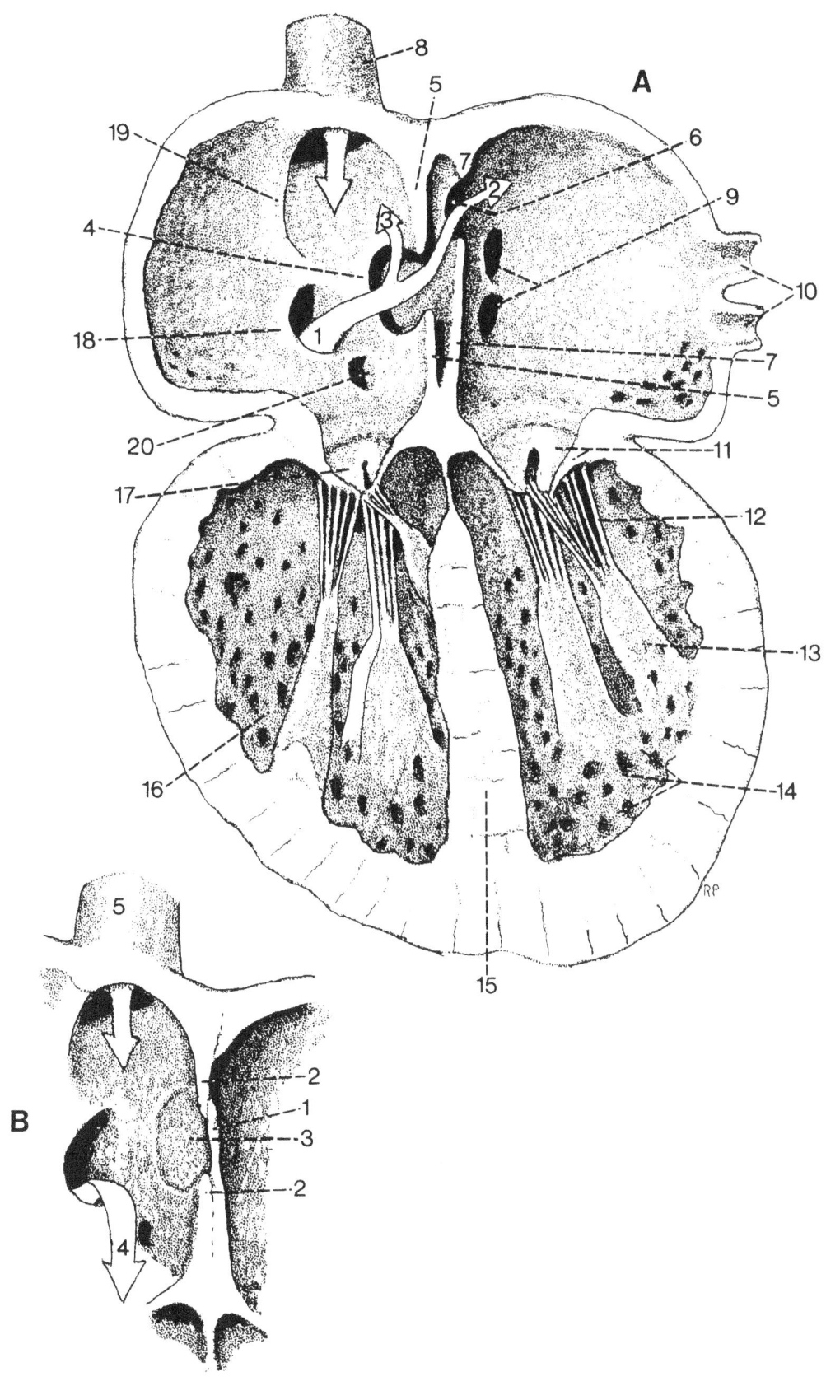

Th-55 Circulatory changes after birth
(opposite page)

From the time of birth until death the volume of blood pumped to the lungs from the right ventricle equals the volume of blood pumped by the left ventricle to the rest of the body. However, during fetal development the lungs contain no air and require only enough blood for their own physical development; consequently the pulmonary circulation is considerably less than circulation to the rest of the body (the systemic circulation). To rectify this imbalance two shunts or "short cuts" develop that allow the left side of the heart to pump a volume of blood equal to that pumped by the right side of the heart, thus insuring a smooth transition at birth from maternal/placental oxygenation of fetal blood to that of oxygenation by air-breathing. These circulatory "short cuts" persist throughout intrauterine life. They close off and cease to function shortly after birth. However, complete anatomical closure may take weeks or months.

Color and label
Figure A
1. Ligamentum arteriosum (postpartum fibrous remnant of ductus arteriosus)
2. Fossa ovalis (postpartum remnant of foramen ovale; L. *fossa*, a depression)
3. Ligamentum venosum (postpartum fibrous remnant of ductus venosus)
4. Left branch of portal vein
5. Round ligament of the liver (ligamentum teres hepatis; postpartum fibrous remnant of intra-abdominal portion of the umbilical vein)
6. Umbilicus
7. Aorta
8. Medial umbilical ligaments in extraperitoneal fat on inside of anterior abdominal wall (postpartum remnants of the intra-abdominal portions of the two umbilical arteries). These close shut just past the origin of their last branch up to the umbilicus.
9. Superior vesical (L. *vesica*, the bladder) arteries; the proximal portions of the umbilical arteries remain patent (open) and function as the beginning lengths of the superior vesical arteries.
10. Bladder
11. Portal vein
12. Inferior vena cava (behind liver)
13. Aortic arch
14. Left pulmonary artery (ductus arteriosus connects the aortic arch to the origin of the left pulmonary artery)

Figure B
Blood flow in the aorta and pulmonary arteries after closure of the ductus arteriosus
1. Ligamentum arteriosum
2. Pulmonary trunk
3. Aortic arch
4. Left pulmonary artery

The foramen ovale becomes the fossa ovalis.
This foramen, along with the foramen secundum (figure 53), conveys blood from the right atrium to the left atrium. A series of three trans-septal foramina develop in the fetus. The first foramen (foramen primum) disappears when the second (foramen secundum) appears. The second and third foramina (foramen secundum and foramen ovale) work together and persist until birth when the increased blood flow from the fully functional lungs and pulmonary veins increases the pressure in the left atrium, forcing shut the valve-like flap and functionally closing off the two foramina in the interatrial septum. Failure to anatomically fuse is not uncommon and is not critical as long the flap covers the foramen ovale.

The ductus arteriosus becomes the ligamentum arteriosum.
This shunt conveys blood from the pulmonary trunk to the aortic arch. With the first breath the lungs expand. Resistance to arterial blood in the pulmonary arteries falls significantly, resulting in a dramatic increase in circulation to the lungs, and blood is no longer forced from the pulmonary trunk to the aorta. Functional closure of the ductus arteriosus occurs a few hours or days after birth, although complete obliteration of the lumen takes 6 to 8 weeks.

The intra-abdominal portion of the umbilical vein becomes the round ligament of the liver. Although no longer functional, the lumen of the round ligament usually persists into adulthood.

The ductus venosus becomes the ligamentum venosum.

The intra-abdominal portion of the umbilical arteries becomes the medial umbilical ligaments or plicae (folds).

Th-55 Circulatory changes after birth

A

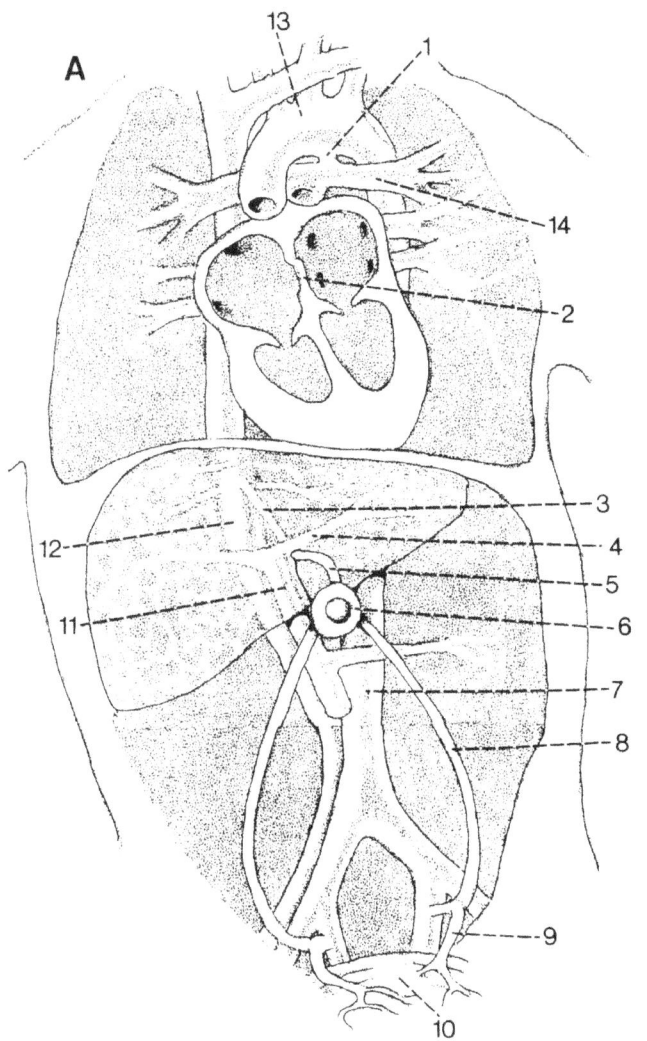

1_____
2_____
3_____
4_____
5_____
6_____
7_____
8_____
9_____
10_____
11_____
12_____
13_____
14_____

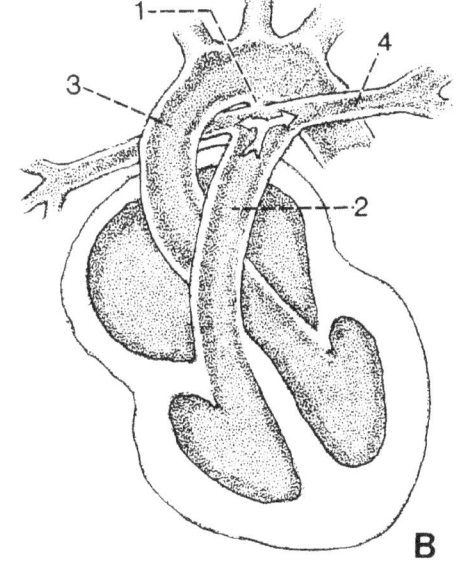

B

1_____
2_____
3_____
4_____

Th-56 Thoracic splanchnic nerves
(opposite page)

Color and label the nerves and ganglia
Label the remaining structures

1. Anterior ramus (also called anterior primary division) of thoracic nerve 5 (= 5th intercostal nerve)
2. Fifth thoracic sympathetic chain ganglion; there are usually 11 thoracic sympathetic chain ganglia on each side of the vertebral column; the sympathetic chain lies beneath the parietal pleura.
3. White communicating ramus; these rami connect the spinal nerves to the adjacent sympathetic chain ganglia; they carry the axons of preganglionic sympathetic neurons from the spinal nerve to the corresponding sympathetic ganglion (see figure 56).
4. Gray communicating ramus; these rami convey the unmyelinated axons of the postganglionic sympathetic neurons in the chain ganglia back to the spinal nerve; there may be more than one gray ramus or a gray ramus may fuse with a white rami; white rami tend to lie more lateral than the gray rami.
5. Ninth thoracic sympathetic chain ganglion; the chain ganglia contain postganglionic sympathetic neurons.
6. Left greater splanchnic nerve; the greater splanchnic nerve usually arises from the coalescence of rami (or roots) from thoracic ganglia 5 through 9. The greater splanchnic nerve is comprised mainly of preganglionic sympathetic fibers* in addition to visceral afferent** fibers (axons).
7. Splanchnic ganglion on greater splanchnic nerve; microscopic studies have indicated that this ganglion is always present.
8. Aorta (cut)
9. Diaphragm (cut)
10. Left greater splanchnic nerve passing through left crus of diaphragm; it sometimes passes through the diaphragm with the aorta.
11. Adrenal (suprarenal) gland (left and right). It receives fibers from the greater splanchnic nerve.
12. Left celiac ganglion; it contains postganglionic sympathetc neurons whose axons innervate abdominal viscera. The axons in the greater splanchnic nerve synapse mainly on postganglionic neurons in the celiac ganglion; however, some greater splanchnic axons also supply the adrenal gland, and other axons continue through the celiac ganglion without synapsing where they form the celiac plexus and synapse in other ganglia. Axons from these ganglia end in various abdominal organs.
13. Lowest splanchnic nerve (not always present) (right and left); it receives fibers from ganglion T12.
14. Lesser splanchnic nerve (right and left); it usually receives fibers (axons) from ganglia T10 and T11, which mainly end in the aorticorenal ganglion.
15. Aorticorenal ganglion (right and left); preganglionic fibers in the lesser splanchnic nerve usually end here upon postganglionic neurons.
16. Renal plexus; axons in the lowest splanchnic (when present) usually terminally synapse on this plexus. Activation of sympathetic fibers to the kidneys causes renal vessels to constrict, thus restricting blood to the kidney and subsequent water loss.
17. Right celiac ganglion; most preganglionic fibers in greater splanchic nerve synapse upon postganglionic sympathetic neurons in this ganglion.
18. Greater splanchnic nerve (right)
19. Ramus (or root) of greater splanchnic nerve from 8th thoracic ganglion; in addition to efferent fibers, these rami contain visceral afferent** fibers traveling back to the spinal cord.
20. Sympathetic trunk; the trunk on each side contains ascending and descending preganglionic axons.

***Fiber** and **axon** are used synonymously here.

****Afferent** and **efferent** applied to nerves mean, respectively, "running toward" and "running away from" the CNS, that is, the brain and spinal cord.

Sympathetic activation causes: conversion of glycogen to glucose in the liver
inhibition of gastric secretion in the stomach
inhibition of intestinal peristalsis
contraction of the spleen, thus expelling more
  blood into the general circulation
contraction of urinary sphincters, thus retaining body water

Th-56 Thoracic splanchnic nerves

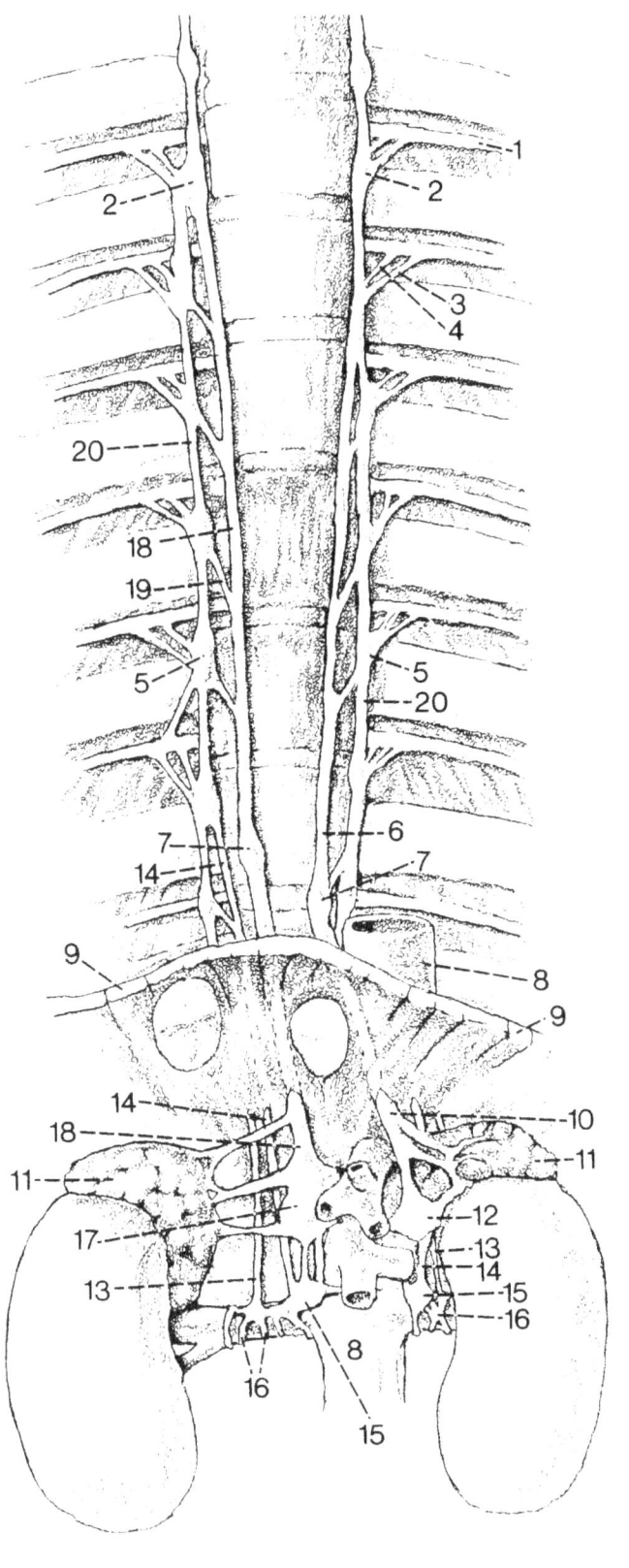

(use abbrevs.)

1 _____
2 _____
3 _____
4 _____
5 _____
6 _____
7 _____
8 _____
9 _____
10 _____
11 _____
12 _____
13 _____
14 _____
15 _____
16 _____
17 _____
18 _____
19 _____
20 _____

Th-57 Autonomic nervous system
(opposite page)

Use a different color for each of the following autonomic neurons and their axons:
Preganglionic sympathetic   Preganglionic parasympathetic   Visceral afferent
Postganglionic sympathetic   Postganglionic parasympathetic

For simplification each category is represented by a single neuron and its axon.
Preganglionic sympathetic neurons 1 and 3 have cell bodies (somata) in the lateral gray column of the thoracic spinal cord where they form two groups, the intermediolateral and intermediomedial. These preganglionic sympathetic neurons are present only in the thoracic and upper lumbar region of the spinal cord (T1-L2). Starting with **preganglionic sympathetic neuron 1**, color its cell body (soma) and its axon as it exits the spinal cord via the anterior root. Trace its axon as it then leaves the thoracic spinal nerve by way of the short white communicating ramus—these axons are lightly myelinated, hence its white appearance—and synapses upon **postganglionic sympathetic neuron 2** in a sympathetic chain ganglion. **Postganglionic neuron 2** sends its axon back to the thoracic spinal nerve via a gray communicating ramus. Postganglionic axons are unmyelinated, hence their gray appearance. The distinction between white (myelinated) and gray (unmyelinated) nerve fibers can be ascertained only by microscopic inspection. However, white communicating branches are usually further lateral than are the gray rami, which may number more than one. Axons of postganglionic sympathetic neurons such as neuron 2 axon will travel within thoracic spinal nerve to the body wall or within nerves to the limbs and eventually end upon and modulate—depending upon the physiologic state and the ambient temperature—sweat glands, blood vessels near the skin, and hair follicles. Return to **preganglionic sympathetic neuron 3**. Color and trace its axon as it enters the sympathetic ganglion, but instead of synapsing in this ganglion, it ascends within the sympathetic trunk to the superior cervical ganglion where it synapses upon **postganglionic sympathetic neurons 4 and 5**. Postganglionic axons of neurons 4 descend to innervate the heart (increase the rate and strength of contraction and dilate coronary vessels) via the cardiac plexus. Postganglionic fibers of **neurons 5** form the **carotid plexus (6)** around the internal carotid artery and ascend into the head where they will affect the size of the pupil in the eye (enlarge it) and inhibit tear production in the lacrimal glands and saliva in the salivary glands. Color and trace the course of **preganglionic neuron 7** into its ganglion where it synapses upon **postganglionic neurons 8, 9, and 10**. The axons of these three neurons re-enter the corresponding spinal nerve and travel in it to its area of distribution. **Sudomotor neuron 8** causes myoepithelial cells on sweat glands to contract, thus expeling sweat. **Pilomotor neuron 9** activates arrector pili muscle of hair on skin. **Neuron 10** modulates cutaneous blood flow. Note that **Neuron 11** passes through its ganglion without synapsing and becomes a **thoracic splanchnic nerve**. These preganglionic fibers pass behind the diaphragm and enter the abdomen where they synapse upon irregular aggregates of sympathetic ganglia (prevertebral ganglia) such as the celiac ganglion (also called solar ganglion). **Postganglionic neurons 12 and 13** in these sympathetic ganglia have a wide distribution to the abdominal viscera where they have a mainly inhibitory effect (constrict abdominal blood vessels, inhibit peristalsis, etc.). The cell body of **visceral afferent neuron 14** is a typical unipolar first-order sensory neuron (with a single process that divides like a T) found in the dorsal root ganglion. It relays diffuse visceral pain (tummy ache) and functions in gastrointestinal reflexes. **Neuron 15** in the opposite lateral gray column gives rise to another preganglionic splanchnic fiber; however, this one ends, not in a ganglion, but in the medulla of the adrenal (suprarenal) gland where it synapses upon **chromaffin cell 16**, which synthesizes epinephrine (adrenalin) and norepinephrine (noradrenalin), which are distributed by blood vessels throughout the body. Thus, should circumstances demand it, these two blood-borne catecholamines can greatly augment the effect of the sympathetic system. **Neuron 17** represents a **preganglionic parasympathetic neuron cell body** in one of the brain stem nuclei* of the vagus nerve. Axons from somata such as 17 travel within the vagus nerve and supply a very wide range of viscera in both the thorax and abdomen. The preganglionic parasympathetic fibers in the vagus nerve are much longer that the postganglionic fibers whose postganglionic cell bodies lie either in plexuses very close to the target organ or within the walls of the organ itself as does **postganglionic parasympathetic neuron 18**. Aggregates of these postganglionic neurons in the walls of target organs are termed intramural (L. within the walls) ganglia . The parasympathetic system tends to conserve and build up free energy. It promotes digestion, assimilation, secretion of glands, peristalsis, and the conversion of glucose to glycogen. Some researchers feel that in addition to the sympathetic and parasympathetic nervous systems, the extensive intrinsic neuronal network in the gastrointestinal tract constitutes a third division of the visceral nervous system, the enteric nervous system. Supportive evidence for a third autonomous division includes experiments demonstrating that transplanted intestine can function after being totally separated from all sympathetic and parasympathetic nervous control.

*A neuroanatomical nucleus is an aggregate of neurons in the CNS.

Th-57 Autonomic nervous system

(use abbrevs.)

1 _____
2 _____
3 _____
4 _____
5 _____
6 _____
7 _____
8 _____
9 _____
10 _____
11 _____
12 _____
13 _____
14 _____
15 _____
16 _____
17 _____
18 _____

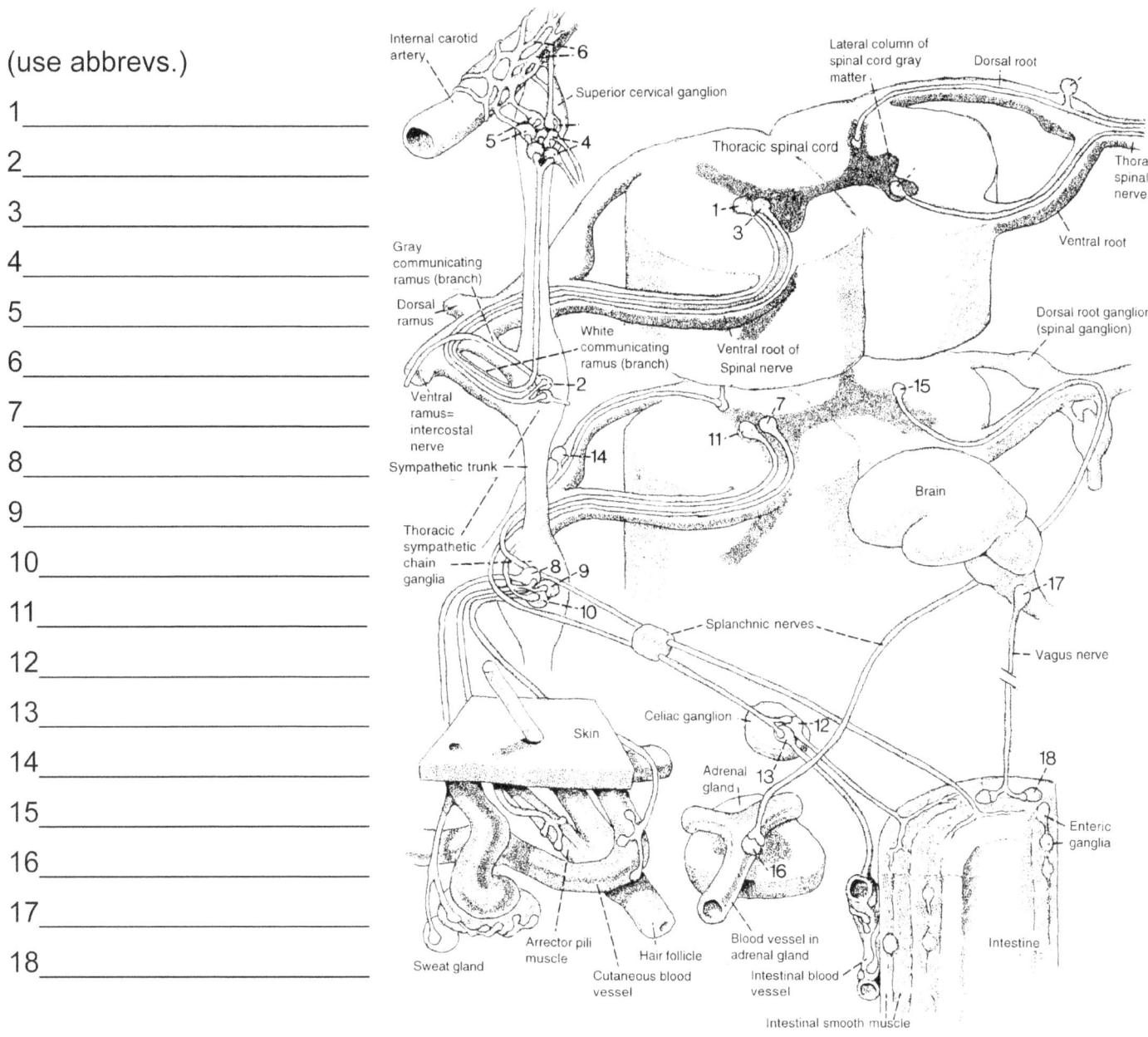

Th-58 Thoracic duct and related structures
(opposite page)

The thoracic duct is the largest lymph vessel in the body. It drains all the lymph from the body except for the right half of the head, the right arm, and the right half of the thorax, which drain into lymphatic duct(s) on the posterior right thoracic wall. Its origin in the upper abdomen has usually been described to be a thin-walled dilation called the cisterna chyli. However, more recent and thorough studies indicate that a "cisternal" dilation occurs in only 1 in 5 bodies. Even when an enlargement is present it tends to assume a wide variety of shapes. It rarely assumes the form of a simple, fusiform, saccular dilation such as that drawn on the opposite page. Thus one should expect to find various patterns and forms at the beginning of the thoracic duct rather than a single saccular swelling. What is important is that at its abdominal origin the thoracic duct receives lymphatic trunks carrying lymph from the legs, the intestines, the stomach, and the abdominal wall. These lymphatic trunks converge and end on the thoracic duct at its origin. The thoracic duct carries the lymph it receives up through the thorax to the base of the neck where it arches to the left and empties into the blood stream through an opening at the junction of the left internal jugular vein with the left subclavian vein. Fat absorbed in the intestines from digested food reaches the venous blood by this route. The duct, which is about 0.5 cm in diameter, reaches the thorax by passing through the aortic hiatus of the diaphragm with the aorta and ascends on the posterior thoracic wall where it lies on the vertebral column between the azygos vein (on its right) and the aorta (on its left). It is easy to overlook the thoracic duct because of its thin walls, which may appear clear. The duct tends to have numerous small dilations that give it a varicose appearance, and as it ascends it takes a somewhat zig-zag course. Should the thoracic duct be cut or damaged, lymph will spill out into the pleural cavity (usually the left). This condition is called chylothorax. Chyle (Gk. *chylos*, juice) is the name for the white milky lymph that appears after a fatty meal. This white lymph contains tiny particles of digested fat called chylomicrons, which were absorbed in the intestines. The greater part of the lymphatic system, with the exception of the thoracic duct and some of the larger lymph nodes, is too small to be seen by gross dissection. One should appreciate that lymphatic vessels accompany blood vessels throughout the body. The lymphatic system serves a vital function in producing lymphocytes and antibodies that fight disease. In addition it returns to the general circulation the protein-laden extracellular fluid that has extravasated from capillaries. As mentioned above, it also transports digested fat from the intestines to the venous blood flow. The term *lymphatics* usually refers to both the lymphatic vessels as well as the lymph nodes situated along their course.

Color and label

1. Cisterna chyli (present only in 20% of cases)
2. Abdominal lymph nodes in afferent lymphatic trunks
3. Outline of aortic hiatus (aorta removed)
4. Thoracic duct
5. Posterior intercostal arteries (cut at origins from aorta, which has been removed)
6. Left subclavian vein
7. Left internal jugular vein
8. Left brachiocephalic vein
9. Superior vena cava
10. Sympathetic trunk
11. Azygos vein

Th-58 Thoracic duct and related structures

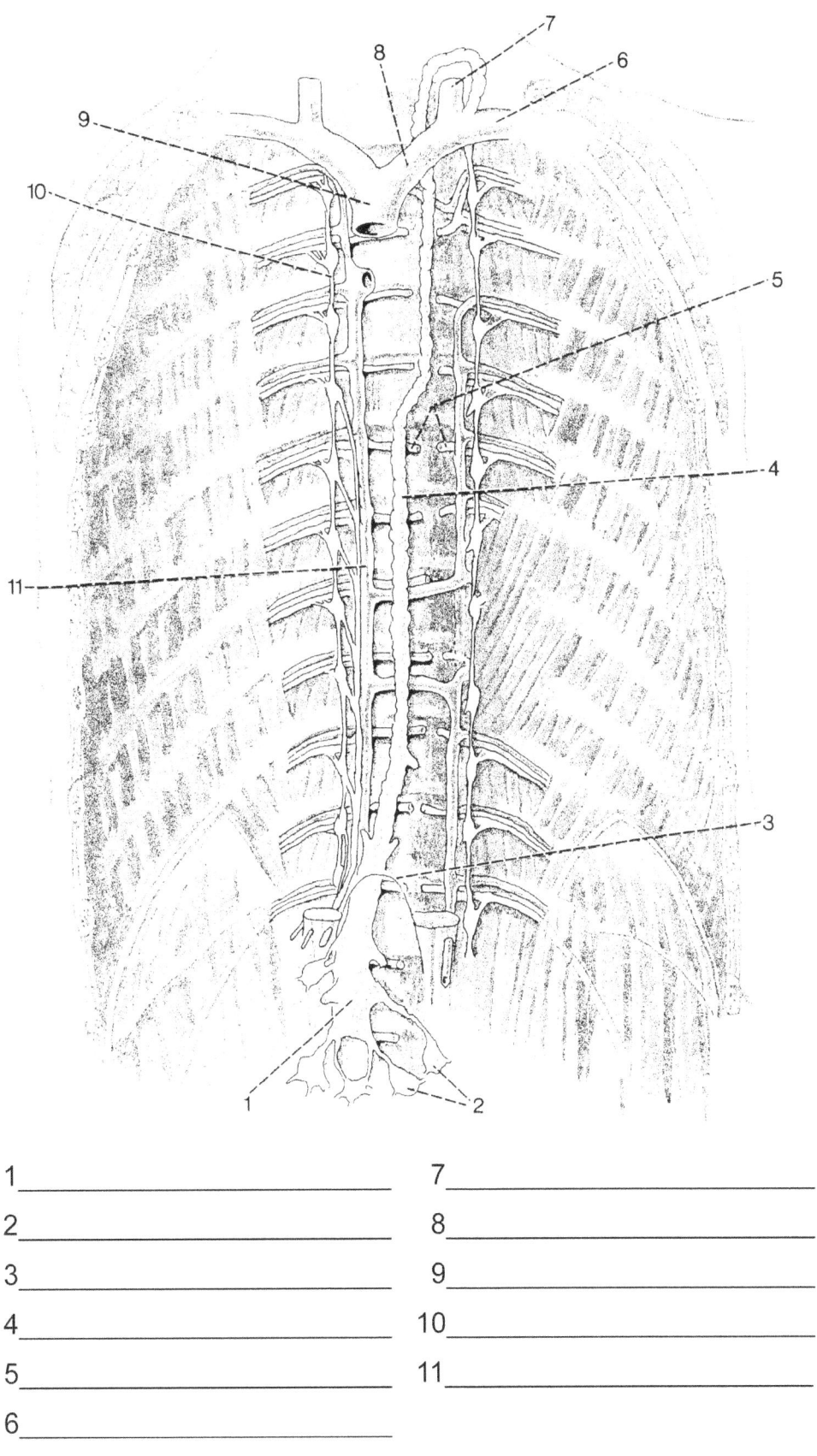

1 _____ 7 _____
2 _____ 8 _____
3 _____ 9 _____
4 _____ 10 _____
5 _____ 11 _____
6 _____

Th-59 Mediastinum after removal of heart and pericardium

The great vessels have been severed.
(opposite page)

Color and label

1. Left internal jugular vein
2. Left middle cervical ganglion (its postganglionic sympathetic axons innervate the cervical region, upper arm, and heart)
3. Thoracic duct (it terminates in the junction of the left internal jugular and subclavian vein)
4. Internal thoracic artery (formerly: internal mammary artery)
5. Thoracic duct
6. Left recurrent laryngeal nerve (a branch of the vagus nerve)
7. Left subclavian artery
8. Vagus nerve
9. Left common carotid artery
10. Arch of the aorta (cut at top of arch)
11. Left recurrent laryngeal nerve (note that as the left recurrent laryngeal nerve leaves the vagus nerve, it winds around the arch of the aorta; it sends motor branches to all the skeletal muscles of the larynx except the cricothyroid; it also sends sensory and autonomic fibers to the cervical esophagus, trachea, and the larynx as far as the vocal cords)
12. Left bronchus
13. Left pulmonary artery
14. Bronchial artery (these vary in number, size, and origin; there is usually one right bronchial artery and two left bronchial arteries; unlike the pulmonary arteries, these carry oxygenated blood to the bronchial tree and the bronchial lymph nodes)
15. Esophageal plexus (a network of parasympathetic fibers partially embedded in the exterior of the esophagus joined by sympathetic fibers from sympathetic ganglia by way of the posterior pulmonary plexus)
16. Descending aorta (thoracic part)
17. Esophagus
18. Thoracic duct
19. Azygos vein (note it receives venous blood from the posterior intercostal veins)
20. Right common carotid artery
21. Right internal jugular vein
22. Right recurrent laryngeal nerve (note the right recurrent laryngeal nerve winds around the right subclavian artery)
23. Right vagus nerve
24. Right subclavian artery
25. Right subclavian vein
26. Right brachial plexus (motor and sensory nerves to the upper extremity)
27. Right phrenic nerve with pericardiacophrenic artery and vein
28. Azygos vein (cut at its junction with the superior vena cava)
29. Right bronchus (note its division into superior, middle, and inferior lobar bronchi)
30. Branches of right pulmonary artery
31. Superior lobar bronchus
32. Right vagus nerve
33. Right middle lobar bronchus
34. Right superior pulmonary vein
35. Right inferior lobar bronchus
36. Right inferior pulmonary vein
37. Greater splanchnic nerve
38. Phrenic nerve with pericardiacophrenic artery and vein (note their "sandwiched" position between the pericardium and mediastinal pleura)
39. Base of pericardium (adherent to central tendon of diaphragm)
40. Inferior vena cava
41. Apex of right
42. left lung

1. _____
2. _____
3. _____
4. _____
5. _____
6. _____
7. _____
8. _____
9. _____
10. _____
11. _____
12. _____
13. _____
14. _____
15. _____
16. _____
17. _____
18. _____
19. _____
20. _____
21. _____
22. _____
23. _____
24. _____
25. _____

Th-59 Mediastinum after removal of heart and pericardium

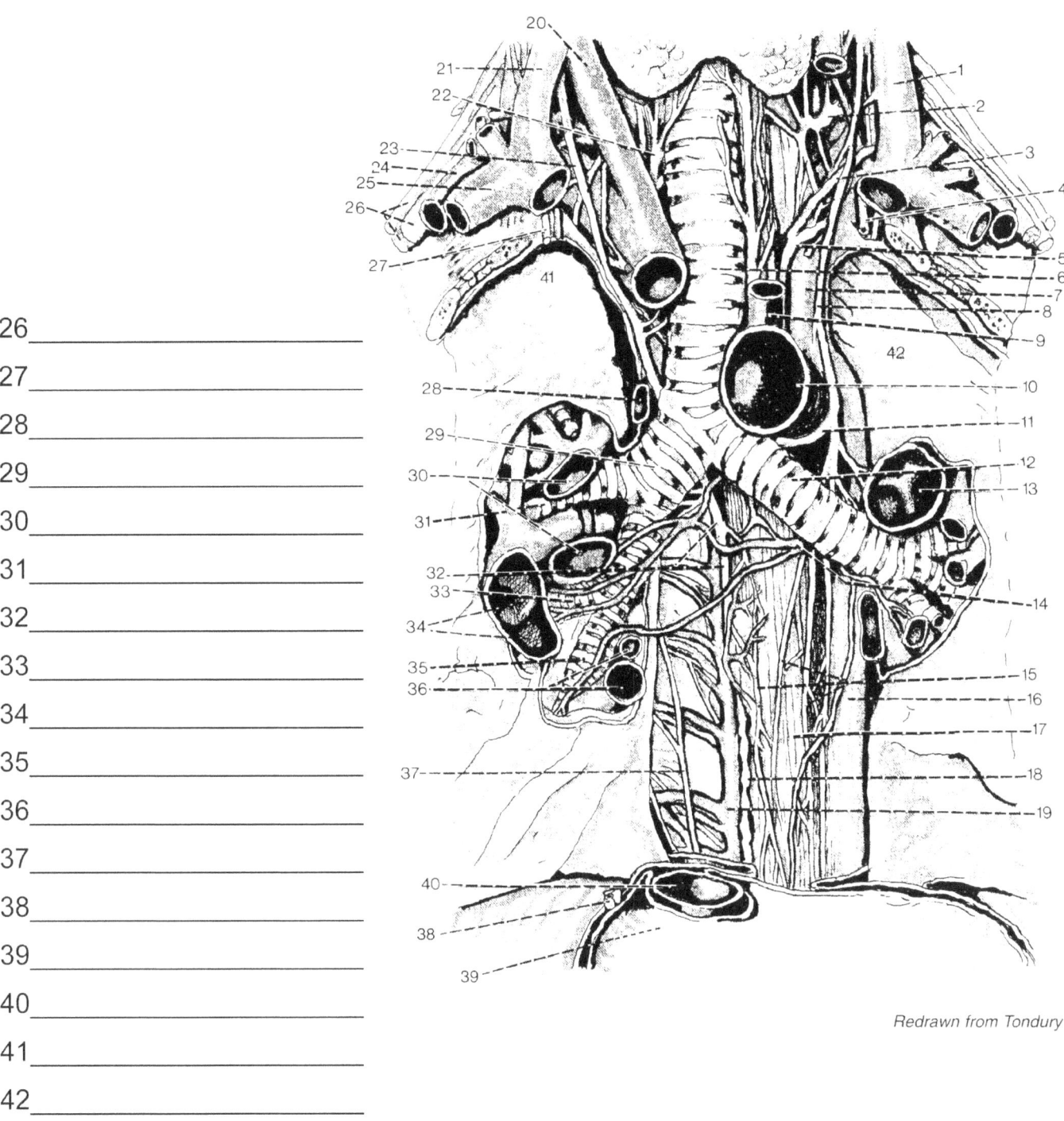

26 ___
27 ___
28 ___
29 ___
30 ___
31 ___
32 ___
33 ___
34 ___
35 ___
36 ___
37 ___
38 ___
39 ___
40 ___
41 ___
42 ___

Redrawn from Tondury

Th-60 Cross section of thorax level of bifurcation of pulmonary trunk

(Looking up from below) (opposite page)

Color and label

1. Remnant of thymus gland and prepericardial fat
2. Sternum (body)
3. Ascending aorta
4. Internal thoracic vein and artery
5. Pulmonary trunk; bifurcation into right and left pulmonary arteries
6. Left main bronchus (note cartilage in walls)
7. Upper lobe of left lung
8. Left phrenic nerve with pericardiacophrenic artery and vein (these three structures lie sandwiched between pericardial sac and mediastinal pleura)
9. Short head of biceps brachii muscle
10. Long head of biceps brachii and tendon
11. Coracobrachialis muscle
12. Humerus of left arm
13. Deltoid muscle
14. Tendon of latissimus dorsi muscle
15. Lateral head of triceps brachii muscle
16. Long head of triceps brachii
17. Radial nerve
18. Brachial artery
19. Basilic vein
20. Ulnar nerve
21. Median nerve
22. Left scapula
23. Subscapularis muscle
24. Serratus anterior muscle
25. Lower lobe of left lung
26. Left pulmonary artery
27. Semispinalis muscle
28. Descending aorta
29. Head of rib sixth rib
30. Body of sixth thoracic vertebra and sympathetic trunk
31. Spinous process of vertebra T5
32. Spinal cord
33. Esophagus, azygos vein, and right vagus nerve (in between)
34. Trapezius muscle
35. Right main bronchus
36. Right pulmonary artery
37. Lower lobe of right lung
38. Right scapula (inferior angle)
39. Teres major muscle
40. Oblique fissure of right lung
41. Pectoralis major muscle
42. Upper lobe of right lung
43. Pectoralis minor muscle
44. Superior vena cava
45. Cartilage forming keel-like carina at bifurcation of trachea
46. Left vagus nerve

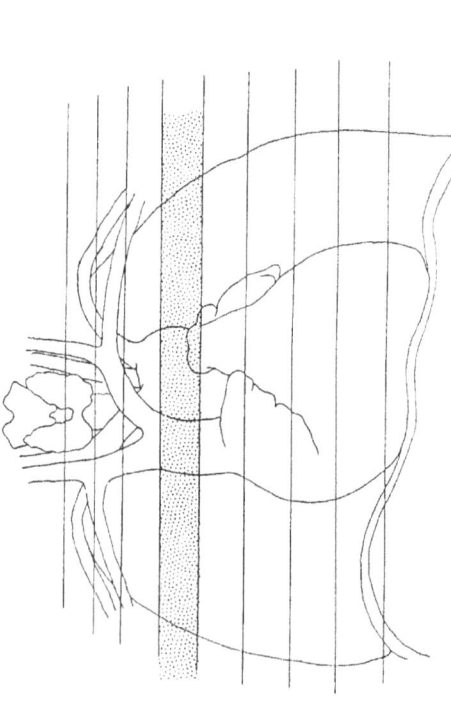

108

Th-60 Cross section of thorax level of bifurcation of pulmonary trunk

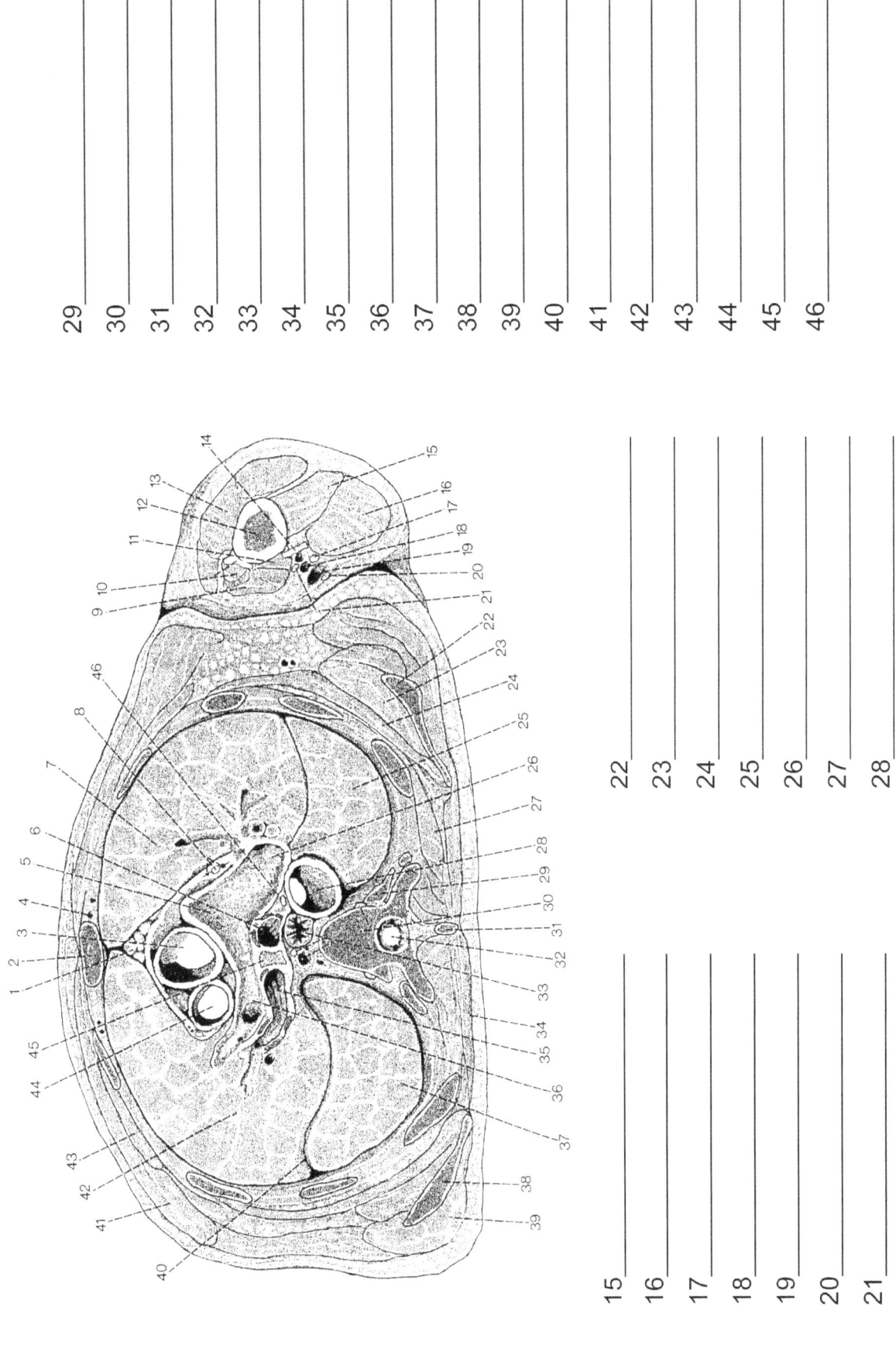

15 ___
16 ___
17 ___
18 ___
19 ___
20 ___
21 ___
22 ___
23 ___
24 ___
25 ___
26 ___
27 ___
28 ___
29 ___
30 ___
31 ___
32 ___
33 ___
34 ___
35 ___
36 ___
37 ___
38 ___
39 ___
40 ___
41 ___
42 ___
43 ___
44 ___
45 ___
46 ___

Th-61 Cross section of thorax just below pulmonary valve

(Looking up from below) (opposite page)

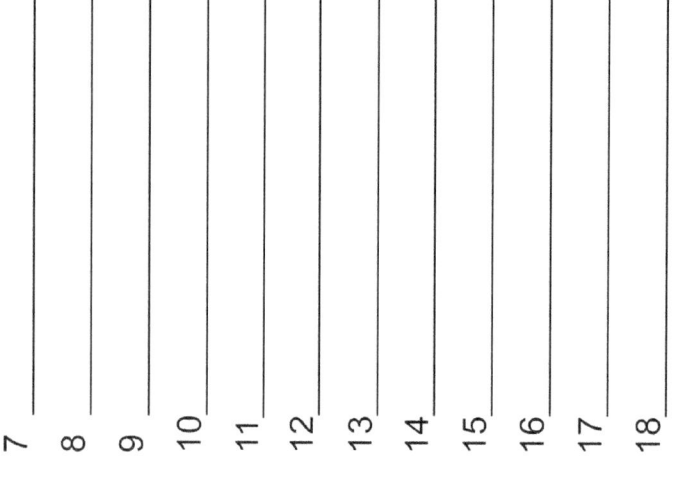

Color and label

1. Sternum (body)
2. Pulmonary valve seen through infundibulum of right ventricle
3. Left phrenic nerve with pericardiacophrenic artery and vein
4. Superior left pulmonary vein leading into left atrium
5. Left inferior lobar bronchus surrounded with bronchial cartilage
6. Superior lobe of left lung
7. Intercostal muscles
8. Lymph nodes
9. Inferior lobe of left lung
10. Serratus anterior muscle
11. Latissimus dorsi muscle
12. Teres major muscle
13. Subscapularis muscle
14. Scapula (inferior angle)
15. Infraspinatus muscle
16. Esophagus (surrounded by anterior and posterior esophageal plexuses formed by left and right vagus nerves)
17. Rhomboideus major muscle
18. Trapezius muscle
19. Aorta (descending thoracic)
20. Sympathetic trunk
21. Azygos vein
22. Spinous process of thoracic vertebra T6
23. Spinal cord
24. Multifidus (deep) and semispinalis (more superficial) back muscles
25. Body of thoracic vertebra T7
26. Right inferior lobar bronchus with cartilage in its wall
27. Pleural space or cavity (bounded externally by parietal pleura on inside of chest wall and internally by visceral pleura on surface of lung; both pleural spaces here are greatly enlarged due to shrinkage of the lungs)
28. Right pulmonary artery dividing into lobar branches
29. Inferior angle of right scapula
30. Inferior lobe of right lung
31. Intercostal vein, artery, and nerve
32. Middle lobe of right lung
33. Oblique fissure
34. Superior lobe of right lung
35. Superior vena cava
36. Pectoralis major muscle
37. Left atrium (superior part)
38. Internal thoracic artery and paired veins
39. Ascending aorta
40. Prepericardial fat with remnants of thymus gland
41. Thoracic duct

Th-61 Cross section of thorax just below pulmonary valve (Looking up from below)

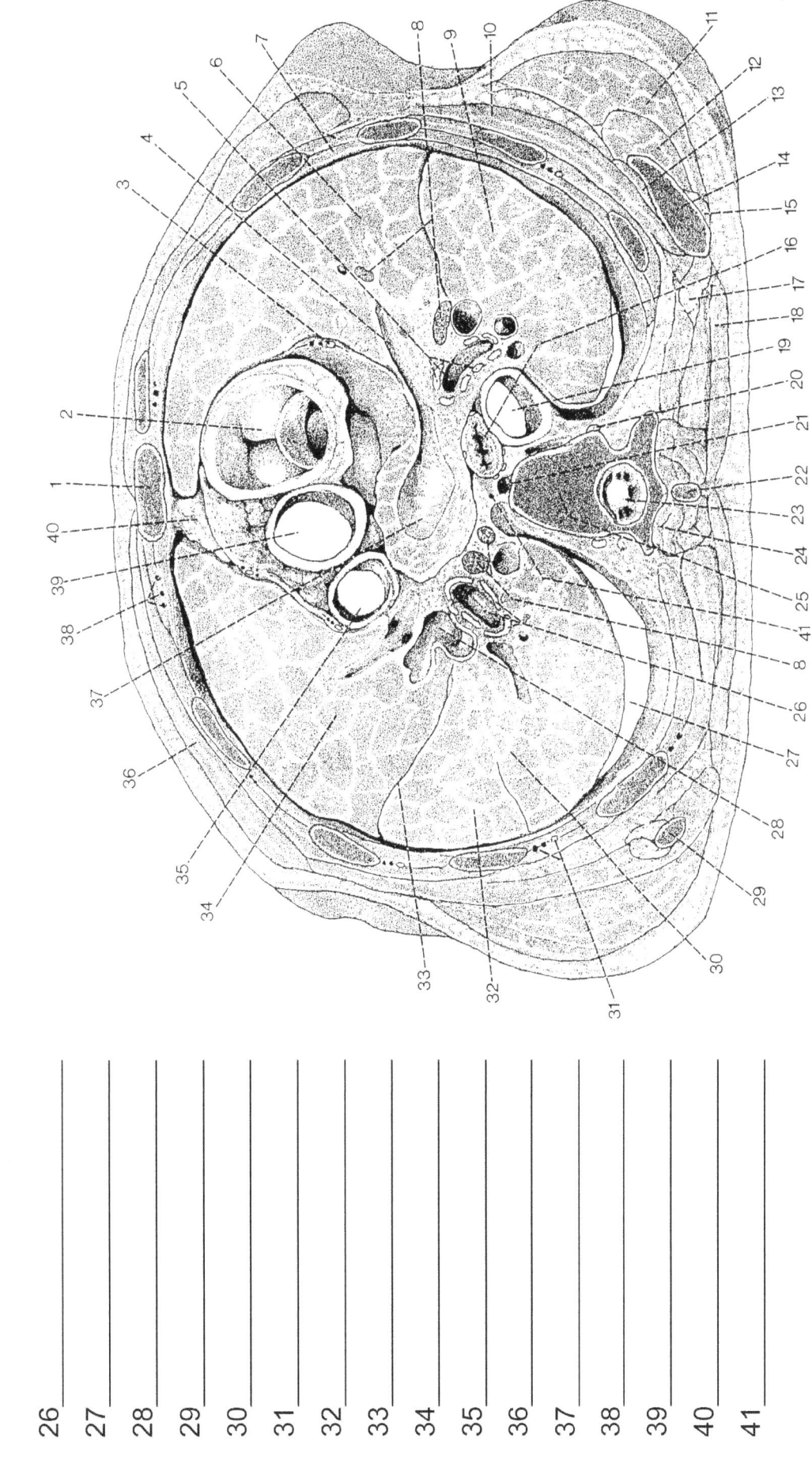

26 _____
27 _____
28 _____
29 _____
30 _____
31 _____
32 _____
33 _____
34 _____
35 _____
36 _____
37 _____
38 _____
39 _____
40 _____
41 _____

Th-62 Cross section of thorax just below aortic valve

(Looking up from below) (opposite page)

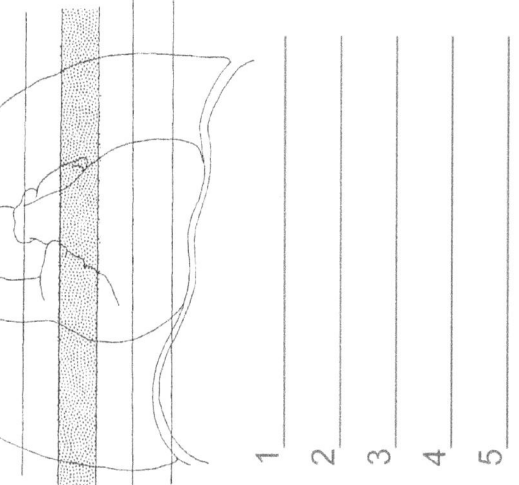

Color and label

1. Body of sternum
2. Right ventricle of heart
3. Fourth costal cartilage
4. Aortic valve (viewed from ventricular side)
5. Great cardiac vein
6. Anterior interventricular branch of left coronary artery; also called left anterior descending or LAD
7. Left ventricle (narrow outflow tract leading to aorta)
8. Wall of left ventricle
9. Superior lobe of left lung
10. Pericardium (fused with pleura)
11. Sixth intercostal vein, artery, and nerve below 6th rib (appear posterior to rib in horizontal section)
12. Portion of anterior cusp of mitral valve (bicuspid or left atrioventricular valve)
13. Lower lobe of left lung
14. Coronary sinus
15. Esophagus
16. Longissimus muscle (part of erector spinae muscle)
17. Aorta (descending thoracic part)
18. Spinal cord
19. Spinous process of vertebra T7
20. Body of thoracic vertebra T8
21. Sympathetic trunk
22. Azygos vein receiving left intercostal vein
23. Right pulmonary veins emptying into left atrium
24. Left atrium
25. Latissimus dorsi
26. Serratus anterior muscle
27. Pleural cavity (greatly expanded due to shrinkage of lung)
28. Middle lobe of right lung
29. Phrenic nerve with pericardiacophrenic artery and vein (between fused pericardium and pleura)
30. Opening of superior vena cava into right atrium
31. Pectinate muscles (musculi pectinati) in right auricle (an out-pouching or appendage of the right atrium)
32. Internal thoracic artery and vein (vein is doubled)
33. Costomediastinal recess of pleural space (parietal pleura is reflected from inside of chest wall onto outside of pericardial sac)
34. Small cardiac vein
35. Right coronary artery
36. Circumflex branch of left coronary artery
37. Crista terminalis (leader points to approximate site of SA node) (pacemaker)
38. Oblique fissure of right lung
39. Thoracic duct

Th-62 Cross section of thorax just below aortic valve (Looking up from below)

26 _____
27 _____
28 _____
29 _____
30 _____
31 _____
32 _____
33 _____
34 _____
35 _____
36 _____
37 _____
38 _____
39 _____

Th-63 Cross section of thorax at level of male nipple

(Looking up from below) (opposite page)

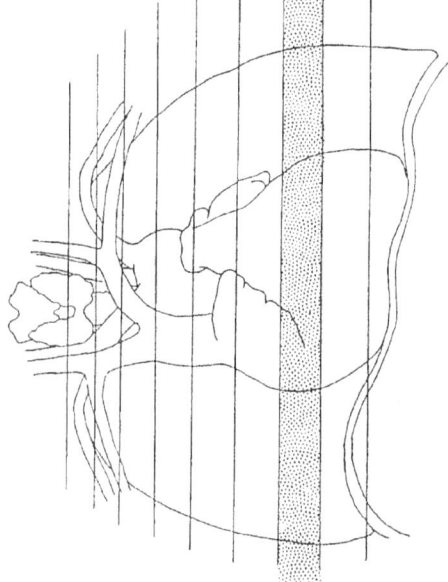

Color and label

1. Right ventricle of heart
2. Body of sternum
3. Interventricular septum
4. Left ventricle and trabeculae carneae (muscular bundles on the inside walls of both ventricles)
5. Male nipple (papilla)
6. Anterior papillary muscle in left ventricle
7. Left phrenic nerve with pericardiacophrenic artery and vein (between pericardium and pleura)
8. Upper lobe of left lung
9. Oblique fissure in left lung
10. Chordae tendineae
11. Serratus anterior muscle
12. Anterior cusp of mitral (bicuspid) valve (left AV valve)
13. Left atrium (small portion)
14. Lower lobe of left lung
15. Coronary sinus (largest intrinsic heart vein)
16. Descending aorta and hemiazygos vein receiving left posterior intercostal vein
17. Semispinalis (superficial) and erector spinae muscles
18. Spinal nerve T8
19. Body and lamina of thoracic vertebra T8
20. Spinal cord and internal venous plexus
21. Spinous process of thoracic vertebra T7
22. Azygos vein and right posterior intercostal vein
23. Sympathetic trunk
24. Trapezius muscle
25. Esophagus (surrounded by esophageal plexus mainly from vagal nerve fibers) and thoracic duct
26. Latissimus dorsi muscle
27. Lower lobe of right lung
28. Intercostal vein, artery, and nerve
29. Intercostal muscles
30. Upper lobe of right lung
31. Pectoralis major muscle
32. Right atrium of heart
33. Internal thoracic artery and veins (doubled)
34. Costal cartilage
35. Anterior cusp of tricusid valve (right AV valve)
36. Pericardium (pericardial sac); made up of internal thin parietal serous pericardium and outer strong fibrous pericardium; on either side the pericardium is fused with the thin parietal (or mediastinal) pleura. Phrenic nerve and accompanying vessels are "sandwiched" between pericardium and pleura
37. Posterior cusp of mitral valve
38. Enlarged pleural cavity due to shrinkage of lungs

Th-63 Cross section of thorax at level of male nipple
(Looking up from below)

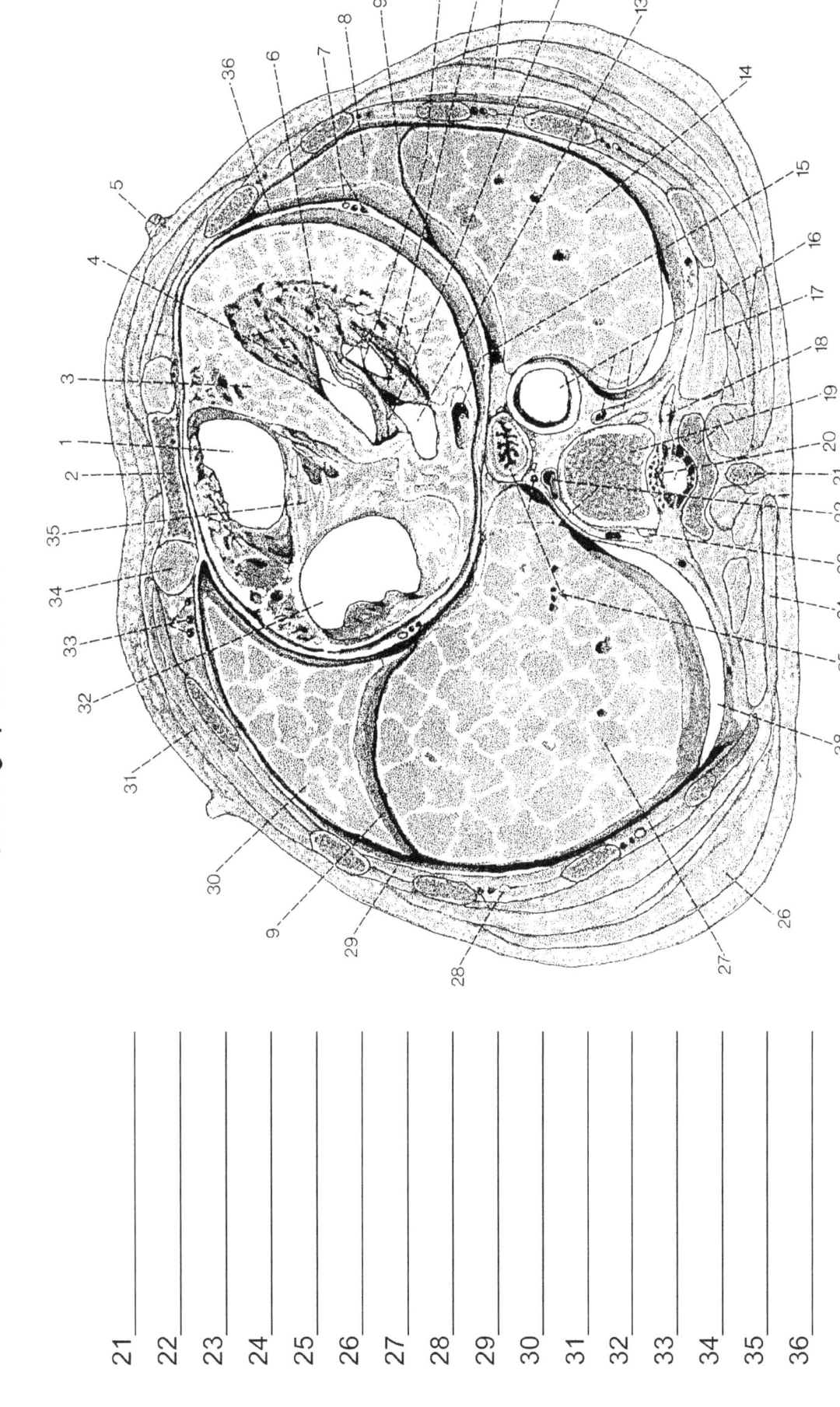

21 _____
22 _____
23 _____
24 _____
25 _____
26 _____
27 _____
28 _____
29 _____
30 _____
31 _____
32 _____
33 _____
34 _____
35 _____
36 _____

Th-64 Cross section of thorax with right dome of diaphragm and right lobe of liver

(Looking up from below) (opposite page)

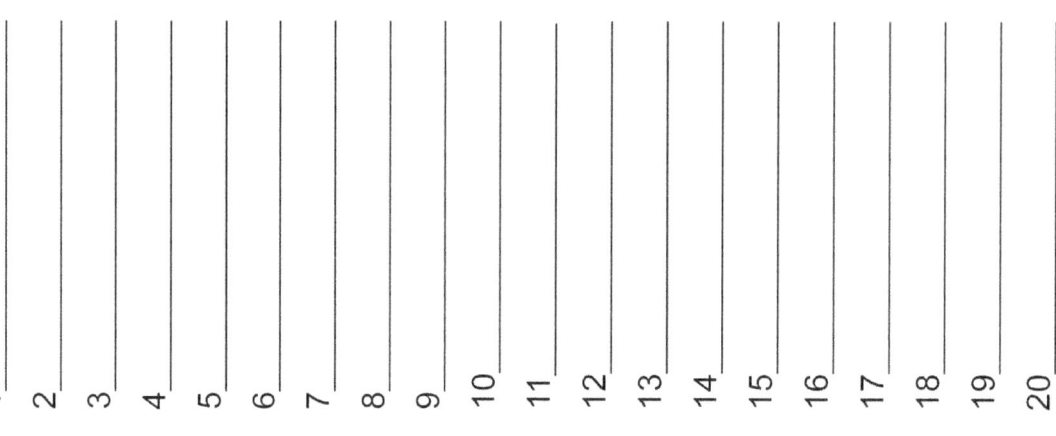

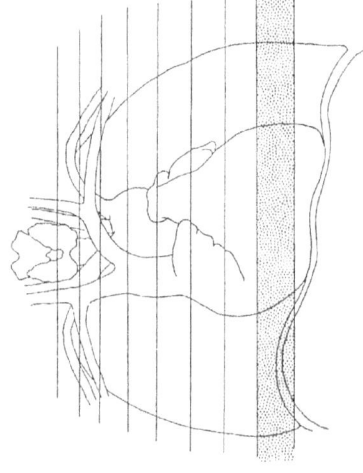

Color and label

1. Inferior vena cava (arrow in right atrium points to superior lip of vena caval "half valve")
2. Thoracic aorta and thoracic duct
3. Right atrium
4. Right ventricle
5. Left ventricle
6. Esophagus (surrounded by esophageal plexus)
7. Pectoralis major muscle
8. Interventricular septum (muscular part)
9. Pleural space (in life it is a potential space containing only a little serous fluid
10. Cusp of mitral valve
11. Lower part (lingula) of upper lobe of left lung
12. Left phrenic nerve, pericardiacophrenic artery and vein
13. Coronary sinus (main vein draining blood from the walls of the heart to the right atrium)
14. External and internal intercostal muscles
15. Lower lobe of left lung
16. Latissimus dorsi muscle
17. Sympathetic trunk
18. Azygos vein receiving posterior intercostal vein
19. Spinous process of thoracic vertebra T8
20. Spinal cord
21. Body of thoracic vertebra T9
22. Intercostal nerve (ventral or anterior ramus) of spinal nerve T9
23. Bare area of liver (not covered with peritoneum and firmly adhering to underside of diaphragm)
24. Right lobe of liver (its most superior part, causing right dome of diaphragm to be higher than left)
25. Diaphragm (right dome)
26. Intercostal vein (nearest to rib), artery, and nerve
27. Ninth rib
28. Serratus anterior muscle
29. Lower lobe of right lung
30. Pericardial sac (fibrous pericardium lined internally with thin serous layer; fused laterally with the pleural membrane)
31. Internal thoracic artery and vein
32. Middle lobe of right lung
33. Costal cartilage
34. Right phrenic nerve with pericardiacophrenic artery and vein (between fused pericardial sac and pleura)
35. Anterior intercostal artery and vein (from internal thoracic artery)
36. Pectinate muscles in right auricle
37. Costal cartilage
38. Sternum
39. Anterior cusp and chordae tendineae of tricuspid valve

Th-64 Cross section of thorax with right dome of diaphragm and right lobe of liver
(Looking up from below)

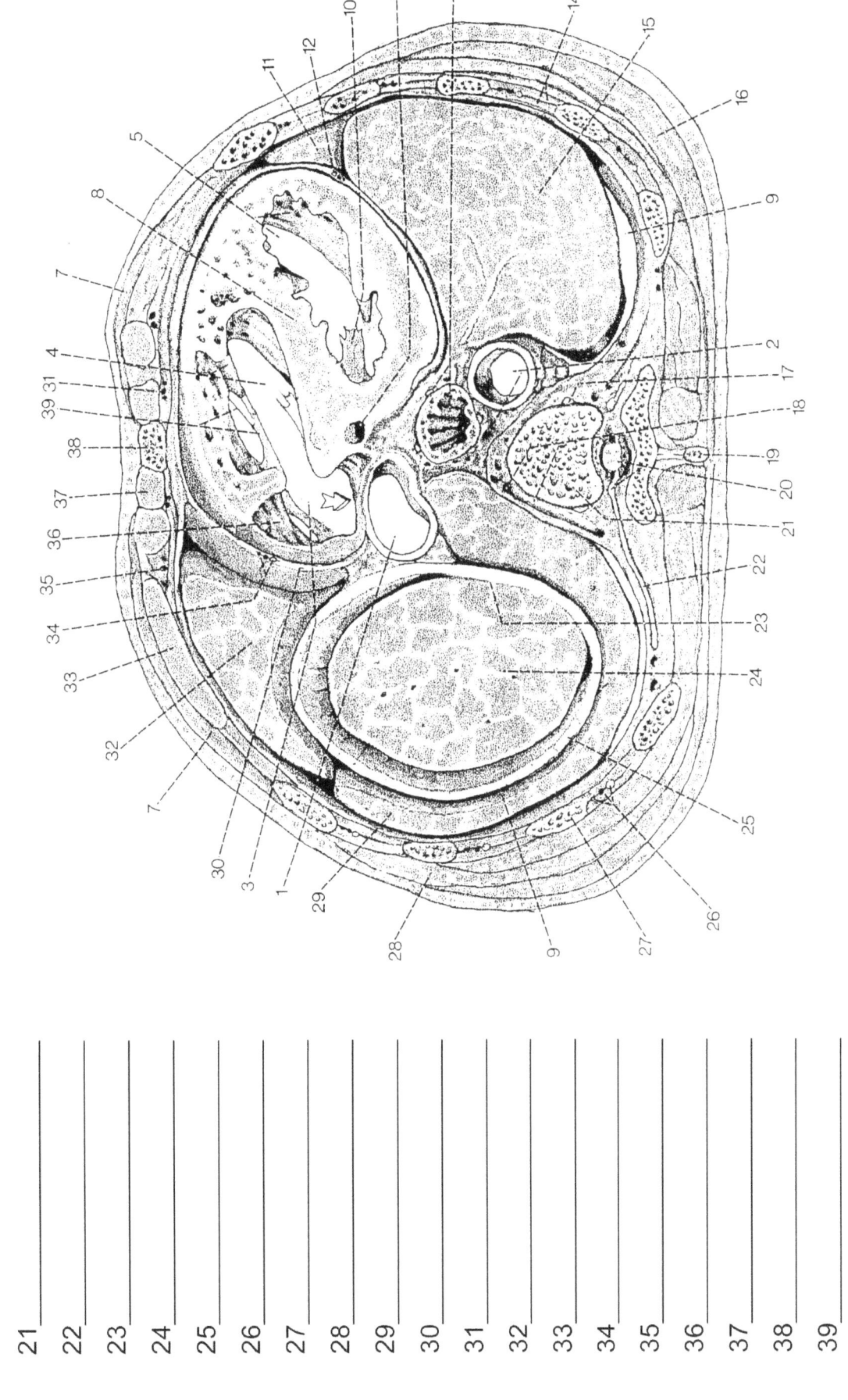

21 _____
22 _____
23 _____
24 _____
25 _____
26 _____
27 _____
28 _____
29 _____
30 _____
31 _____
32 _____
33 _____
34 _____
35 _____
36 _____
37 _____
38 _____
39 _____

The Abdomen
Duodenum (etymological cartoon)

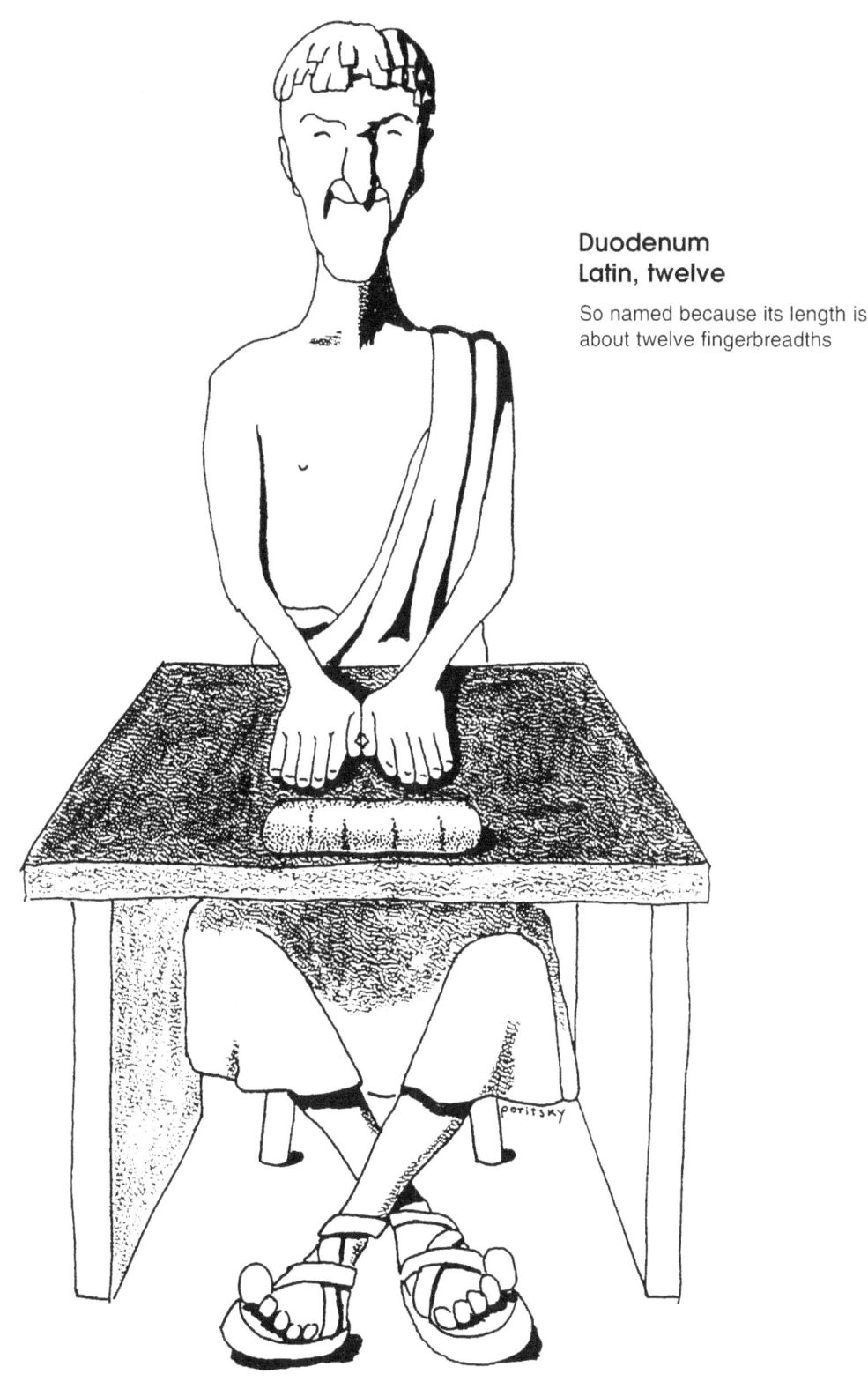

Duodenum
Latin, twelve

So named because its length is about twelve fingerbreadths

Ab-1 Segmental innervation of the skin of the anterior trunk
(opposite page)

The right side (viewer's left) shows the bands of skin called dermatomes, each of which is supplied by the cutaneous* branches of a single spinal nerve. The cutaneous fibers in each nerve pass through the underlying muscles and deep fascia and enter the superficial fascia in 2 sites: as medial anterior branches and as lateral branches (shown on left side). Each branch emerges from the deep fascia as a white cord about 2 mm thick. It then ramifies in the superficial fascia into smaller and smaller branches which eventually become microscopic. These spread out and supply the deep layer of the skin with sensory fibers (pain, touch, and temperature) along with fibers to sweat glands (sudomotor), hair follicles (pilomotor), and cutaneous blood vessels (vasomotor). There is considerable overlap in the distribution of each spinal nerve, which sends branches into adjacent dermatomes, so that injury to a single spinal nerve will not result in a loss of sensation to skin area in question. Note that the nipple is usually supplied by the anterior branch of the 4th thoracic verve (T4), and the umbilicus (belly button) is supplied by the 10th thoracic nerve (T10). The lower 5 thoracic nerves (intercostal nerves T7–T11) along with the subcostal nerve (T12) and the first lumbar nerve (L1) innervate the anterolateral abdominal wall muscles. These nerves begin as ventral (primary) rami of spinal nerves and travel between the muscles of the body wall which they supply. Nerves T5-T11 supply the lower intercostal muscles including the muscles of the innermost layer. They then continue downward and medially and supply the transversus abdominis, the internal and external oblique muscles, and finally the rectus abdominis. Should the nerve to a muscle be accidentally severed, the muscle will be paralyzed, and if the damaged nerve is unable to regenerate into the affected muscle, the muscle will eventually atrophy and be replaced by connective tissue. Herpes zoster† (shingles)‡ is an acute viral disease which attacks the sensory cells in a dorsal root ganglia. One of its most striking symptoms is the eruption of smallpox-like vesicles in a dermatomic distribution that corresponds to the distribution of the affected sensory nerve cells.

SC, supraclavicular nerves; these are small and difficult to find by blunt dissection.

VAL, ventral axial line; the original midline in the embryonic developing arm; note there is a "jump" from cervical nerve C4 to thoracic nerve T2 along this line, leaving out skin areas supplied by cervical nerves C6,C7, C8, and thoracic nerve T1. In the embryo these nerves supplied the distal tip of the arm bud which was to become the future hand and forelimb. As the developing arm grew out, the strips of cutaneous innervation no longer kept the original band-like pattern. These nerves elongated with their cutaneous endings supplying discrete dermatomes that encompassed just the hand or the forelimb and no longer extended as a continuous band back to the thorax.

*Cutaneous, pertaining to the skin, L. *cutis*, skin

†Herpes is Greek for to creep, to crawl; zoster is Greek for a belt, a girdle.

‡The word shingles is derived from the Middle English schingles, an alteration of the medieval Latin *cingulus* from the Latin *cingulum*, a belt, a girdle; from *cingere*, to tie about, to gird.

Ab-1 Segmental innervation of the skin of the anterior trunk

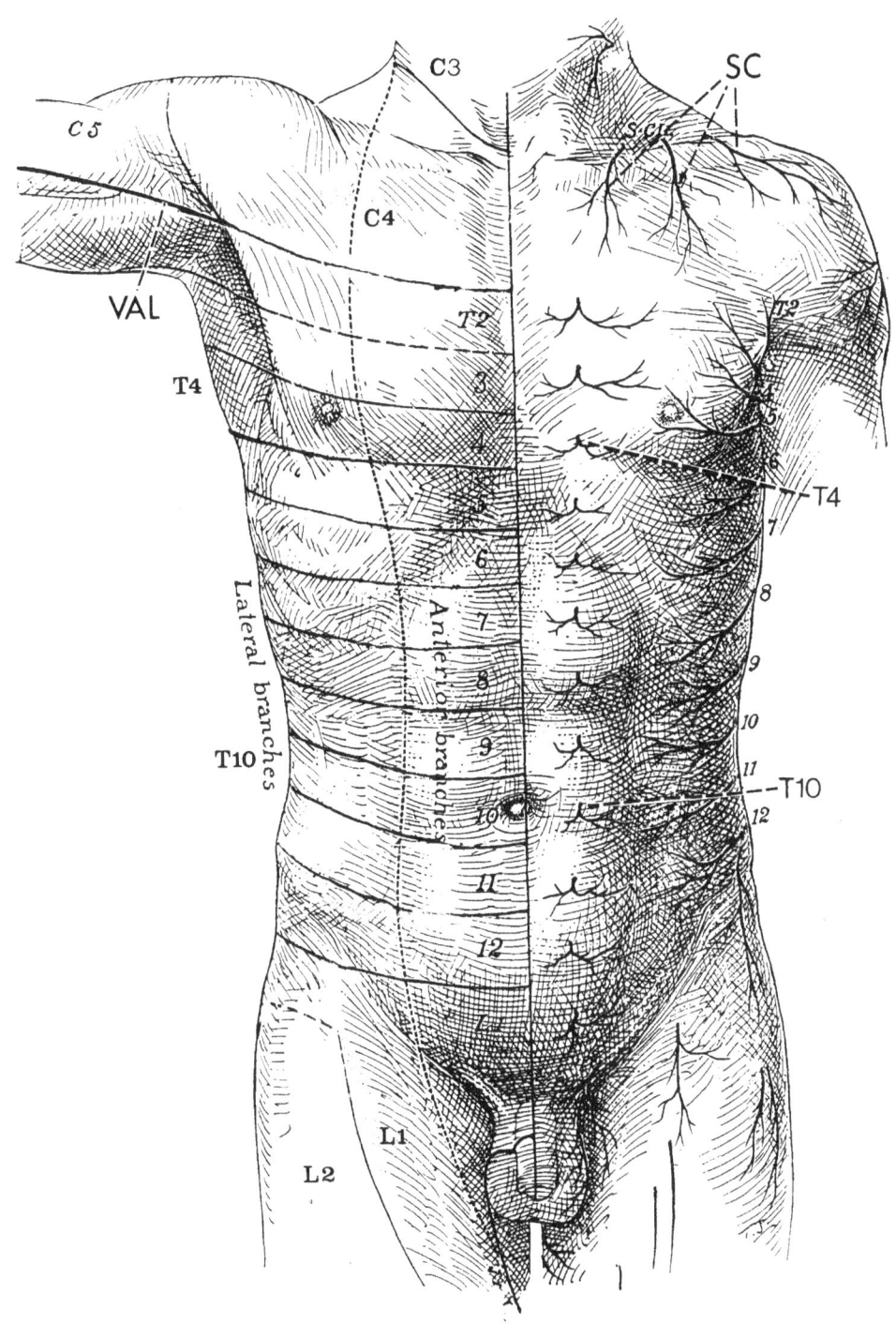

Eycleshymer and Jones

Ab-2 Muscles of the anterior and lateral abdominal walls I
(opposite page)

Color and label

1. Rectus abdominis; note its segmental arrangement with (usually) 3 fibrous bands between the segments (tendinous intersections). In well-developed individuals, the enlarged muscular segments often give the anterior abdomen wall a "washboard" appearance.
2. Tendinous intersection
3. Transversus abdominis muscle
4. Internal abdominal oblique muscle (cut)
5. External abdominal oblique muscle (cut)
6. Aponeurosis* of external abdominal oblique; medially it fuses with the anterior layer of the aponeurosis of the internal oblique to form the anterior wall of the rectus sheath.
7. Anterior layer of the aponeurosis of the internal oblique which divides into anterior and posterior layers
8. Inguinal ligament; traditionally described as the "thickened" lower border of external oblique aponeurosis; it extends from the anterior superior iliac spine to the pubic tubercle; recent reports have questioned any thickening.
9. Superficial inguinal ring in external oblique aponeurosis; opening for the spermatic cord in males and the round ligament in females; bigger on males
10. Pubic tubercle
11. Pubic symphysis and pubic crest; origin of rectus abdominis muscle
12. Conjoint tendon; formed by the fused aponeuroses of the internal oblique and the transversus abdominis muscles
13. Anterior superior iliac spine
14. Insertion of the rectus abdominis on the costal cartilages of ribs 5-7 and xiphoid process
15. Origin of external abdominal oblique muscle from ribs 5-12
16. Anterior cutaneous branch of intercostal nerve T12; note that it supplies a band of skin that includes the umbilicus. The rectus abdominis and the 3 lateral abdominal muscles are innervated by thoracic (intercostal) nerves T5-T12 (subcostal nerve) plus L1 (iliohypogastric nerve). Cutaneous branches of these nerves also supply strips of skin; for example, cutaneous branches of nerve T4 supply the nipple.
17. Linea semilunaris; a curved depression that indicates the lateral border of the rectus abdominis muscle and the rectus sheath.
18. Linea alba; all three lateral abdominal muscles insert on the linea alba by way of their aponeuroses. All 6 muscles working together will draw in the abdominal wall (suck in the gut).

*An aponeurosis is a strong flat tendinous sheet which acts as an extension of its attached muscle.

1 _____
2 _____
3 _____
4 _____
5 _____
6 _____
7 _____
8 _____
9 _____
10 _____
11 _____

Ab-2 Muscles of the anterior and lateral abdominal walls I

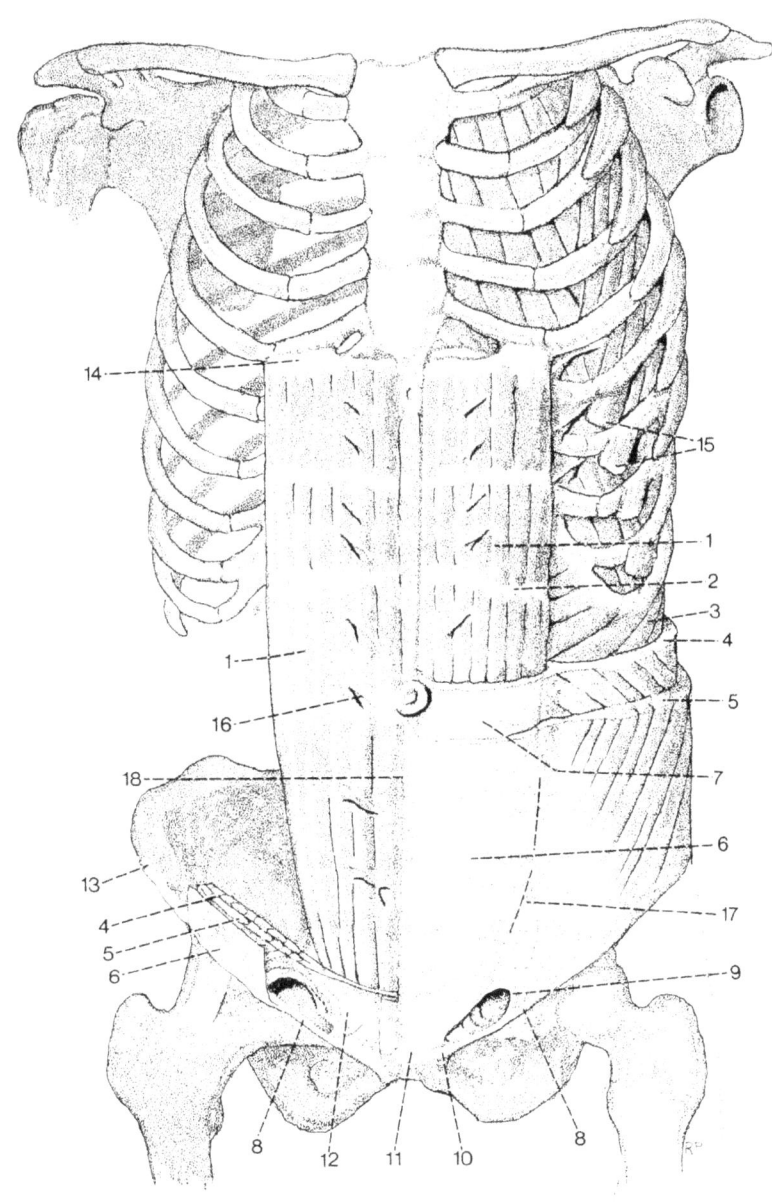

12 _____
13 _____
14 _____
15 _____
16 _____
17 _____
18 _____

Ab-3 Muscles of the anterior and lateral abdominal walls II
(opposite page)

Color and label

1. Rectus abdominis muscle
2. Tendinous intersection
3. External abdominal oblique muscle
4. Aponeurosis of external abdominal oblique (a small piece; fusing with aponeurosis of internal oblique)
5. Internal abdominal oblique muscle
6. Anterior and posterior layers of rectus sheath formed by the splitting of the aponeurosis of the internal oblique
7. Transversus abdominis muscle
8. Aponeurosis of transversus abdominis (cut; at this level all 3 aponeuroses pass in front of the rectus abdominis)
9. Arcuate line (*linea arcuata*; a crescentic line, not always clearly defined, which marks the lower border of the posterior layer of the rectus sheath)
10. Linea alba; midline fibrous insertion of the 3 aponeuroses from the 3 flat abdominal muscles on each side; this avascular strip extends from the xiphoid process to the pubic symphysis; it is free of all but the tiniest blood vessels, and a surgical incision in the midline will sever no nerves to muscles since the nerves travel from the posterior spinal cord within the body wall to the anterior midline.
11. Transversalis fascia; a layer of connective tissue lying just beneath the transversus abdominis muscle and external to the peritoneum; in the lower third of the rectus abdominis sheath, where there is no posterior fibrous layer, the transversalis fascia forms the posterior layer of the rectus sheath.
12. Superior epigastric artery; accompanied by 2 or more veins (not shown)
13. Inferior epigastric artery; the inferior and superior epigastric arteries, along with their accompanying veins, anastomose within the rectus abdominis muscle, thus providing potential side channels (collateral circulation) for blood to reach the legs and lower trunk in the case of an obstructed aorta.
14. Inguinal ligament
15. Conjoined tendon; formed by the fused aponeuroses of the internal oblique and the transversus muscles
16. Opening in the internal oblique for the spermatic cord
17. Superficial inguinal ring in the external oblique aponeurosis
18. Spermatic cord with fibers of cremaster muscle
19. Testis
20. Pyramidalis muscle; absent in approximately 20% of cases
21. Posterior layer of rectus sheath

1 _____
2 _____
3 _____
4 _____
5 _____
6 _____
7 _____
8 _____
9 _____
10 _____
11 _____
12 _____

Ab-3 Muscles of the anterior and lateral abdominal walls II

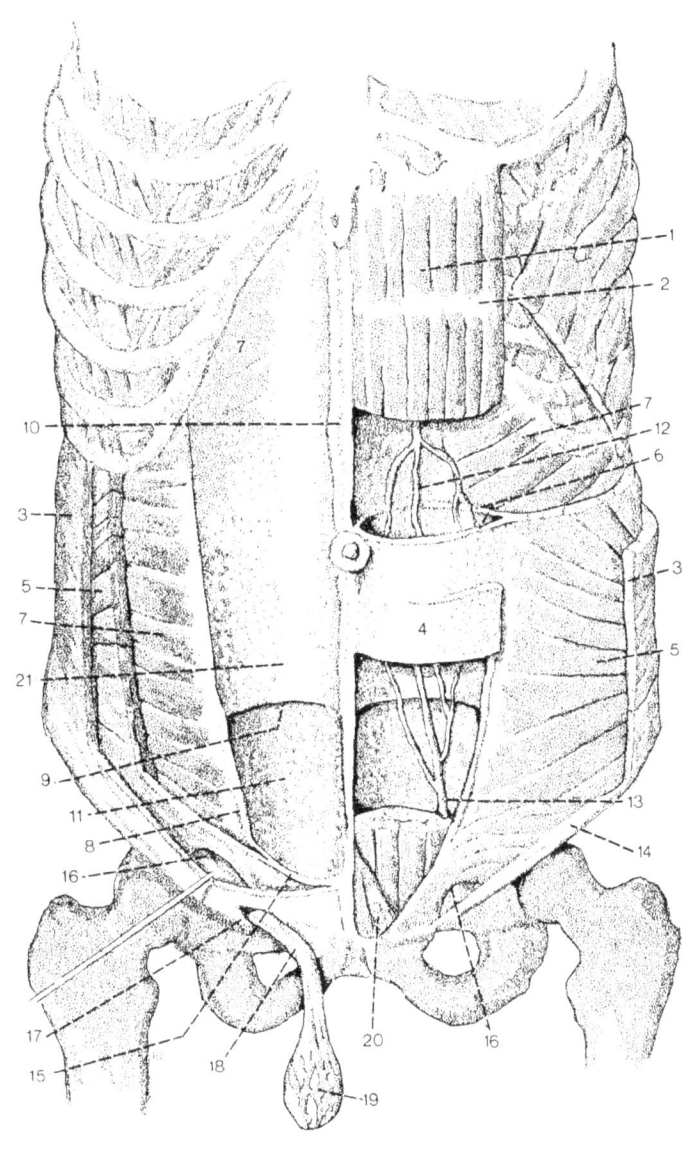

13 _____
14 _____
15 _____
16 _____
17 _____
18 _____
19 _____
20 _____
21 _____

Ab-4 Muscles and layers of the anterior abdominal wall
(opposite page)

Color and label

Figure A. Muscles of the anterior abdominal wall

1. Umbilicus
2. Rectus abdominis muscle
3. Tendinous intersection
4. Aponeurosis of the external abdominal oblique muscle; note that it combines with the aponeurosis of the internal oblique to form the anterior layer of the rectus sheath.
5. External abdominal oblique muscle
6. Internal abdominal oblique muscle
7. Transversus abdominis muscle
8. Aponeurosis of the internal oblique; note that it splits into an anterior and a posterior layer with the former becoming the anterior layer of the rectus sheath and the latter becoming the posterior layer.
9. Posterior layer of the rectus sheath; formed by the posterior layer of the internal oblique aponeurosis and the aponeurosis of the transversus abdominis; the posterior layer is present in only the upper two-thirds of the abdominal wall; in the lower one-third, all 3 aponeuroses pass to the front of the rectus abdominis muscles.
10. Anterior layer of the rectus sheath

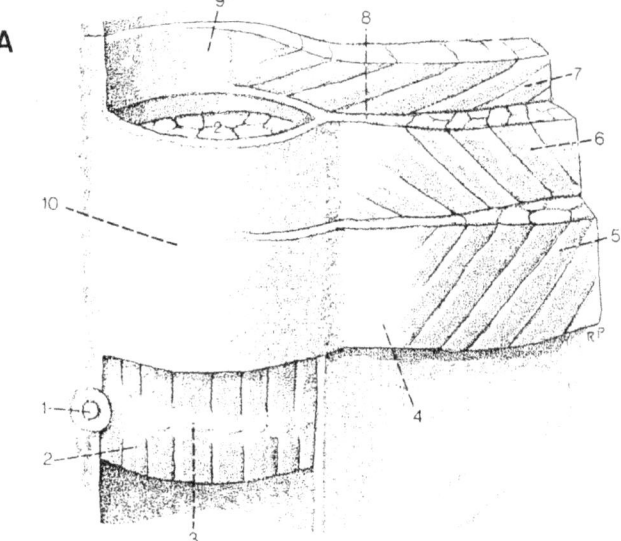

Figure B. The 9 layers of the anterior abdominal wall

The deep fascia surrounding the muscles has been exaggerated in thickness and partially removed on the right side (viewer's left).

1. Skin
2. Superficial fascia fatty layer (Camper's)
3. Superficial fascia fibrous layer (Scarpa's)
4. External abdominal oblique muscle
5. Internal abdominal oblique muscle
6. Transversus abdominis muscle
7. Transversalis fascia
8. Extraperitoneal (preperitoneal) fat
9. Peritoneum (parietal layer which lines the inside of the walls)
10. Rectus abdominis muscles
11. Anterior layer of the rectus sheath
12. Posterior layer of the rectus sheath
13. Linea alba
14. Aponeurosis of the external oblique muscle
15. Intestine; covered with visceral peritoneum or serosa

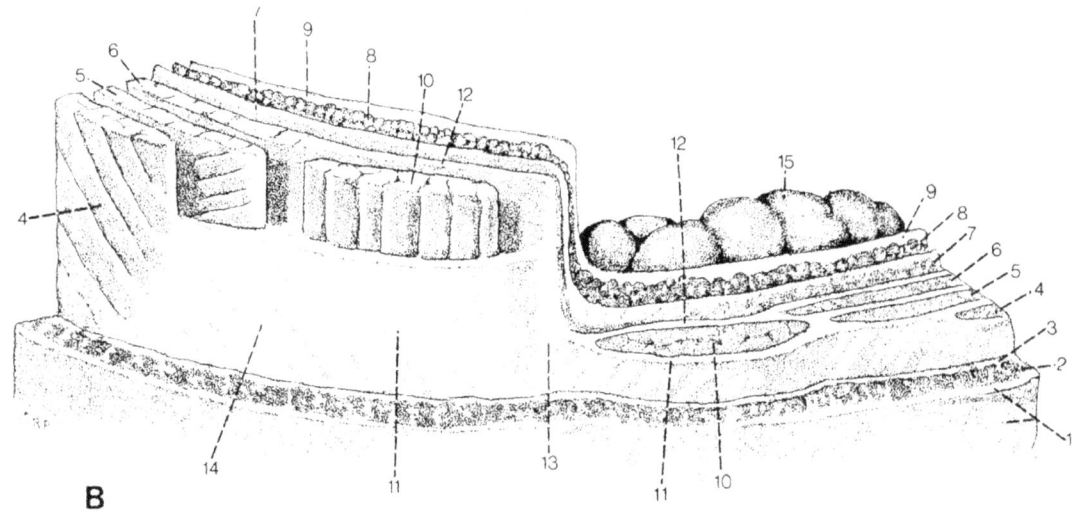

Ab-4 Muscles and layers of the anterior abdominal wall

FIG A

1_____
2_____
3_____
4_____
5_____
6_____
7_____
8_____
9_____
10_____

FIG B

1_____   10_____
2_____   11_____
3_____   12_____
4_____   13_____
5_____   14_____
6_____   15_____
7_____
8_____
9_____

Ab-5 External abdominal oblique aponeurosis and superficial inguinal ring

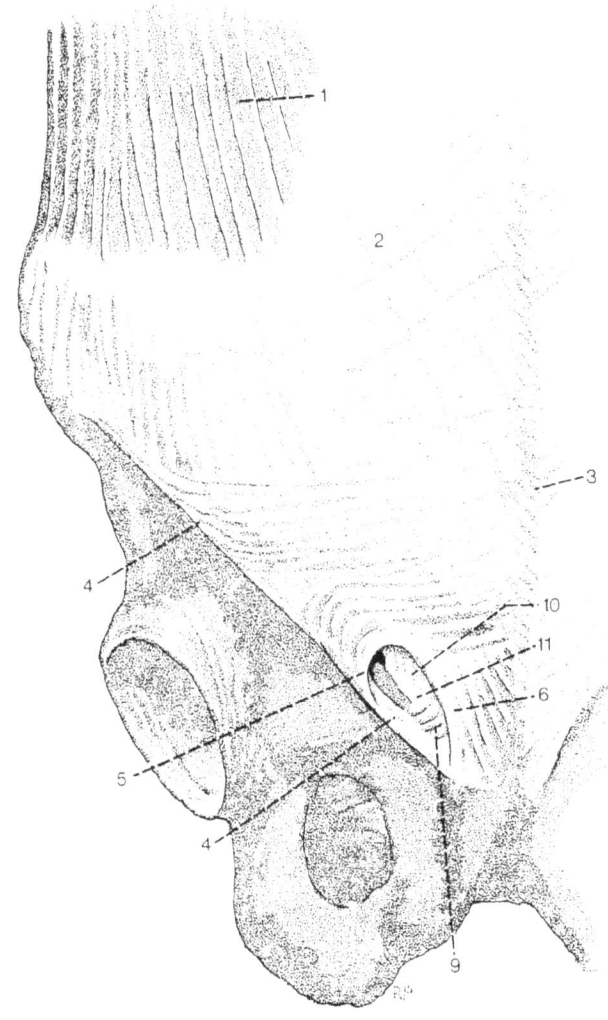

Redrawn from Moore

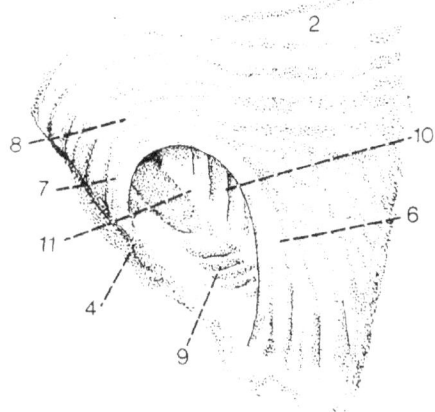

Color and label
1. External abdominal oblique muscle
2. Aponeurosis of external oblique
3. Linea alba
4. Inguinal ligament
5. Superficial inguinal ring; opening for spermatic cord in males; for round ligament of uterus in females
6. Medial crus; attached to the pubic crest and in front of the pubic symphysis
7. Lateral crus; attached to the pubic tubercle
8. Intercrural fibers
9. Lacunar ligament
10. Conjoint tendon attached to pectineal ligament
11. Pectineal ligament

1_____
2_____
3_____
4_____
5_____
6_____
7_____
8_____
9_____
10_____
11_____

Ab-6 Inguinal canal dissection

Color and label

1. Aponeurosis of external abdominal oblique (cut)
2. Inguinal ligament; lower border of external oblique aponeurosis
3. Aponeurosis of internal abdominal oblique (cut)
4. Aponeurosis of transversus abdominis; note that all 3 aponeuroses pass in front of the rectus abdominis muscle at this level.
5. Anterior layer of rectus sheath
6. Conjoint tendon; formed by the arched lower borders of the aponeuroses of the internal oblique and the transversus abdominis
7. Spermatic cord; round ligament of the uterus in the female
8. Deep inguinal ring in the transversalis fascia
9. Transversalis fascia
10. Interfoveolar ligament
11. Internal abdominal oblique muscle
12. Transversus abdominis muscle
13. Extraperitoneal fat
14. Rectus abdominis muscle
15. Peritoneum
16. External spermatic fascia; continuous with deep fascia of external oblique
17. Cremasteric fascia and cremasteric muscle; continuous with internal oblique
18. Internal spermatic fascia; continuous with transversalis fascia
19. Vas (ductus) deferens
20. Testicular artery surrounded by pampiniform plexus of testicular vein; countercurrent heat exchange cools blood to the testis
21. Inferior epigastric artery and vein(s)
22. Femoral vein
23. Femoral artery
24. Great saphenous vein
25. Saphenous hiatus (opening)
26. Fascia lata (deep fascia of the thigh)
27. Subcutaneous fat (superficial fascia)
28. Superficial inguinal ring

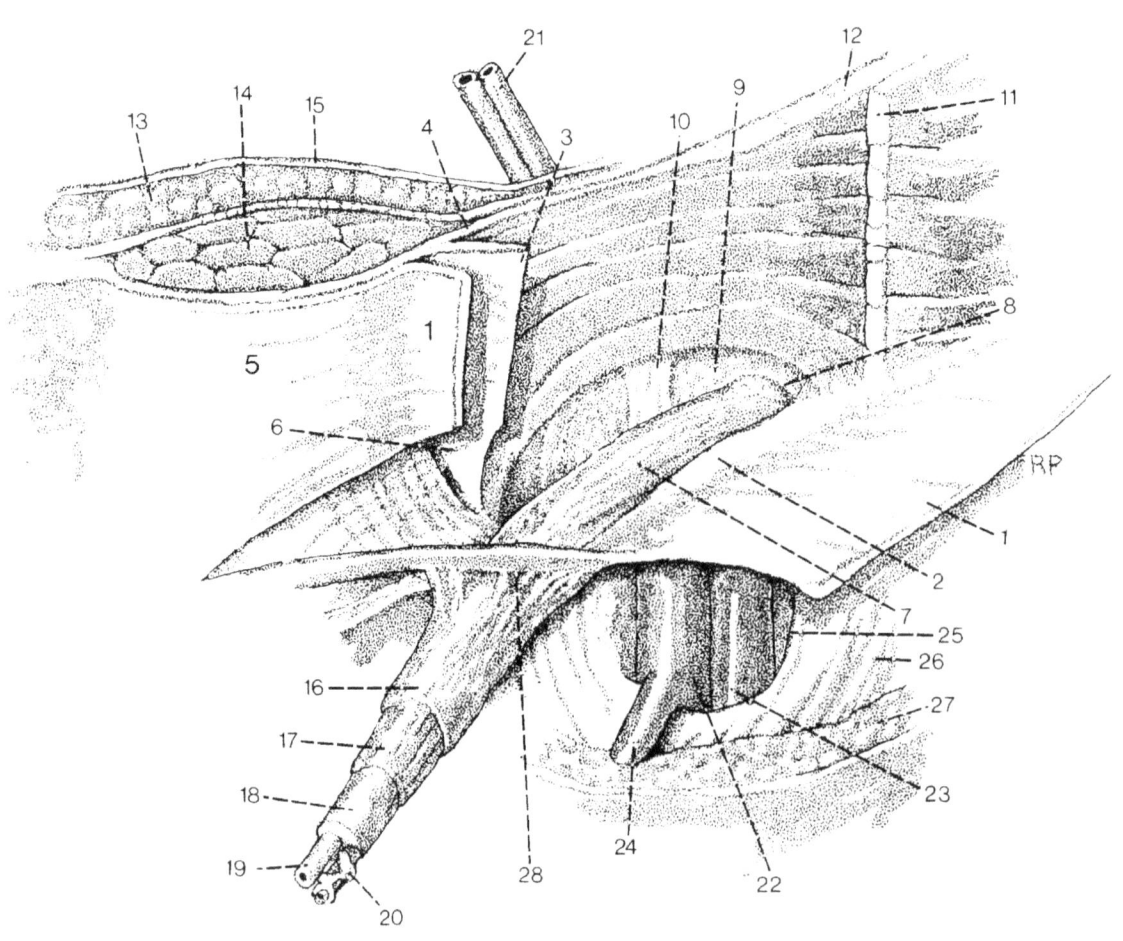

Ab-6 Inguinal canal dissection
(opposite page)

1. _____
2. _____
3. _____
4. _____
5. _____
6. _____
7. _____
8. _____
9. _____
10. _____
13. _____
14. _____
15. _____
16. _____
17. _____
18. _____
19. _____
20. _____
21. _____
22. _____
23. _____
24. _____
25. _____
26. _____
27. _____
28. _____

Ab-7 Inguinal ligament and related structures
(opposite page)

Color and label
Figure A

1. Inguinal ligament; hammock-like free lower edge of the aponeurosis of the external abdominal oblique muscle; it extends from the anterior superior iliac spine to the pubic tubercle; attached to the deep fascia of thigh (fascia lata).
2. Aponeurosis of the external abdominal oblique; it has been cut above the inguinal ligament, pulled forward, and partially dissected free of the inguinal ligament on the left.
3. Lacunar ligament; triangular extension of the medial end of the inguinal ligament extending to the pectineal ligament; its apex is attached medially to the pubic tubercle and its lateral concave base forms the medial border of the femoral ring; the spermatic cord passes over it; its superior surface forms the floor of the inguinal canal medially.
4. Reflex ligament; a poorly developed triangular band usually fused with either the conjoint tendon directly behind it or with the aponeurosis of the external oblique directly in front of it;* it has been reflected backwards on the left side.
5. Pectineal ligament; a strong fibrous band extending laterally from the base of the lacunar ligament along the pecten pubis (*pecten*, Latin, a comb); the conjoint tendon inserts upon it.
6. Superficial inguinal ring; the spermatic cord in the male and the round ligament of the uterus in the female and the ilioinguinal nerve in both sexes pass through it.
7. Lateral (inferior) crus of superficial inguinal ring
8. Medial (superior) crus of superficial inguinal ring

Figure B

1. Inguinal ligament (cut on left side)
2. Aponeurosis of external oblique
3. Lacunar ligament
4. Reflex ligament (see above)
5. Conjoint tendon (falx** inguinalis); formed by the joined tendons of the medial inferior borders of the aponeuroses of both the transversus abdominis and internal oblique muscles; it arches over the spermatic cord in males and the round ligament of the uterus in the female and inserts on the pectineal ligament.
6. Superficial inguinal ring
7. Lateral crus of the superficial inguinal ring
8. Medial crus of the superficial inguinal ring
9. Aponeurosis of transversus abdominis muscle
10. Aponeurosis of internal abdominal oblique muscle

*The reflex ligament has been decribed by some authors as a poorly developed expansion of the lateral crus of the inguinal ligament which passes medially and upward behind the medial end of the superficial inguinal ring in front of the conjoint tendon, feebly reinforcing the posterior wall of the inguinal canal and interweaving with similar fibers from the opposite side. Others describe it as a poorly developed triangular band of the external oblique aponeurosis of one side that crosses the midline, passes behind the superficial inguinal ring of the opposite, and inserts on the pectineal line. Churchill's Medical Dictionary, New York, Churchill Livingstone, 1989.

**Falx*, Latin, a sickle, a scythe (falciform, arched, in the form of a sickle or scythe)

Ab-7 Inguinal ligament and related structures

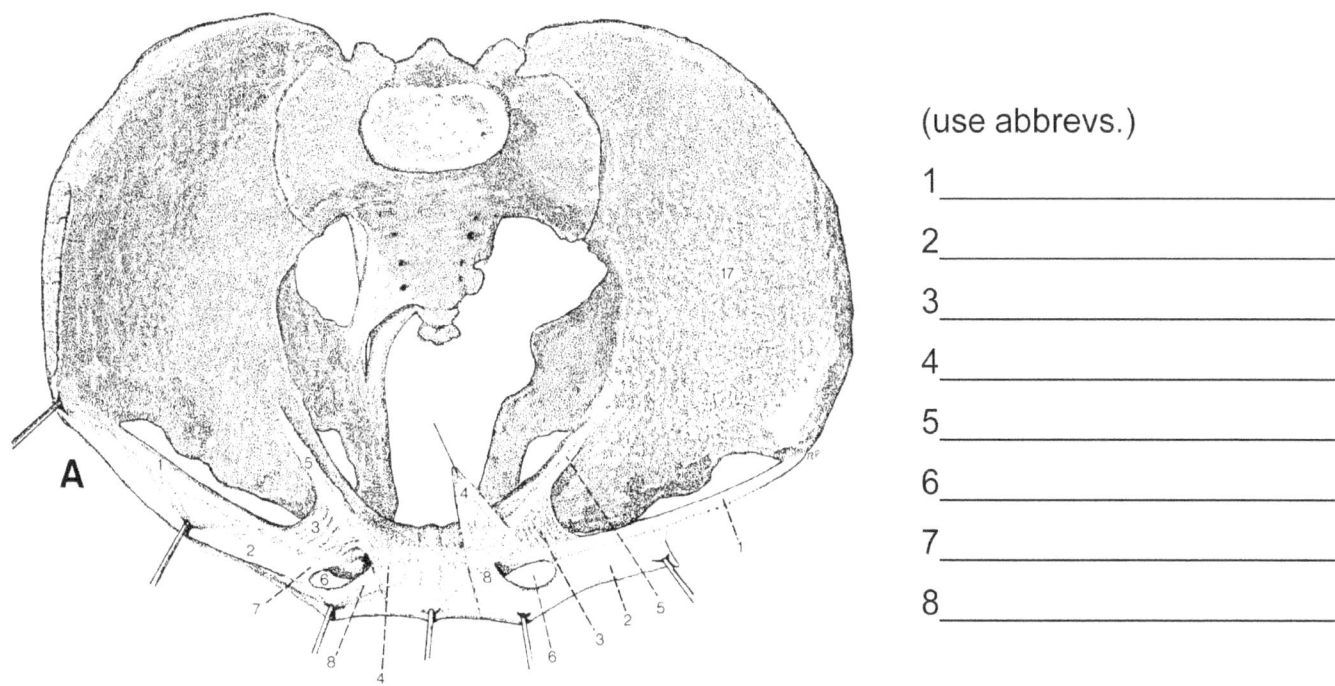

(use abbrevs.)

1_____
2_____
3_____
4_____
5_____
6_____
7_____
8_____

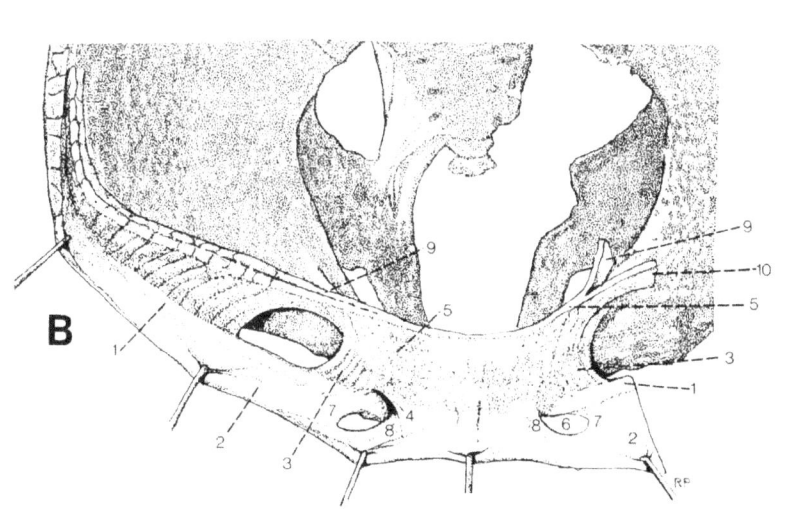

(use abbrevs.)

1_____
2_____
3_____
4_____
5_____
6_____
7_____
8_____
9_____
10_____

Ab-8 Lower anterior abdomen wall viewed from the inside
(opposite page)

Color and label

1. Median umbilical fold (or *plica*, Latin, fold); a raised fold of peritoneum formed by the ligamentous remains of the embryologic urachus,* extending in the midline from the apex of the urinary bladder to the umbilicus.
2. Medial umbilical fold (or plica); formed by the obliterated umbilical artery extending from the superior vesical (*vesica*, Latin, a bladder) artery to the umbilicus
3. Lateral umbilical fold (or plica); formed by inferior epigastric artery and vein
4. Rectus abdominis muscle
5. Umbilicus
6. Lateral border of rectus abdominis muscle
7. Inferior epigastric artery and vein(s); the vein is often doubled; these will anastomose with the superior epigastric vessels
8. Inguinal trigone, Hesselbach's triangle; formed by lateral border of rectus abdominis medially, by inguinal ligament inferiorly, and by inferior epigastric vessels laterally; **site of direct inguinal hernia**.
9. Parietal peritoneum partially stripped away
10. Deep inguinal ring; **site of indirect inguinal hernia**; this tends to be much larger in males than in females.
11. Testicular artery and vein
12. Ureter; conveys urine from the kidney to the bladder
13. Vas (ductus) deferens; conveys semen from the testis to the protate gland
14. Seminal vesicle; secretes part of the seminal fluid
15. Prostate gland
16. Urinary bladder; under parietal peritoneum
17. External iliac vein; becomes femoral vein in thigh
18. External iliac artery; becomes femoral artery in thigh; the external iliac artery and vein give rise to the inferior epigastric artery and vein.
19. Iliopsoas muscle
20. Femoral nerve
21. Deep inguinal ring
22. Parietal peritoneum

*Urachus: the vestigial distal part of the embryonic allantois. The lumen of the urachus is obliterated early in human embryos and becomes the cord-like median umbilical fold. The proximal part of the sausage-like allantois forms the bladder.

1 _____
2 _____
3 _____
4 _____
5 _____
6 _____
7 _____
8 _____
9 _____
10 _____

Ab-8 Lower anterior abdomen wall viewed from the inside

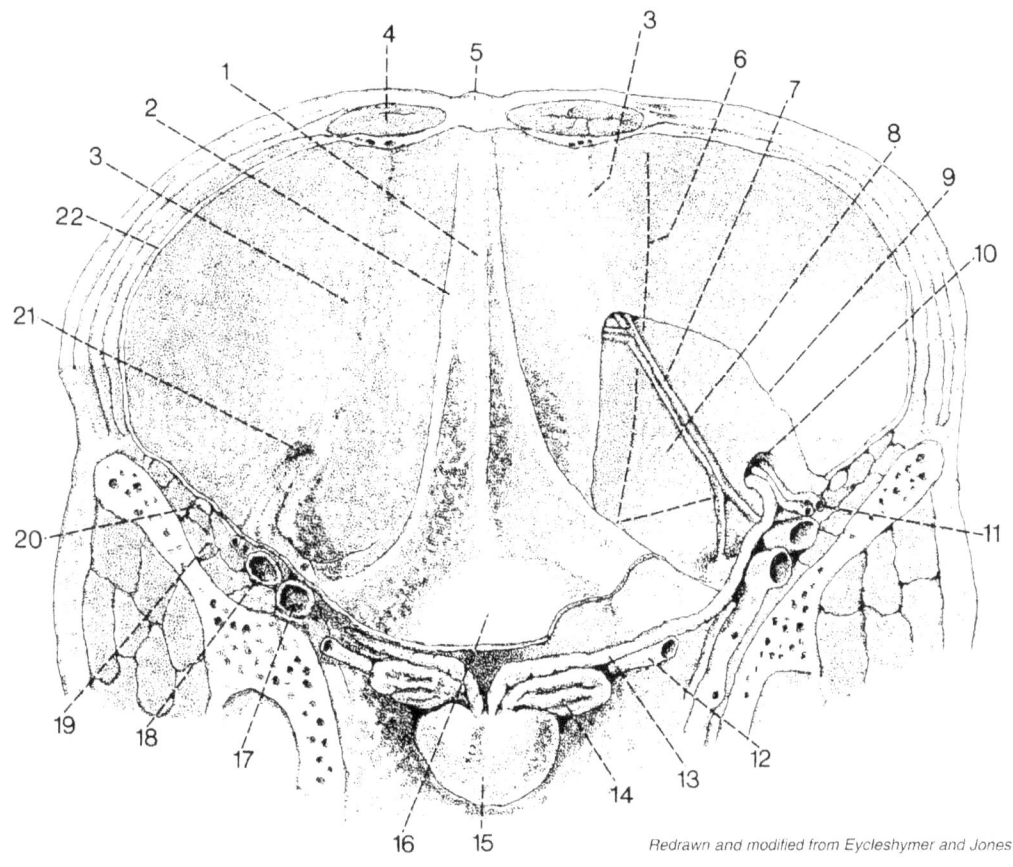

Redrawn and modified from Eycleshymer and Jones

11 _____
12 _____
13 _____
14 _____
15 _____
16 _____
17 _____
18 _____
19 _____
20 _____
21 _____
22 _____

Ab-9 Thoracic and abdominal viscera after removal of anterior thoracic and abdominal walls
(opposite page)

1_____
2_____
3_____
4_____
5_____
6_____
7_____
8_____
9_____
10_____

Ab-9 Thoracic and abdominal viscera after removal of anterior thoracic and abdominal walls

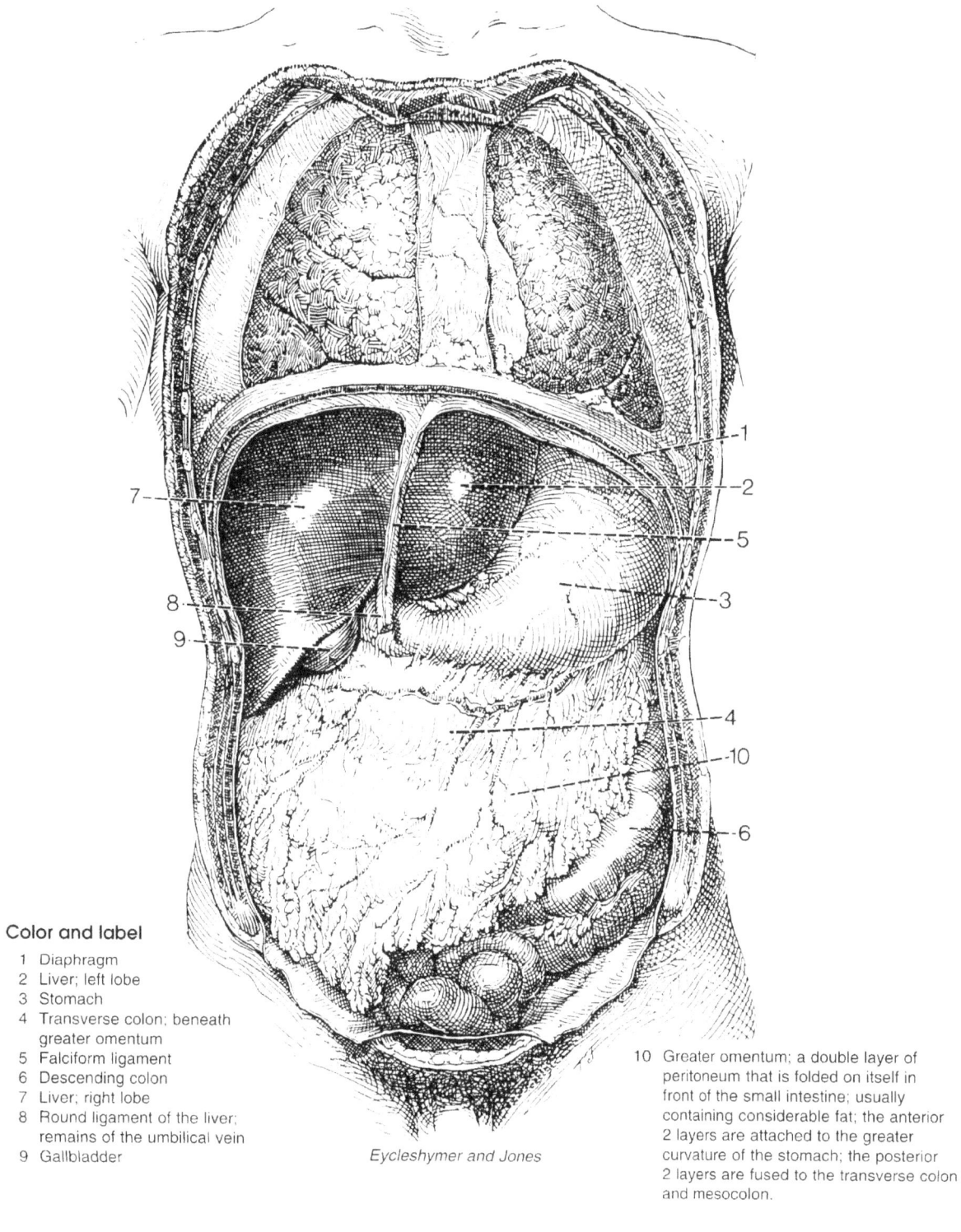

Color and label
1. Diaphragm
2. Liver; left lobe
3. Stomach
4. Transverse colon; beneath greater omentum
5. Falciform ligament
6. Descending colon
7. Liver; right lobe
8. Round ligament of the liver; remains of the umbilical vein
9. Gallbladder
10. Greater omentum; a double layer of peritoneum that is folded on itself in front of the small intestine; usually containing considerable fat; the anterior 2 layers are attached to the greater curvature of the stomach; the posterior 2 layers are fused to the transverse colon and mesocolon.

Eycleshymer and Jones

Ab-10 Thorax and abdominal viscera

In relation to the skeleton - Anterior view
(opposite page)

Color and label

1. Trachea
2. Esophagus
3. Left common carotid artery
4. Left subclavian artery
5. Clavicle
6. Manubrium
7. Pericardium covering heart
8. Left lung; lower lobe
9. Diaphragm
10. Spleen
11. Stomach
12. Transverse colon (tenia coli)
13. Descending colon
14. Inguinal ligament
15. Femoral nerve
16. Femoral artery (lateral) and femoral vein (medial)
17. Peritoneum (external surface)
18. Bladder
19. Spermatic cord
20. Small intestine
21. Ascending colon
22. Gallbladder
23. Falciform ligament
24. Liver (right lobe)
25. Right lung; lower lobe
26. Middle lobe of right lung
27. Superior lobe of right lung
28. Humerus
29. Coracoid process of scapula
30. Acromion of scapula
31. Clavicle

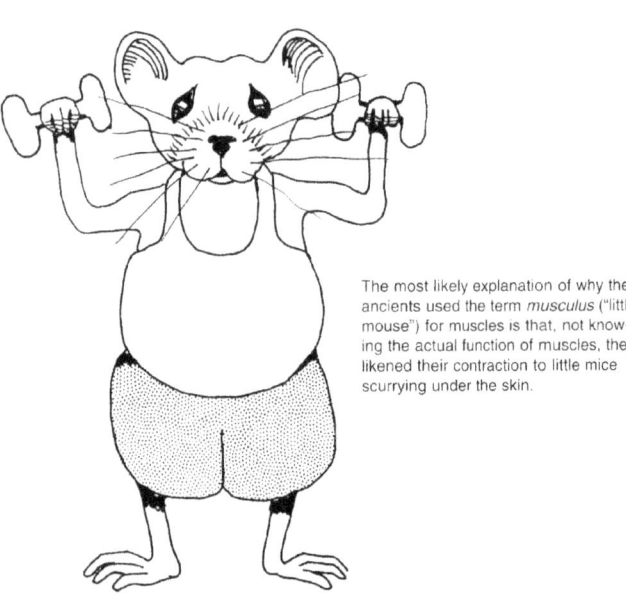

The most likely explanation of why the ancients used the term *musculus* ("little mouse") for muscles is that, not knowing the actual function of muscles, they likened their contraction to little mice scurrying under the skin.

The word **muscle** originally meant "little mouse"
(Latin, *mus*, mouse; *musculus*, little mouse)

1 _____
2 _____
3 _____
4 _____
5 _____
6 _____

7 _____
8 _____
9 _____
10 _____
11 _____
12 _____
13 _____
14 _____
15 _____
16 _____
17 _____
18 _____
19 _____
20 _____
21 _____
22 _____
23 _____
24 _____
25 _____
26 _____
27 _____
28 _____
29 _____
30 _____
31 _____

Ab-10 Thorax and abdominal viscera
In relation to the skeleton

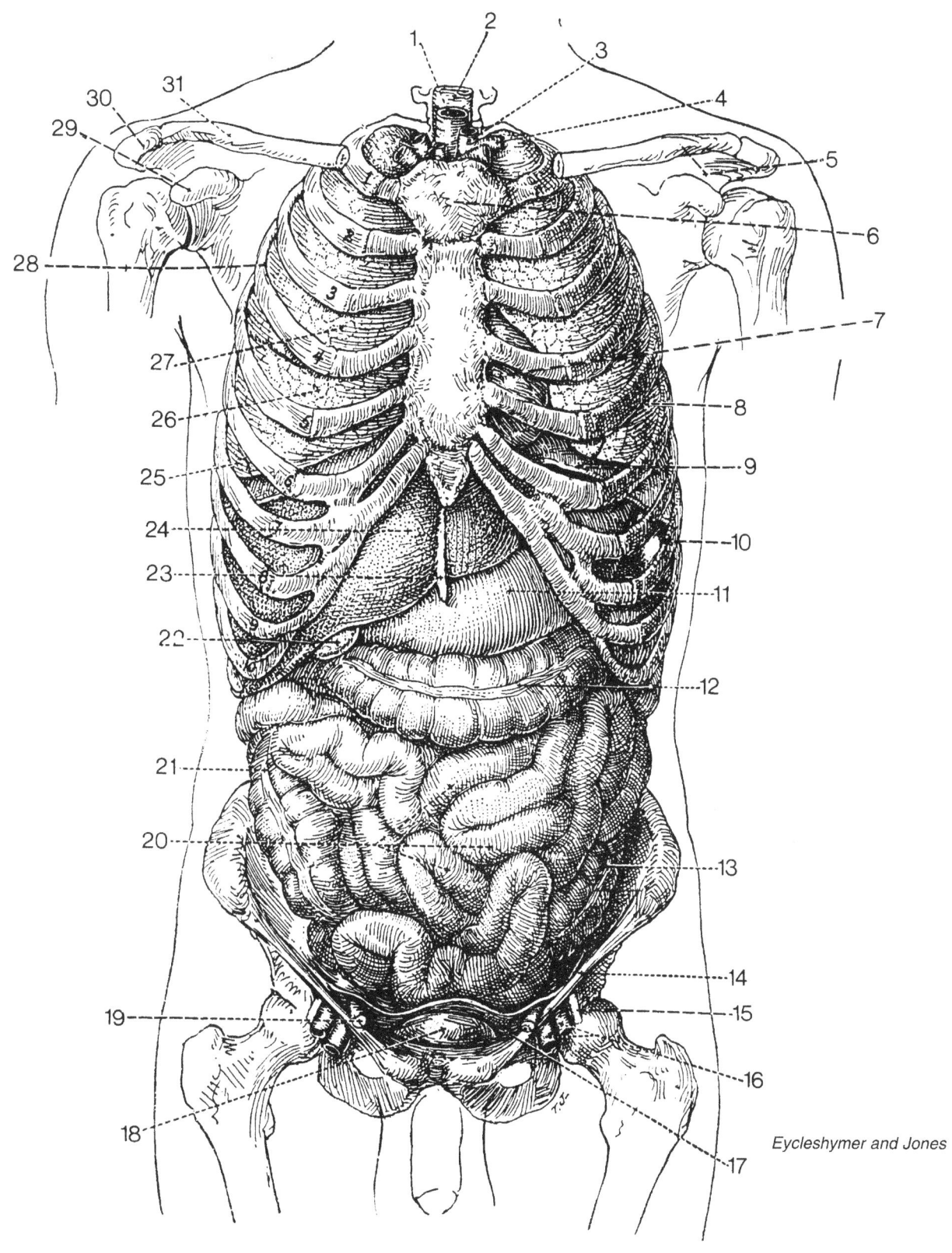

Eycleshymer and Jones

Ab-11 Frontal (coronal) section of the trunk

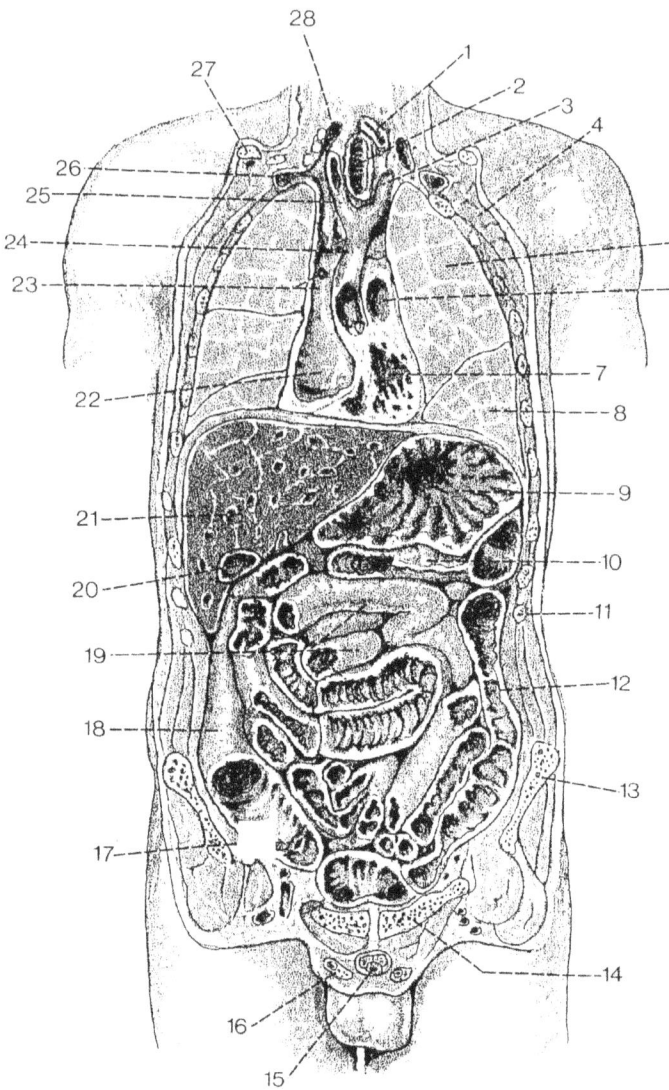

Redrawn and modified from Eycleshymer and Jones

Color and label

1. Esophagus
2. Trachea
3. Left common carotid artery
4. Pectoralis major muscle
5. Superior lobe of left lung
6. Pulmonary trunk
7. Left ventricle
8. Lower (inferior) lobe of left lung
9. Stomach
10. Transverse colon
11. Rib 10
12. Descending colon
13. Ilium
14. Pubis
15. Penile (spongy) urethra
16. Spermatic cord
17. Ileocecal valve
18. Ascending colon
19. Small intestine
20. Gallbladder
21. Liver
22. Right atrium
23. Superior vena cava with opening of azygos vein
24. Aorta (ascending)
25. Brachiocephalic artery
26. Subclavian vein
27. Clavicle (cut)
28. Internal jugular vein

1. _____
2. _____
3. _____
4. _____
5. _____
6. _____
7. _____
8. _____
9. _____
10. _____
11. _____
12. _____
13. _____
14. _____
15. _____
16. _____
17. _____
18. _____
19. _____
20. _____
21. _____
22. _____
23. _____
24. _____
25. _____
26. _____
27. _____
28. _____

Ab-12 Thoracic and abdominal viscera

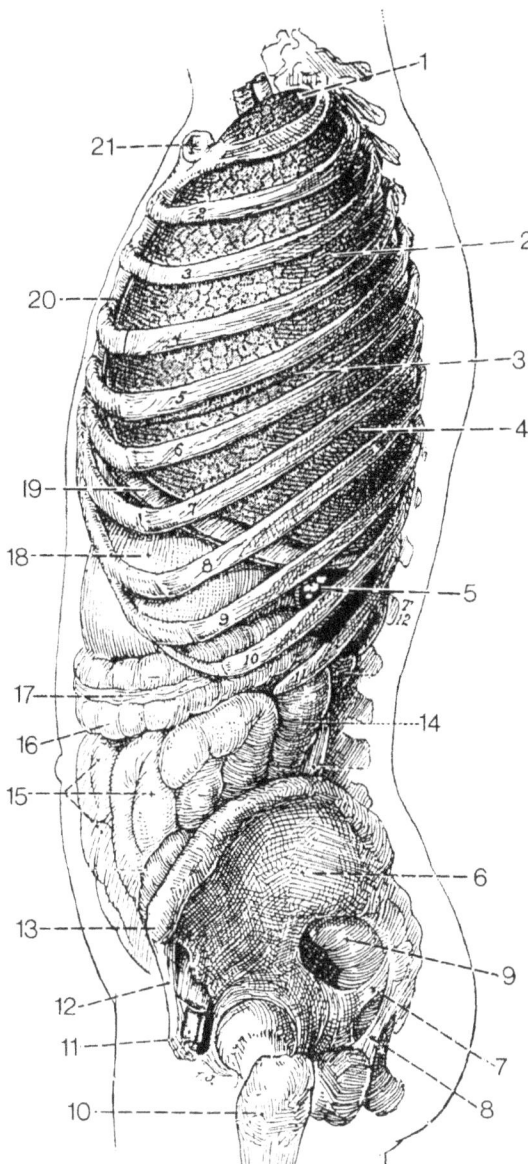

Eycleshymer and Jones

Color and label
1 Apex
2 Upper lobe of lung
3 Oblique fissure
4 Lower lobe of lung
5 Spleen
6 Ilium
7 Sacrospinous ligament
8 Sacrotuberous ligament
9 Rectum (viewed through greater sciatic foramen)
10 Femur; greater trochanter
11 Pubic tubercle
12 Inguinal ligament
13 Anterior superior iliac spine
14 Descending colon
15 Small intestine
16 Saccules (haustra) of transverse colon
17 Tenia coli
18 Stomach
19 Diaphragm
20 Sternum
21 Manubrium; clavicular notch

1_____
2_____
3_____
4_____
5_____
6_____
7_____
8_____
9_____
10_____
11_____
12_____
13_____
14_____
15_____
16_____
17_____
18_____
19_____
20_____
21_____

Ab-13 Thoracic and abdominal viscera

Right aspect

Color and label

1. Cervical vertebra 7
2. Apex of right lung
3. Upper lobe of right lung
4. Middle lobe
5. Oblique fissure
6. Lower lobe
7. Gallbladder
8. Stomach
9. Transverse colon
10. Small intestine
11. Anterior superior iliac spine
12. Femur; greater trochanter
13. Ischial tuberosity
14. External anal sphincter
15. Sacrotuberous ligament
16. Sacrospinous ligament
17. Ilium
18. Ascending colon; tenia coli
19. Right kidney
20. Head of femur
21. Liver
22. Diaphragm
23. Horizontal fissure

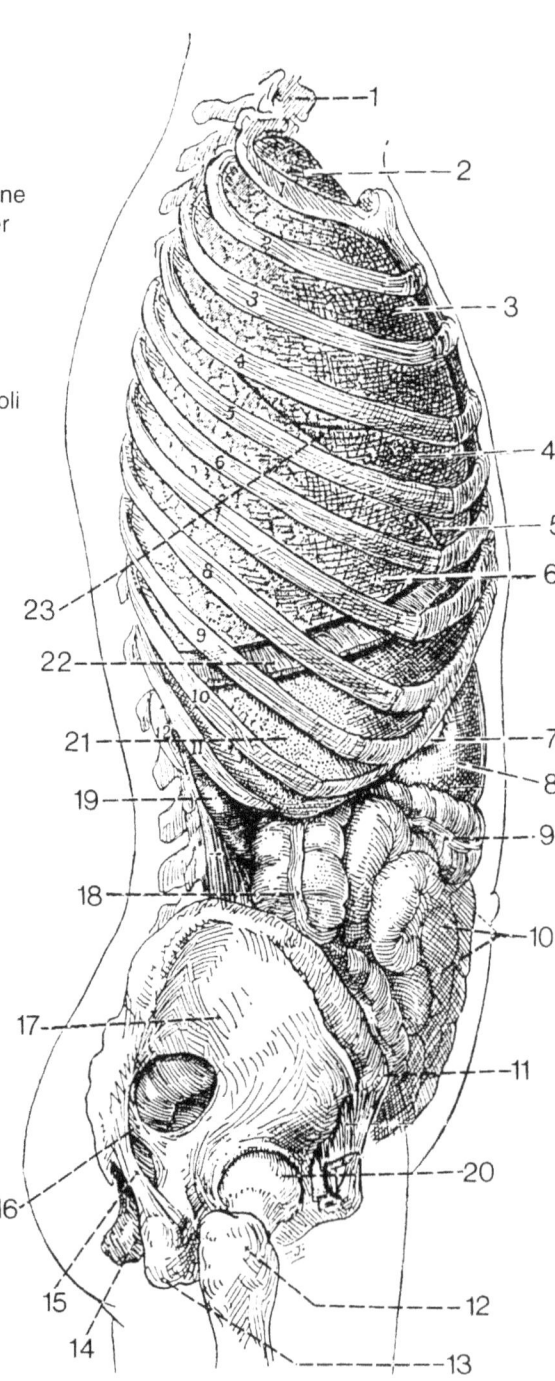

1. _____
2. _____
3. _____
4. _____
5. _____
6. _____
7. _____
8. _____
9. _____
10. _____
11. _____
12. _____
13. _____
14. _____
15. _____
16. _____
17. _____
18. _____
19. _____
20. _____
21. _____
22. _____
23. _____

Ab-14 Thoracic and abdominal viscera

In relation to the skeleton — Posterior view

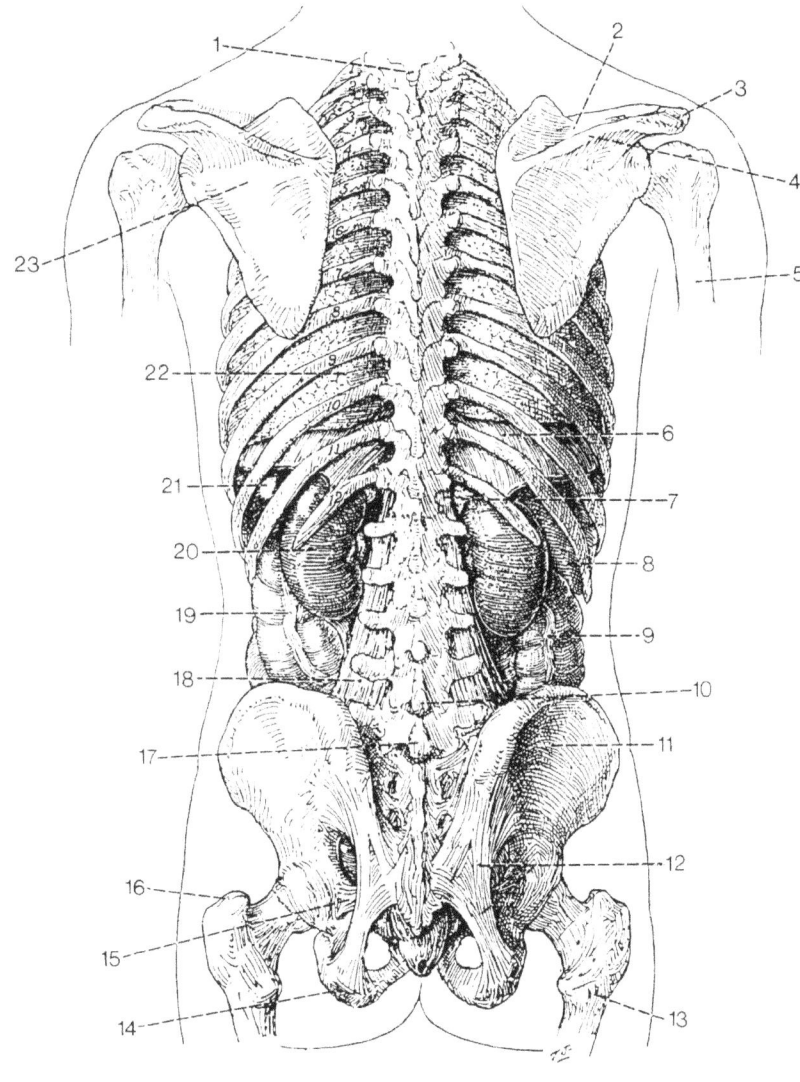

Color and label

1. Thoracic vertebra 1
2. Scapula (supraspinous fossa)
3. Acromion
4. Spine of scapula
5. Humerus
6. Diaphragm
7. Adrenal gland
8. Liver
9. Ascending colon
10. Fifth lumbar vertebra spinous process
11. Ilium of coxal (hip) bone
12. Sacrospinous ligament
13. Femur
14. Ischial tuberosity
15. Sacrospinous ligament
16. Greater trochanter
17. Median sacral crest (fused spinous processes)
18. Psoas major muscle
19. Tenia coli of descending colon
20. Left kidney
21. Spleen
22. Left lung; lower lung
23. Infraspinous fossa of scapula

1_____
2_____
3_____
4_____
5_____
6_____
7_____
8_____
9_____
10_____
11_____
12_____
13_____
14_____
15_____
16_____
17_____
18_____
19_____
20_____
21_____
22_____
23_____

Ab-15 Midsagittal section of the female peritoneal cavity

(opposite page)

Trace the lining and covering of the peritoneum

1. Parietal peritoneum; lines the inner surface of the walls of the abdominopelvic cavity; the free surface of the peritoneum is lined with a single layer of flattened mesothelial cells that secrete serous fluid that allows the peritoneal-covered organs, such as the stomach, small intestines, and transverse colon, to freely slide against each other.
2. Peritoneum (parietal) lining inferior surface of the diaphragm
3. Peritoneum (visceral) covering the liver; its reflection (folding) from the liver on to the inferior surface of the diaphragm forms the **coronary ligament,** which attaches the liver to the diaphragm. The **bare area** of the liver is that portion of the liver surface not covered with peritoneum.
4. Lesser omentum; a double layer of peritoneum extending from the liver to the lesser curvature of the stomach; it forms part of the anterior wall of the lesser bursa (lesser sac).
5. Peritoneum (visceral); forming the outermost layer (serosa) of the stomach; the stomach, like the liver, is almost completely covered with peritoneum.
6. Greater omentum; anterior layer; note that the greater omentum consists of a double layer of peritoneum that is folded on itself in front of the small intestines; the anterior layer is suspended from the greater curvature of the stomach.
7. Greater omentum; posterior layer; note that the posterior layer ascends and adheres to the transverse colon and the anterior layer of the transverse mesocolon. In early embryonic development, a cavity is present between the anterior and posterior layers of the greater omentum as indicated in the accompanying illustration. However, in late pregnancy this cavity is obliterated below the level of the transverse colon as the layers fuse, the internal layers of mesothelium disappear, and fat is deposited in the greater omentum.
8. Transverse mesocolon; the mesentery of the large intestine is called the **mesocolon**. Like the mesentery of the small intestine, it is a double layer of peritoneum. Here it attaches the transverse colon to the posterior abdominal wall. It contains blood vessels, nerves, lymph nodes, and lymphatic vessels that supply the transverse colon, and varying amounts of fat. Unlike the ascending and descending colon, which are both fused to the posterior abdominal wall and have no mesocolon, the transverse meso colon gives the transverse colon has a certain amount of mobility.
9. Peritoneum (parietal) lining the posterior abdominal wall; here covering the pancreas; organs such as the kidneys, which lie behind the peritoneum, or are covered with peritoneum only on their anterior surface such as the pancreas, are considered to be **retroperitoneal**.
10. Mesentery; this is a double layer of peritoneum with connective tissue support that attaches the major part of the small intestines (the jejunum and ileum) to the posterior abdominal wall. It contains a rich network of blood vessels, nerves, lymph nodes, and lymph vessels (here called lacteals).
11. Serosal layer of peritoneum on the small intestine
12. Peritoneum covering anterior surface of the duodenum; this part of the duodenum is retroperitoneal.
13. Peritoneum (parietal) on posterior abdominal wall
14. Peritoneum covering the uterus (tunica serosa, perimetrium)
15. Omental bursa (lesser sac); this is the peritoneal-enclosed space behind the liver and stomach (indicated by the vertical arrow).
16. Omental foramen (epiploic foramen, foramen of Winslow); connects the omental bursa with the remainder of the peritoneal cavity.
17. Rectouterine pouch (excavatio rectouterine, pouch of Douglas)
18. Vesicouterine pouch (excavatio vesicouterina)

1 _____
2 _____
3 _____
4 _____
5 _____
6 _____

Ab-15 Midsagittal section of the female peritoneal cavity

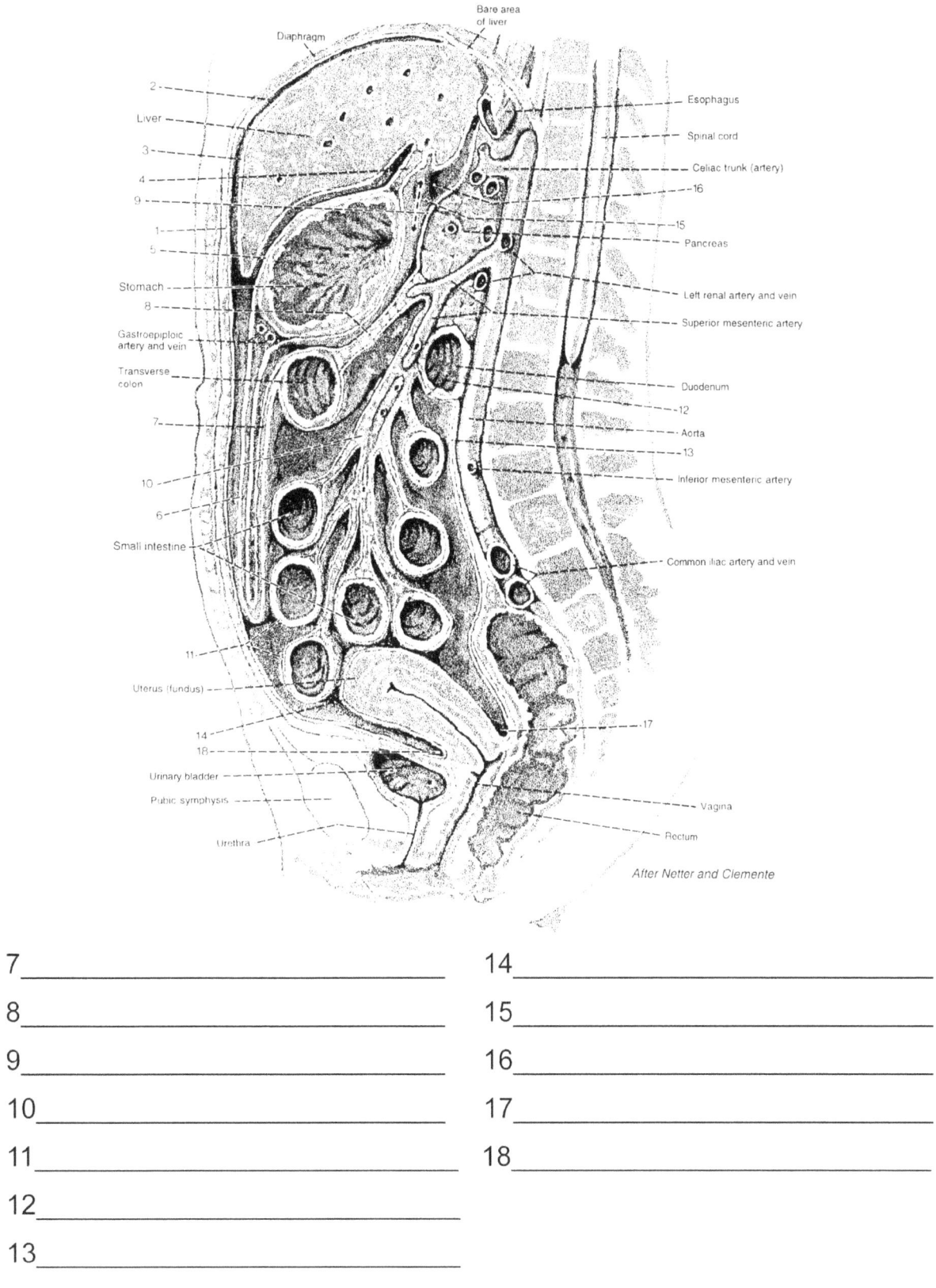

After Netter and Clemente

7 _____
8 _____
9 _____
10 _____
11 _____
12 _____
13 _____
14 _____
15 _____
16 _____
17 _____
18 _____

Ab-16 The stomach

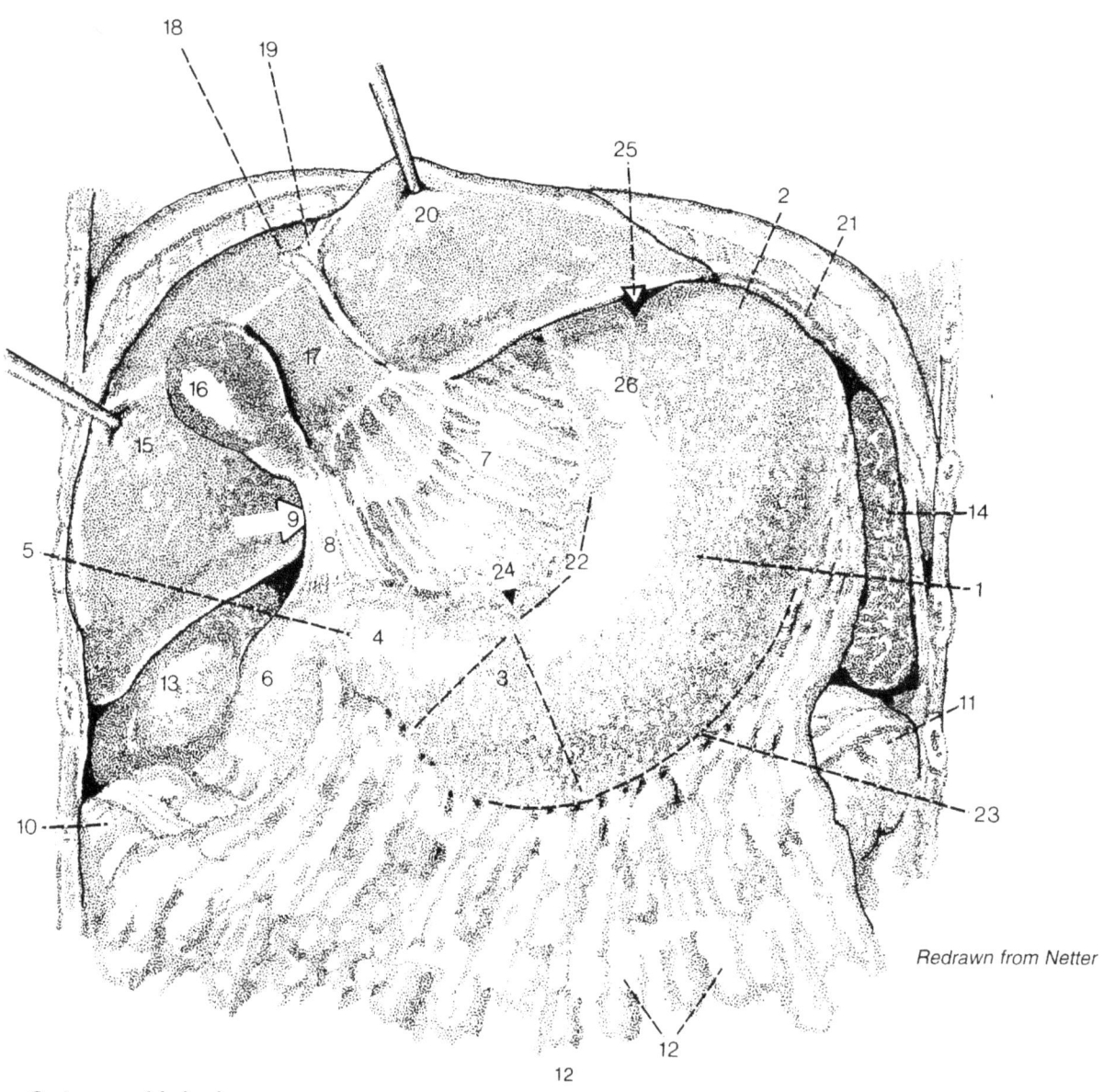

Redrawn from Netter

Color and label

1. Stomach (body, corpus)
2. Stomach (fundus)
3. Stomach (pyloric antrum)
4. Stomach (pyloric canal)
5. Stomach (pyloric sphincter)
6. Duodenum
7. Lesser omentum; peritoneum extending from the liver to the lesser curvature of stomach; this part of the lesser omentum is also called the hepatogastric ligament.
8. Hepatoduodenal ligament; part of the lesser omentum; consists of peritoneum surrounding the common bile duct, the proper hepatic artery, and the portal vein.
9. Arrow in omental foramen (former names: epiploic foramen, foramen of Winslow)
10. Right (hepatic) flexure of colon
11. Left (splenic) flexure of colon
12. Greater omentum
13. Right kidney
14. Spleen
15. Liver; right lobe
16. Gallbladder
17. Liver; quadrate lobe
18. Round ligament of the liver; remnant of umbilical vein
19. Falciform ligament
20. Liver; left lobe
21. Diaphragm
22. Lesser curvature of stomach
23. Greater curvature of stomach
24. Angular incisure (notch, indentation) of stomach
25. Cardiac incisure of stomach
26. Cardiac part of stomach; pars cardiaca gastris; an area 3-4 cm wide that surrounds and includes the esophageal opening (cardiac orifice) into the stomach.

Ab-16 The stomach
(opposite page)

1. _____
2. _____
3. _____
4. _____
5. _____
6. _____
7. _____
8. _____
9. _____
10. _____
11. _____
12. _____
13. _____
14. _____
15. _____
16. _____
17. _____
18. _____
19. _____
20. _____
21. _____
22. _____
23. _____
24. _____
25. _____
26. _____

Ab-17 Blood supply of the stomach

Color and label

1. Abdominal aorta
2. Celiac trunk; a very short artery that immediately divides into 3 branches; it is the sole source of arterial blood to the stomach.
3. Common hepatic artery
4. Proper hepatic artery
5. Right gastric artery; note its origin from the proper hepatic artery
6. Gastroduodenal artery
7. Superior pancreaticoduodenal arteries (anterior and posterior); these supply both the head of the pancreas (not shown) and the upper duodenum.
8. Left gastric artery
9. Esophageal branch of left gastric artery
10. Splenic artery (posterior to stomach)
11. Short gastric arteries
12. Left gastro-epiploic artery (its new name is gastro-omental artery)
13. Spleen
14. Esophagus
15. Right gastro-omental (gastro-epiploic) artery

Note the anastomoses between the right and left gastric arteries as well as between the right and left gastroepiploic arteries.

After Hollinshead and Rosse

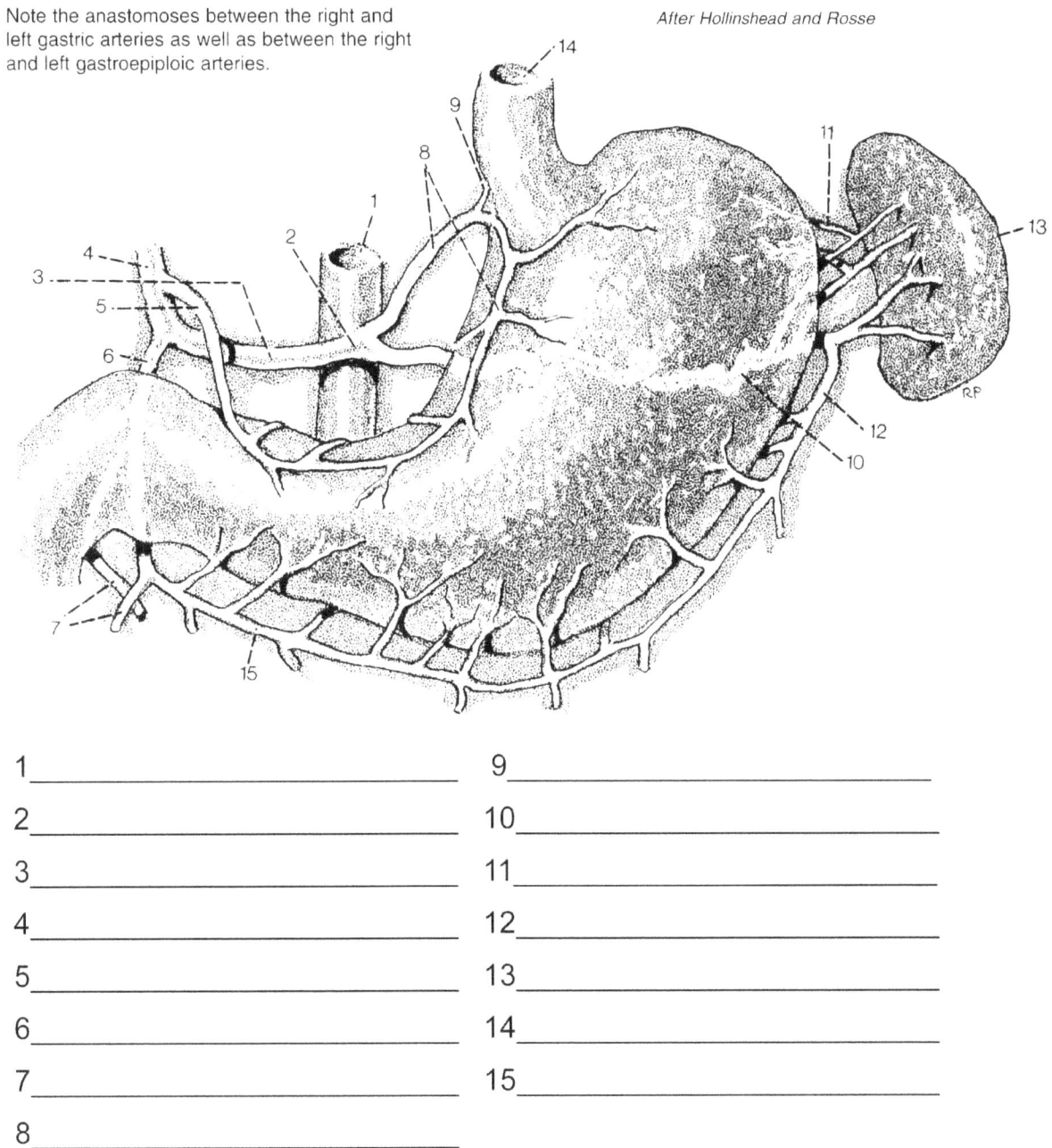

1 _____
2 _____
3 _____
4 _____
5 _____
6 _____
7 _____
8 _____
9 _____
10 _____
11 _____
12 _____
13 _____
14 _____
15 _____

Ab-18 Stomach, duodenum, and pancreas
(opposite page)

Color and label

1. Esophagus
2. Cardiac orifice and cardiac region of stomach
3. Fundus of stomach; left dome-shaped part of stomach superior to horizontal plane X—X; usually filled with air.
4. Body of stomach
5. Pyloric antrum
6. Pyloric canal
7. Pyloric opening
8. Pyloric sphincter (*pylorus*, Greek for gatekeeper)
9. Duodenum; first or superior part, "duodenal bulb"
10. Duodenum; second or descending part
11. Duodenum; third or horizontal part
12. Duodenum; fourth or ascending part
13. Probe in greater duodenal papilla; opening for common bile duct and pancreatic duct; these 2 ducts may unite and end as a single duct or they may end as 2 very close but separate ducts within the papilla.
14. Lesser duodenal papilla; opening of accesssory pancreatic duct
15. Pancreatic duct; the head of the pancreas, which "nestles" into the C-shape of the duodenum, has been partially removed to reveal the 2 pancreatic ducts.
16. Accessory pancreatic duct
17. Pancreas
18. Circular folds of duodenal mucosa (plicae circulares)*
19. Common bile duct
20. Cystic duct
21. Common hepatic duct
22. Right hepatic duct
23. Left hepatic duct
24. Gallbladder
25. Gastric folds (rugae, plicae, ridges); these flatten out and partially disappear when stomach is full and distended.
26. Aorta
27. Celiac trunk
28. Left gastric artery
29. Splenic artery
30. Common bile duct
31. Proper hepatic artery
32. Left hepatic artery
33. Right hepatic artery
34. Middle hepatic artery
35. Right gastric artery
36. Gastroduodenal artery
37. Superior mesenteric vein
38. Superior mesenteric artery

1 _____
2 _____
3 _____
4 _____
5 _____
6 _____
7 _____
8 _____
9 _____
10 _____
11 _____
12 _____
13 _____
14 _____
15 _____
16 _____
17 _____
18 _____
19 _____
20 _____
21 _____
22 _____

* Plicae circulares: circular folds of mucous membrane which project into the lumen of the small intestine whether it is empty or distended. They may extend partly or totally around the circumference of the lumen. They first appear in the second part of the duodenum. They are most numerous in the proximal half of the jejunum, after which they decrease in both size and in number so that they are absent in the end of the ileum. They were formerly called valves of Kerckring. Churchill's Illustrated Medical Dictionary, New York, Churchill Livingstone, 1989.

Ab-18 Stomach, duodenum, and pancreas

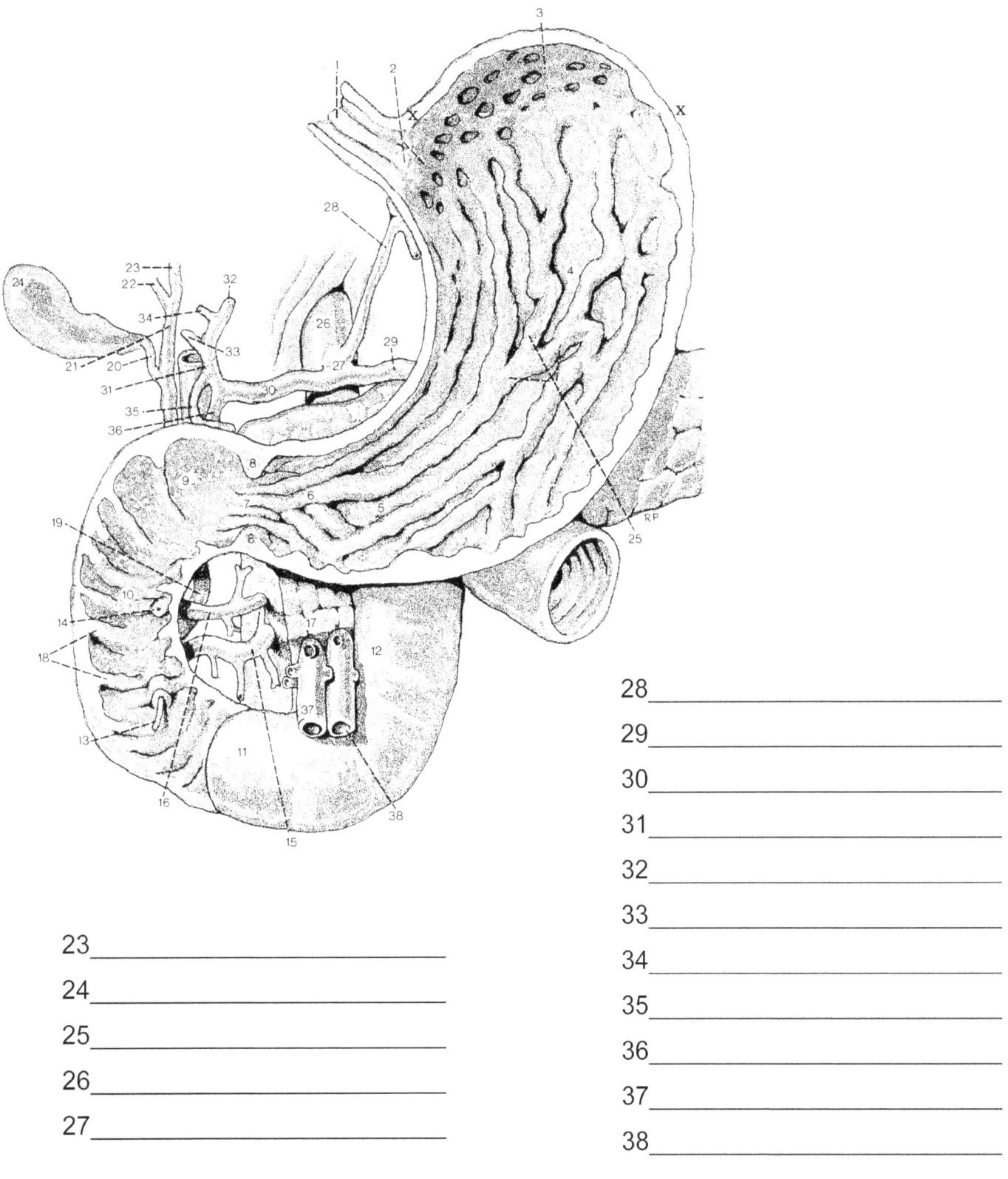

23 _____
24 _____
25 _____
26 _____
27 _____

28 _____
29 _____
30 _____
31 _____
32 _____
33 _____
34 _____
35 _____
36 _____
37 _____
38 _____

Ab-19 Pancreas, duodenum, and spleen

Stomach has been removed and the liver raised
(opposite page)

Color and label

1. Portal vein (hepatic portal vein, vena portae hepatis); notice that the portal vein is rather large in diameter but short in length, being formed by the union of the superior mesenteric vein and the splenic vein. It carries practically all the venous blood rich in digested and absorbed food from the stomach and intestines to the liver, with the exception of absorbed fat, which is conveyed by the lymphatic vessels to one of the large veins in the neck. The spleen sends products from the breakdown of red blood cells to the liver. Unlike regular veins, the hepatic portal vein terminates in the liver by dividing into smaller and smaller veins.
2. Superior mesenteric vein
3. Splenic vein
4. Celiac trunk (celiac artery)
5. Left gastric artery
6. Common hepatic artery
7. Splenic artery
8. Common bile duct; note it is formed by the union of the cystic duct and the common hepatic duct.
9. Cystic duct (duct of gallbladder)
10. Common hepatic duct
11. Proper hepatic artery; in anatomic terminology, the word proper implies exclusivity or specifically "its own" artery, that is, not to be shared with other organs; whereas *common* implies, in spite of its name, *hepatic*—it goes to other organs in addition to the liver
12. Gastroduodenal artery
13. Duodenum; superior part
14. Major duodenal papilla
15. Duodenum; descending part
16. Duodenum; horizontal part
17. Beginning of jejunum; just distal (nearer to the anus) to the duodenojejunal flexture
18. Head of pancreas
19. Pancreatic duct (partially dissected free)
20. Tail of pancreas
21. Liver (underside of right lobe)
22. Cystic artery
23. Gallbladder (fundus)
24. Inferior vena cava
25. Abdominal aorta
26. Adrenal (suprarenal) gland
27. Splenic artery and vein
28. Spleen
29. Left kidney
30. Superior mesenteric artery
31. Right kidney

Ab-19 Pancreas, duodenum, and spleen

Stomach has been removed and the liver raised

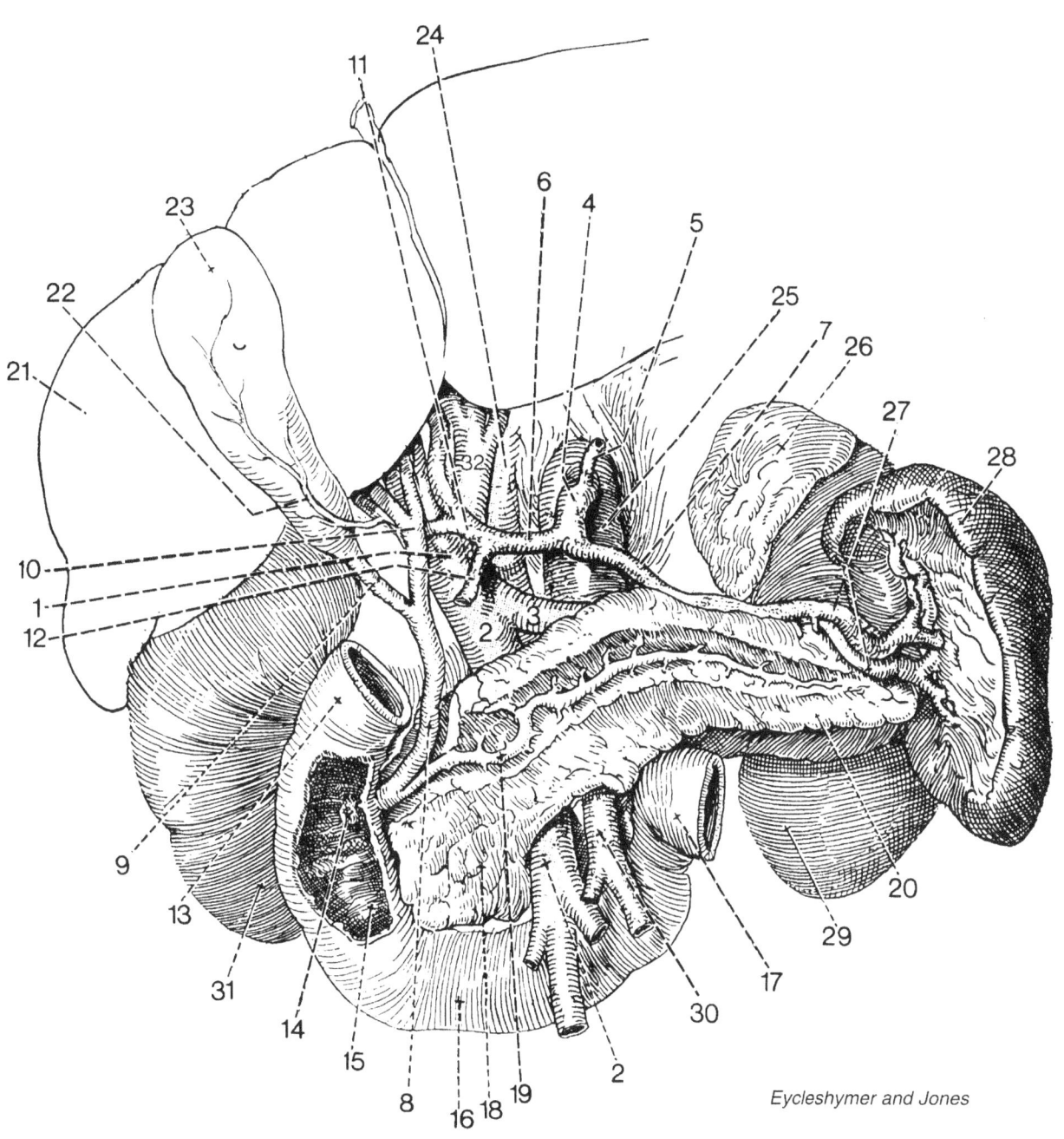

Eycleshymer and Jones

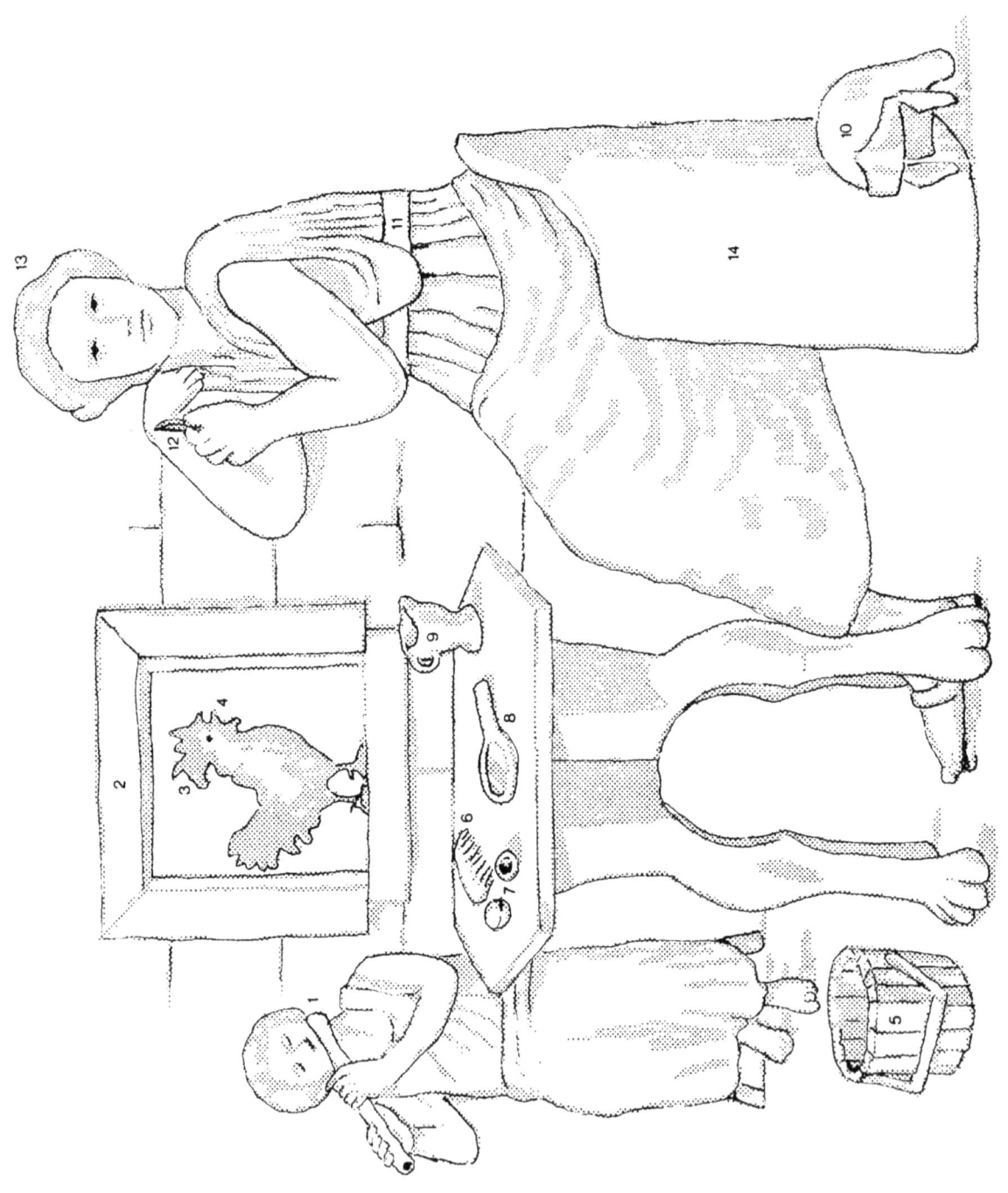

Some Latin anatomic terms

1. Tibia means a flute or pipe as well as the shinbone. The ancients probably made flutelike instruments from the shinbones of animals.

2. Fenestra is Latin for window. Fenestrated means to contain little windows, as in fenestrated capillaries.

3. Crista galli is Latin for cock's comb and is the name of the bony ridge at the top of the ethmoid bone.

4. Rostrum means a beak or snout, or a ship's prow. The speaker's platform in the forum was decorated with the prows of ships captured in battle. Rostral means toward the nose.

5. Alveolus is Latin for a little hollow or bucket and is the diminutive of alveus, which could mean a trough, boat, hold of a ship, bathtub, bed of a stream, beehive, or gaming table.

6. Pecten is Latin for comb. Pectinate means comb-like. The pectinate muscles in the heart suggested a comb to earlier anatomists.

7. Putamen is Latin for "that which falls off with paring," such as a husk or a shell. The putamen is a mass of nerve cells in the brain in the shape of a shell.

8. Speculum is Latin for mirror. A speculum in medicine is an instrument with which a physician can examine passages and the interior of the body.

9. Acetabulum is the bony socket of the hip joint. It is derived from *acetum*, vinegar, and probably *poculum*, cup; hence, it means vinegar cup.

10. Galea means helmet. The galea aponeurotica is a tough membrane that covers the top of the skull somewhat like the furry animal skins used as head coverings by ancient soldiers.

11. Cingulum means a girdle or sword belt. The cinch is a girth or a saddle or pack. To an experienced hand it was an easy job; so easy, in fact, that "it was a cinch" to tie.

12. Fibula means clasp, brooch, or buckle; in particular, the needle of the clasp or the tongue of the buckle. The long, thin fibula bone in the leg resembled the needle of a clasp to the Romans. Poorer Romans probably used the fibulas of animals as straight pins to hold clothes in place.

13. Capillus is Latin for hair of the head, being derived from *caput*, head, and *pilus*, hair. Capillaries are blood vessels so thin they were likened to the hair of the head.

14. Sella means a chair or stool. The sella turcica, which houses the pituitary gland, suggested a Turkish saddle to the ancient anatomists.

Ab-20 Celiac trunk and its branches
(opposite page)

Color and label

1. Gallbladder
2. Fundus of stomach (most of stomach removed)
3. Spleen
4. Duodenum
5. Jejunum
6. Pancreas
7. Celiac trunk
8. Left gastric artery
9. Splenic artery
10. Common hepatic artery
11. Proper hepatic artery
12. Right gastric artery (cut)
13. Right branch of proper hepatic artery
14. Middle branch of proper hepatic artery
15. Left branch of proper hepatic artery
16. Supraduodenal artery
17. Gastroduodenal artery
18. Anterior superior pancreaticoduodenal artery
19. Posterior superior pancreaticoduodenal artery
20. Dorsal pancreatic artery
21. Great pancreatic artery
22. Artery of tail of pancreas
23. Short gastric artery
24. Left gastro-epiploic (gastro-omental) artery
25. Inferior pancreatic artery
26. Inferior phrenic artery
27. Inferior pancreaticoduodenal artery
28. Posterior inferior pancreaticoduodenal artery
29. Anterior inferior pancreaticoduodenal artery
30. Right gastro-epiploic (gastro-omental) artery
31. Cystic artery
32. Common bile duct
33. Cystic duct
34. Common hepatic duct
35. Portal vein
36. Superior mesenteric vein
37. Superior mesenteric artery
38. Middle colic artery
39. Cut edge of transverse mesocolon and dorsal layer of greater omentum
40. Cut edge of root of mesentery

1 _____
2 _____
3 _____
4 _____
5 _____
6 _____
7 _____
8 _____
9 _____
10 _____
11 _____
12 _____
13 _____
14 _____
15 _____
16 _____
17 _____
18 _____
19 _____
20 _____
21 _____
22 _____
23 _____
24 _____
25 _____
26 _____
27 _____
28 _____
29 _____
30 _____
31 _____
32 _____
33 _____
34 _____
35 _____
36 _____
37 _____
38 _____
39 _____
40 _____

Ab-20 Celiac trunk and its branches

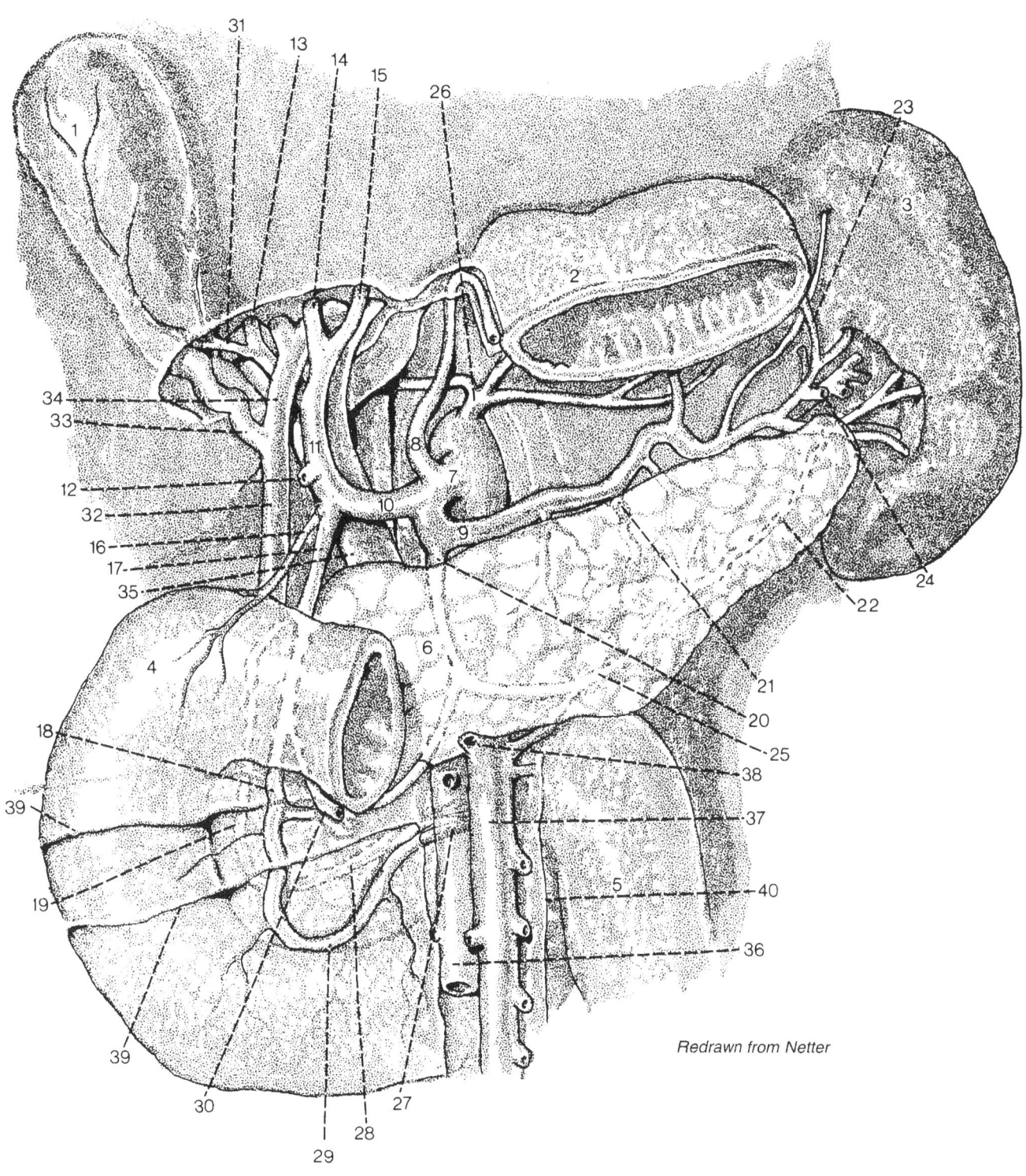

Redrawn from Netter

Ab-21 Nerve supply of the stomach
(opposite page)

Color and label

1. Anterior vagal trunk; made up of mainly nerve fibers from the the left vagus nerve. The vagus nerve is the main outflow of the **parasympathetic nervous system**. Note that it enters the abdomen as 2 trunks, an anterior and a posterior, the latter formed mainly by the right vagus nerve, both closely applied to the esophagus. It consists of preganglionic parasympathetic fibers headed to postganglionic neurons within the walls of the stomach and intestines, which in turn will send their axons to digestive glands and smooth muscle of the alimentary tract. Vagal stimulation causes secretion of the gastric glands and motility (peristalsis) of the musculature in the walls of the stomach.
2. Hepatic branch of anterior vagal trunk; note that it lies between the two layers of peritoneum that comprise the lesser omentum.
3. Celiac branch of posterior vagal trunk. Here parasympathetic fibers from the vagus nerve intermingle with, and subsequently travel with, sympathetic neurons as part of the celiac plexus.
4. Celiac ganglia. Note that these 2 ganglia lie on the aorta on either side of the (arterial) celiac trunk. These ganglia contain postganglionic **sympathetic** neuron cell bodies. Unlike vagal fibers, which stimulate the digestive glands to secrete and promote peristalsis, the sympathetic fibers arising from these ganglia have an inhibitory effect on the digestive tract. These postganglionic neurons receive preganglionic sympathetic fibers by way of the thoracic greater splanchnic nerves (7) and also from some lumbar splanchnic nerves. Stimulation of sympathetic fibers to the liver causes breakdown of glycogen to glucose, thus affording more readily available energy to the body as would be required during physical exertion.
5. Aorticorenal ganglion; postganglionic sympathetic neurons receive preganglionic fibers from the lesser thoracic splanchnic nerve and in turn send their fibers to the kidney where they have the effect of inhibiting the production of urine and conserving water.
6. Superior mesenteric ganglion
7. Greater splanchnic nerve. These fibers arise from preganglionic sympathetic cell bodies at levels T5-T9 in the thoracic spinal cord and pass through the diaphragm to end in the celiac ganglia.
8. Lesser splanchnic nerve
9. Greater anterior gastric nerve
10. Vagal branch to pylorus via hepatic plexus
11. Plexus on left gastric artery
12. Plexus on splenic artery
13. Plexus on common hepatic artery
14. Hepatic plexus
15. Plexus on gastro-epiploic artery
16. Superior mesenteric plexus
17. Lesser omentum, anterior leaf
18. Right crus of diaphragm
19. Inferior vena cava
20. Aorta and subphrenic arteries on underside of diaphragm

The autonomic nerve fibers, such as those derived from the vagus nerve and the celiac ganglia, are extremely thin and difficult to find by gross dissection.

1 _____
2 _____
3 _____
4 _____
5 _____
6 _____
7 _____
8 _____

Ab-21 Nerve supply of the stomach

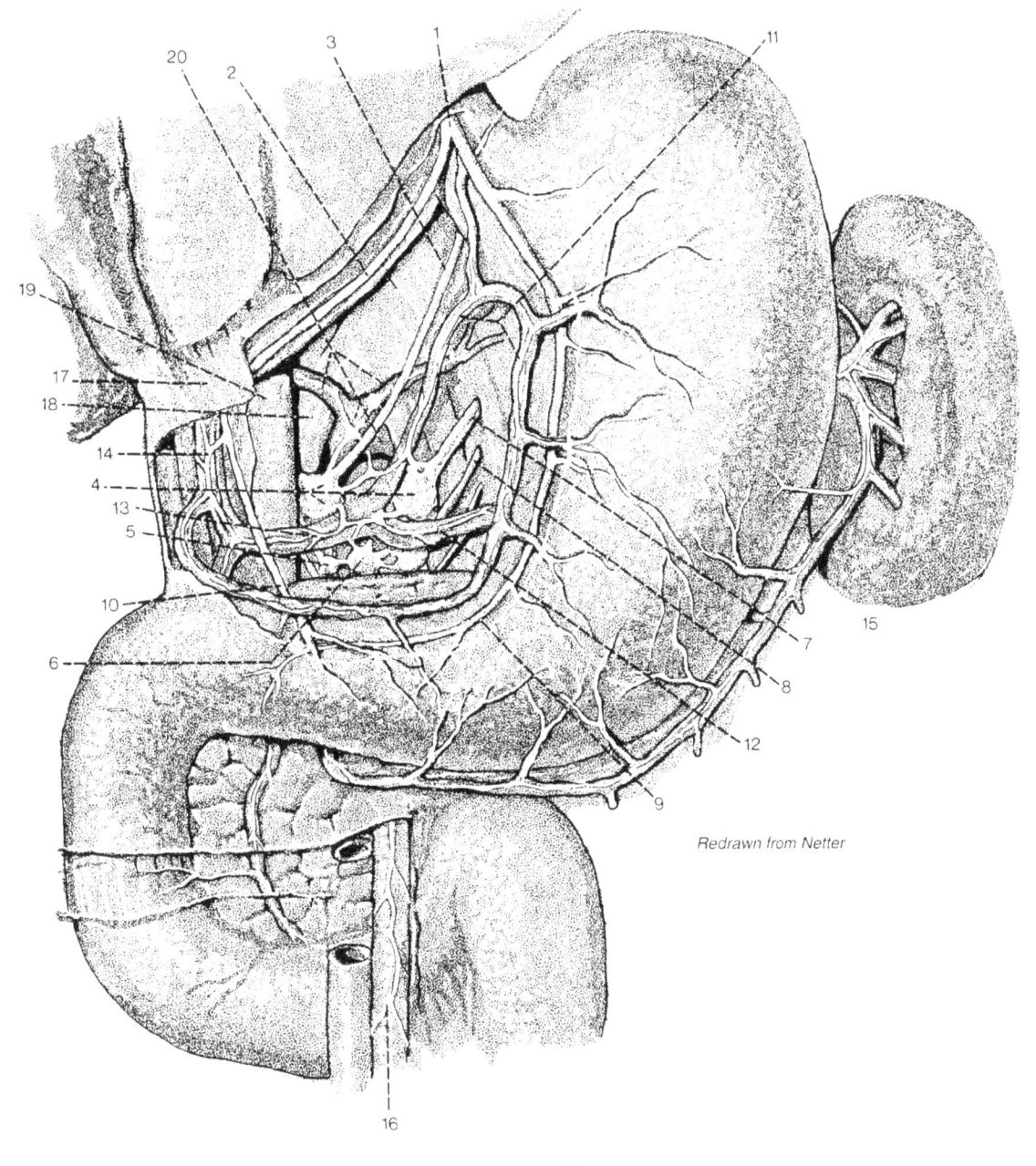

Redrawn from Netter

9_____
10_____
11_____
12_____
13_____
14_____
15_____

16_____
17_____
18_____
19_____
20_____

Ab-22 The liver (hepar)

(opposite page)

Color and label

Figure A. Diaphragmatic surface (anterior/superior surface)

1. Round ligament of the liver; intra-abdominal portion of the obliterated umbilical vein. This part of the umbilical vein extends from the umbilicus to the liver where it forms a fissure on the underside of the liver. During fetal life the umbilical vein conveyed oxygenated blood and nutrients from the mother's placenta to the fetal liver where the major portion of its blood flowed into the ductus venosus, which in turn emptied directly into the inferior vena. Although nonfunctional after birth, the lumen of the round ligament persists and may be used to inject substances directly into the liver.
2. Falciform ligament (sickle-shaped, *falx*, Latin, a sickle or scythe). The round ligament forms its inferior border.
3. Anterior leaf (peritoneal reflection) of coronary ligament extending from right lobe of liver to the diaphragm; also called upper layer of coronary ligament.
4. Left coronary ligament extending from left lobe of liver to the diaphram; on the left lobe, the anterior and posterior layers tend to fuse into a single layer (see figure B below)
5. Right triangular ligament
6. Left triangular ligament
7. Fibrous hepatic annex; this may contain liver tissue.
8. Right lobe* of liver
9. Left lobe* of liver
10. Fundus of gallbladder
11. Bare area of the liver; not covered by peritoneum and adhering to diaphragm by areolar tissue

Figure B. Posterior surface of liver

1. Falciform ligament
2. Anterior (or superior layer) of right coronary ligament
3. Right triangular ligament
4. Left triangular ligament
5. Fibrous hepatic annex
6. Bare area of liver
7. Inferior vena cava; notice that it is held firmly against the liver in a deep groove by the ligament of the inferior vena cava (13), which surrounds it posteriorly, and also by the 3 hepatic veins that empty into it.
8. Left lobe*
9. Right lobe*
10. Caudate lobe; the caudate lobe is so named not because it is more caudal than the quadrate lobe, which it is actually superior to, but rather because it has a tail-like extension or *cauda* (Latin, tail).
11. Right hepatic vein emptying into the inferior vena cava
12. Esophageal impression
13. Ligament of inferior vena; may contain liver tissue.

*The long-held anatomical description of the liver as consisting of 4 lobes was based upon its gross appearance. However, this designation of 4 lobes does not coincide with or accurately relate to the internal distribution of the hepatic veins and the branches of the portal vein.

Ab-22 The liver (hepar)

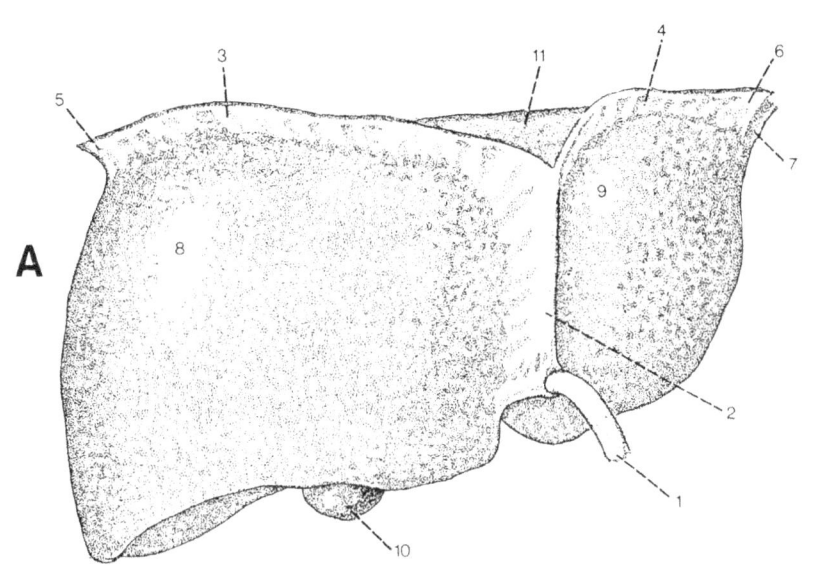

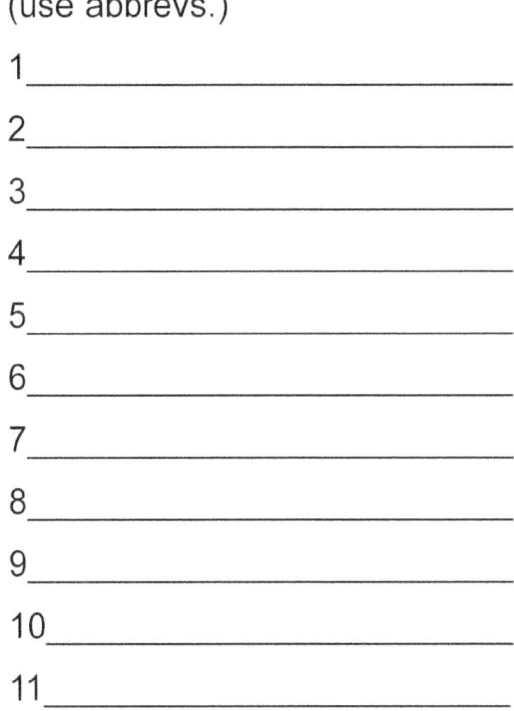

A

(use abbrevs.)

1 _____
2 _____
3 _____
4 _____
5 _____
6 _____
7 _____
8 _____
9 _____
10 _____
11 _____

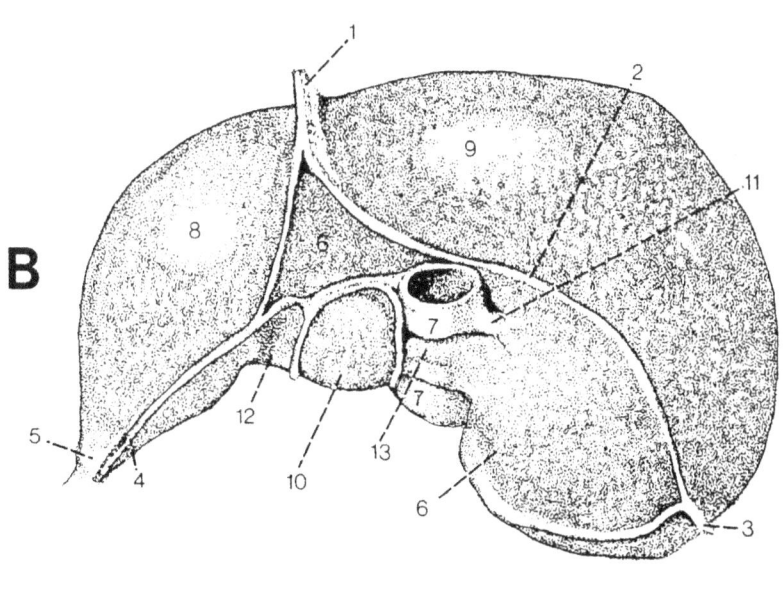

B

(use abbrevs.)

1 _____
2 _____
3 _____
4 _____
5 _____
6 _____
7 _____
8 _____
9 _____
10 _____
11 _____
12 _____
13 _____

Ab-23 Liver

Visceral (posterior/inferior) surface
(opposite page)

Color and label
Figure A

1. Right lobe
2. Left lobe
3. Caudate lobe (so named because of its tail-like process)
4. Quadrate lobe
5. Caudate process of caudate lobe
6. Gallbladder
7. Inferior vena cava
8. Hepatic veins terminating in the inferior vena cava
9. Ligament of the inferior vena cava
10. Round ligament of the liver
11. Ligamentum venosum; obliterated ductus venosus which shunted placental blood from the umbilical vein to the inferior vena cava.
12. Portal vein; carries blood from the stomach, spleen, and intestines to the liver. Notice that the portal vein, unlike other veins, ends by divding into smaller and smaller branches within the liver.
13. Left branch of the portal vein; notice that in the fetus the umbilical vein (round ligament after birth) empties into both the left branch of the portal vein and the ductus venosus (ligamentum venosum after birth), thus allowing a portion of oxygen-rich and nutrient-rich placental blood to be diverted to the fetal liver as needs arise.
14. Common bile duct; formed by the joining of the cystic duct and the common hepatic duct.
15. Cystic duct
16. Aorta
17. Celiac trunk (actually arising from the **front** of the aorta)
18. Common hepatic artery
19. Proper hepatic artery (*proper* here means "its own"; that is, it supplies just the liver)
20. Right posterior layer of the coronary ligament
21. Left posterior layer of the coronary ligament
22. Right triangular ligament
23. Left triangular ligament
24. Lesser omentum (cut, vertical part, hepatogastric ligament). This extends from the liver to the lesser curvature of the stomach.
25. Lesser omentum (cut, horizontal part, hepatoduodenal ligament); this part contains the portal vein, proper hepatic artery, and the bile ducts between its two layers. It extends from the transverse porta hepatis to the duodenum.

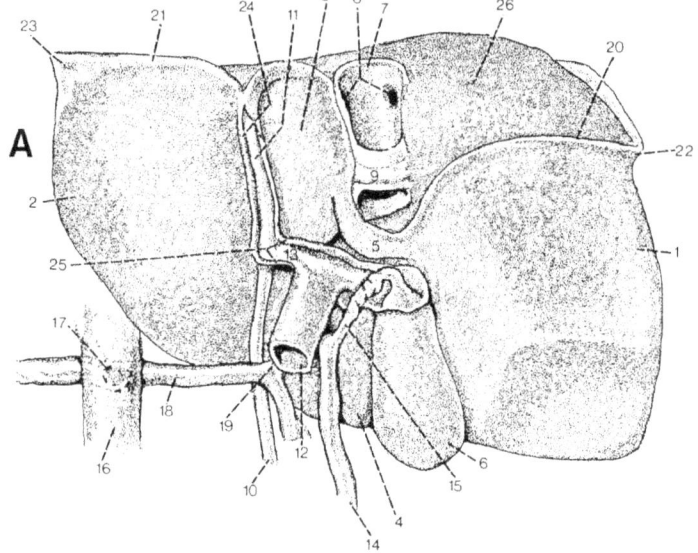

Figure B

1. Right lobe
2. Left lobe
3. Caudate lobe
4. Quadrate lobe
5. Round ligament of the liver
6. Ligamentum venosum
7. Portal vein
8. Left branch of portal vein
9. Inferior vena cava
10. Bare area of liver
11. Porta hepatis (gate of the liver, Latin); this transverse fissure forms the horizontal bar of the H-shape on the visceral surface of the liver. The hepatic ducts, portal vein, and proper hepatic artery pass through it.
12. Proper hepatic artery
13. Hepatic duct
14. Fossa for gallbladder (gallbladder removed)

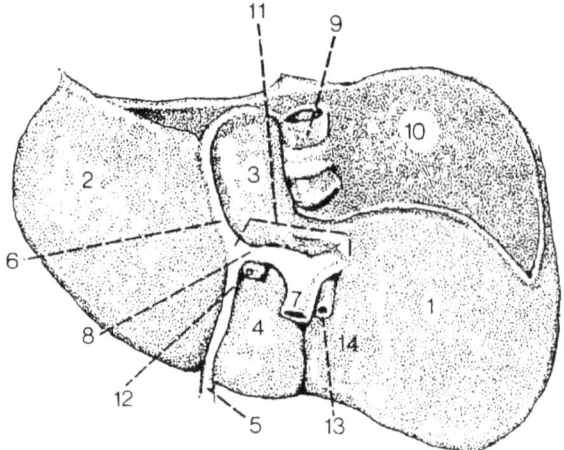

Ab-23 Liver
(visceral surface)

FIG A

1. _____
2. _____
3. _____
4. _____
5. _____
6. _____
7. _____
8. _____
9. _____
10. _____
11. _____
12. _____
13. _____
14. _____
15. _____
16. _____
17. _____
18. _____
19. _____
20. _____
21. _____
22. _____
23. _____
24. _____
25. _____

FIG B

1. _____
2. _____
3. _____
4. _____
5. _____
6. _____
7. _____
8. _____
9. _____
10. _____
11. _____
12. _____
13. _____
14. _____

Ab-24A The intestines I

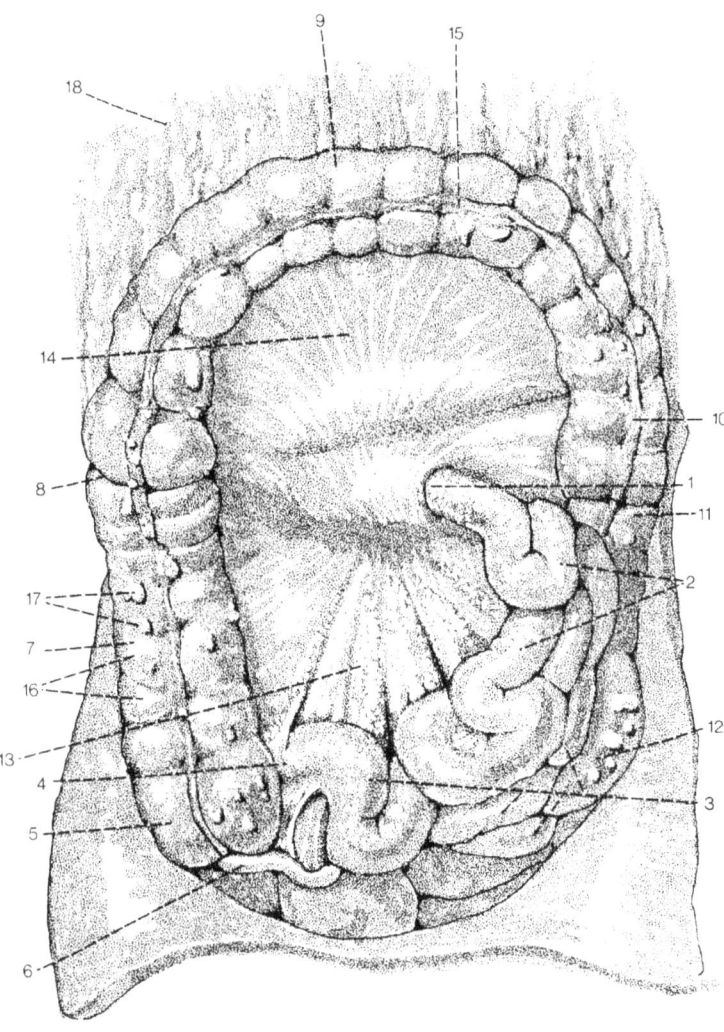

Color and label

1. Duodenojejunal flexure; beginning of mesenteric small intestine (jejunum and ileum)
2. Jejunum (second part of small intestine; Latin, *jejunus*, empty or fasting, from the early anatomists' finding that it was always empty when examined after death)
3. Ileum (third part of small intestine; Greek, *eileo*, to twist or roll up)
4. Ileocolic junction (end of small intestine)
5. Cecum (Latin, *caecus*, blind, as in a blind passageway or dead end)
6. Vermiform appendix (worm-like, Latin, *vermis*, worm)

7. Ascending colon (the large intestine or bowel is also called the colon)
8. Right colic flexture
9. Transverse colon
10. Left colic flexture
11. Descending colon
12. Sigmoid colon (named by its supposed resemblance to the Greek letter sigma)
13. Mesentery; attaches the jejunum and ileum to the posterior abdominal wall.
14. Transverse mesocolon; attaches transverse colon posteriorly.
15. Tenia coli (longitudinal strip of smooth muscle)
16. Haustra coli (outpouchings on colon)
17. Epiploic appendices (new name: omental appendices). These are small fatty appendices unique to the large intestine.
18. Greater omentum (raised up)

1. _____
2. _____
3. _____
4. _____
5. _____
6. _____
7. _____
8. _____
9. _____
10. _____
11. _____
12. _____
13. _____
14. _____
15. _____
16. _____
17. _____
18. _____

Ab-24B The intestines II

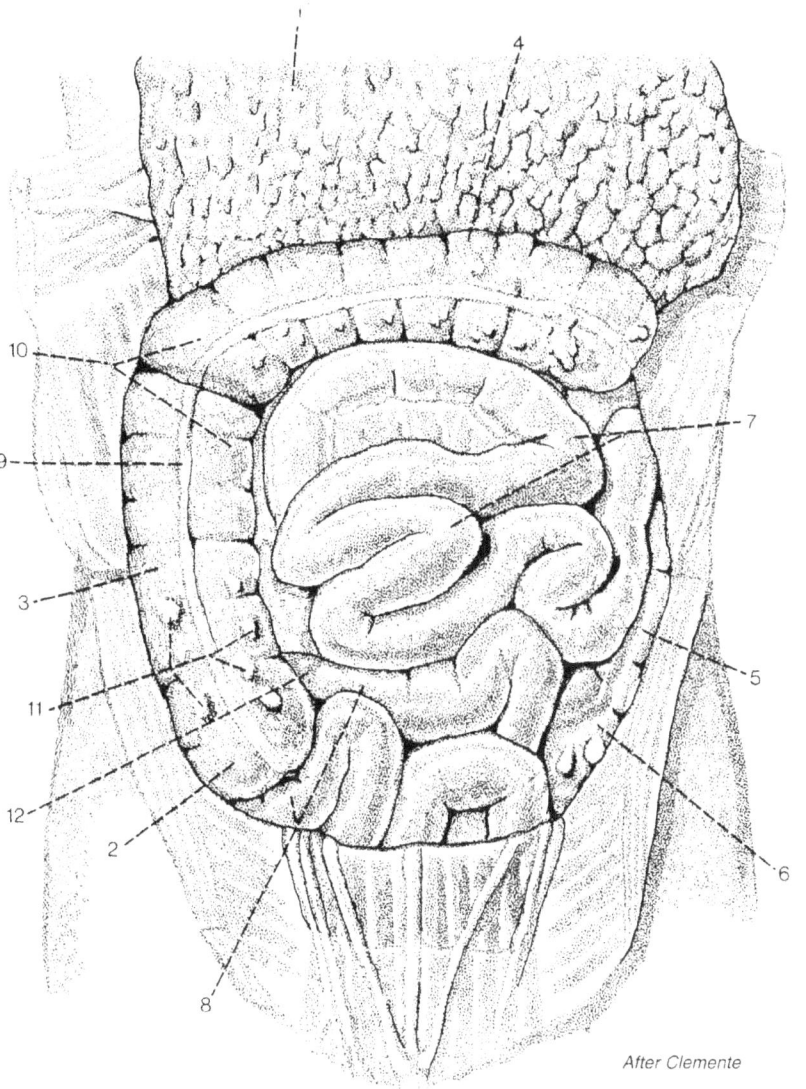

After Clemente

Color and label

1. Greater omentum (raised up)
2. Cecum (beginning of large intestine)
3. Ascending colon (large intestine)
4. Transverse colon
5. Descending colon
6. Sigmoid colon
7. Jejunum (second part of small intestine)
8. Ileum (third part of small intestine)
9. Teniae coli (three longitudinal strips of smooth muscle on the large intestine)*
10. Haustra coli (outpouchings or sacculations)*
11. Appendices epiploicae (small fatty globs)*
12. Termination of the ileum (emptying into the large intestine)

* These are found only on the large intestine or colon.

1_____
2_____
3_____
4_____
5_____
6_____

7_____
8_____
9_____
10_____
11_____
12_____

Ab-25 Distribution of the superior mesenteric artery and vein

The mesentery has been stripped away to expose the blood vessels
(opposite page)

Color and label

1. Superior mesenteric artery. Branches of this large artery supply the major portion of the intestines: the lower half of the duodenum*, all of the jejunum and ileum, the ascending colon, and the right half of the transverse colon. The remainder of the large intestine (left half of transverse colon, descending colon, and sigmoid colon) is supplied by branches of the smaller inferior mesenteric artery. Branches of the latter anastomose with those of the superior mesenteric artery within the transverse mesocolon (the mesentery of the large intestine).
2. Superior mesenteric vein. This vein is the major contributor of venous blood to the hepatic portal system. It carries the digested and absorbed food from the intestine to the portal vein, which then empties into the liver. The relatively short portal vein is formed by the joining of the splenic vein with the superior mesenteric vein behind the pancreas (not shown).
3. Jejunal vessels
4. Ileal vessels
5. Ileocolic artery and vein
6. Right colic artery and vein
7. Midcolic artery and vein (branches)
8. Left colic artery and vein. These are branches of the inferior mesenteric artery and vein.
9. Jejunum; the proximal (upper) two-fifths of the small intestine. It forms coils and loops mainly in the upper left quadrant of the abdominal cavity. It is suspended from the posterior abdominal wall by its mesentery, which allows its coils enough mobility to slide past each other.
10. Ileum. The distal (lower) three-fifths of the small intestine. Like the jejunum, it has a mesentery, which permits its coils and loops to change their shape and position.
11. Cecum; the beginning of the colon or large intestine
12. Termination of the ileum at the cecum
13. Appendix epiploica: these small fatty appendages are present only on the large intestine and are helpful in identifying it.
14. Lymph node; the interconnecting lymph channels (lymphatics) are too small to be seen with the naked eye unless specially stained.
15. Transverse colon (raised up)
16. Greater omentum (raised up)
17. Transverse mesocolon. The transverse colon and the sigmoid colon retain their mesocolons, which allows them greater mobility than the ascending colon and descending colon, which have fused with the posterior abdominal wall along with their mesocolons and the blood vessels that coursed through their meocolons. However, a gentle pulling of the ascending or descending colon will free them from the posterior abdominal wall along with their mesocolons and contained blood vessels with no breakage of the vessels.
18. Descending colon (partly hidden)
19. Haustrum (Latin, a water wheel, so named because of its fancied resemblance to the buckets on a water wheel). These are the outpouchings or sacculations of the colon. Haustra are unique to the large intestine.†
20. Tenia coli (Latin, worm of the colon); there are 3 of these longitudinal tape-like bands of smooth muscle that make up the outer longitudinal layer of smooth muscle. Being shorter than the wall of the large intestine, they cause the characteristic outpouching or sacculations of the colon.

*The 10-inch long duodenum (not shown here) is retroperitoneal, having fused to the rear wall, rendering it immobile.

†The empty large intestine may at times appear narrower than the small intestine should the latter be distended. The teniae, the appendices epiploica, and the haustra are helpful in distinguishing the large intestine from the small intestine.

1. _____
2. _____
3. _____
4. _____
5. _____
6. _____

Ab-25 Distribution of the superior mesenteric artery and vein

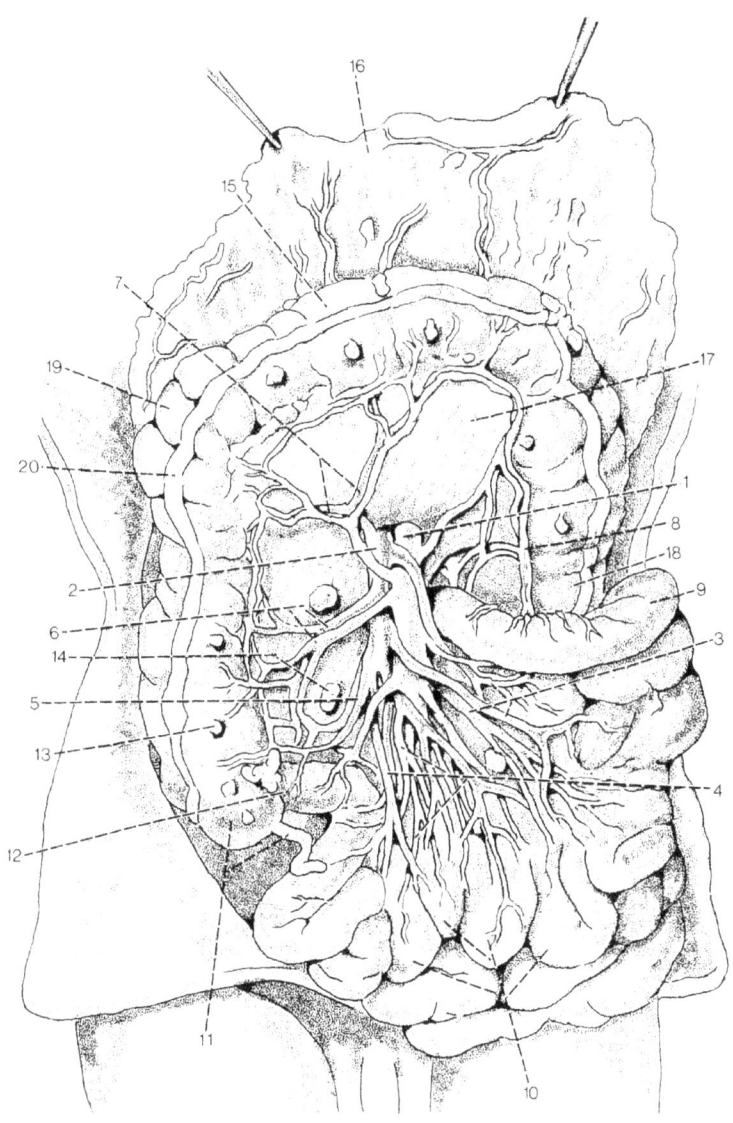

Redrawn and modified from Eycleshymer and Jones

(use abbrevs.)

7_____
8_____
9_____
10_____
11_____
12_____
13_____

14_____
15_____
16_____
17_____
18_____
19_____
20_____

Ab-26 Blood supply of the jejunum
(opposite page)

Color and label

1. Superior mesenteric artery; the mesentery has been stripped away from both the superior mesenteric artery and vein.
2. Superior mesenteric vein; all the vessels that supply the jejunum and ileum travel within the mesentery where they are enclosed by the 2 layers of peritoneum.
3. Jejunal arteries
4. Jejunal arteries and veins within the mesentery
5. Fat within mesentery
6. Translucent fat-free "windows" in the mesentery adjacent to the intestine; these are a distinguishing feature of the jejunal mesentery as opposed to the mesentery in the ileum where these "windows" are absent and where the fat extends right up to the intestine.
7. Arcades (1st tier); formed by the branching blood vessels as they approach the intestine.
8. Arcades (2nd tier)
9. Arcades (3rd tier); 3 tiers or rows of U-shaped vascular arcades in the mesentery is characteristic of the jejunum, as opposed to the ileum, which may have 5 or more rows of arcades.
10. Straight arteries (arteriae rectae). Here the veins and arteries together comprise the **vasae rectae** (straight vessels). Long vasae rectae are typical of the jejunum, whereas short vasae rectae and more arcades are characteristic of the ileum.
11. Jejunum (cut open)
12. Circular folds (*plicae circulares*; old name: valves of Kerckring). These folds greatly increase the internal (luminal) surface. They are more plentiful in the jejunum than in the ileum where they are fewer and farther between.
13. Cut edge of the peritoneum. On the right (13) *visceral* peritoneum encloses the intestine, forming its outermost layer or serosa. The mesenteric peritoneum connects the *visceral* peritoneum with the *parietal* peritoneum, thus forming a continuous unbroken sheet of peritoneum that lines the abdominal cavity and covers all the organs that protrude into the peritoneal cavity.
14. Two layers of peritoneum form the mesentery* and enclose the structures that pass through it. Part of one layer has been removed. In addition to fat and blood vessels, the mesentery carries lymphatic vessels, lymph nodes, sympathetic and parasympathetic nerves, and visceral afferent fibers.

* The double layer of peritoneum that anchors the large intestine to the posterior abdominal wall is called **mesocolon**.

1. _____
2. _____
3. _____
4. _____
5. _____
6. _____
7. _____
8. _____
9. _____
10. _____
11. _____
12. _____
13. _____
14. _____

Ab-26 Blood supply of the jejunum

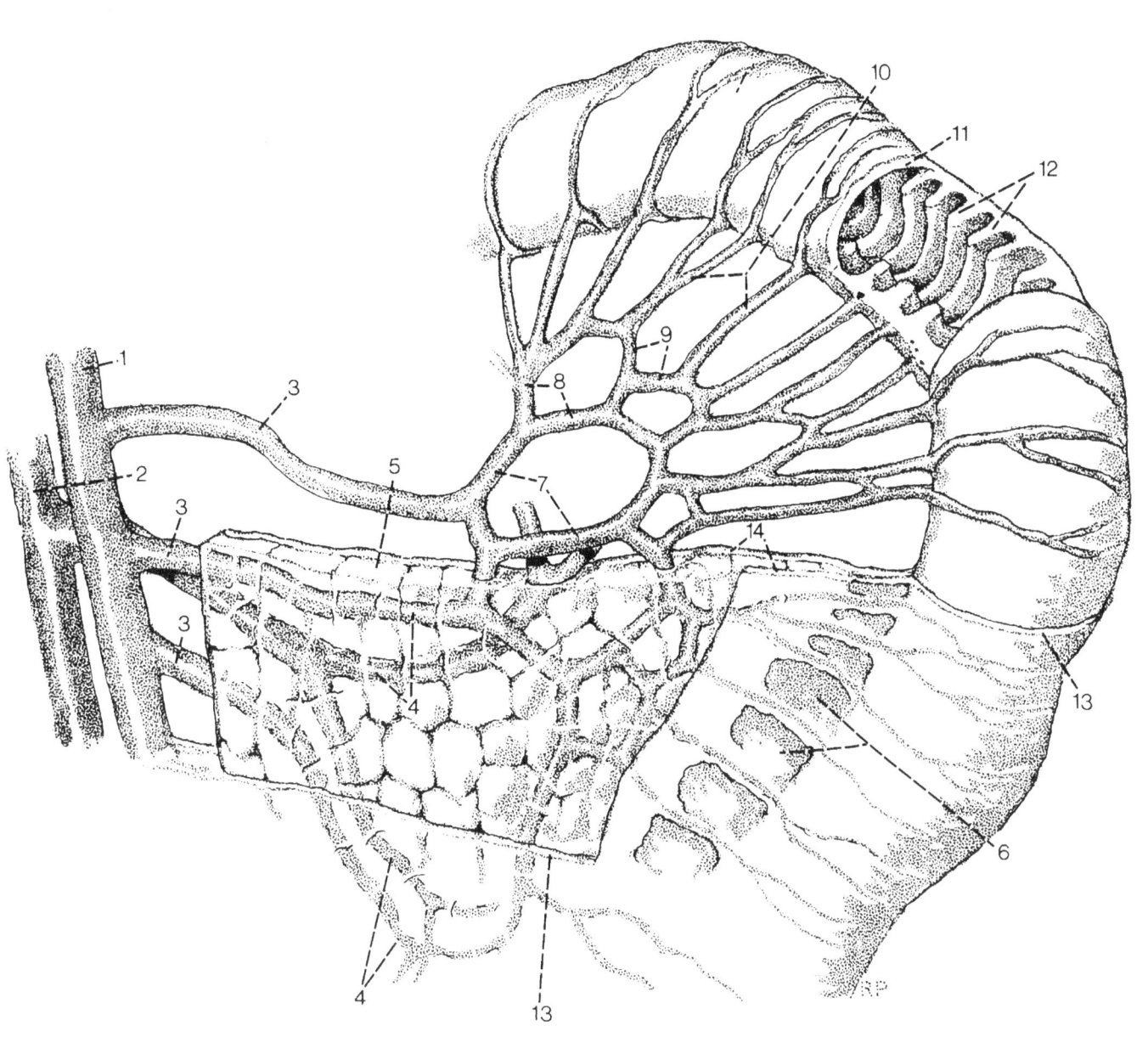

Ab-27 Blood supply to the small intestine

(opposite page)

A. Jejunum. The second part of the small intestine is the jejunum. It is the cranial two-fifths of the *mesenteric portion* of the small intestine. In general it is of greater diameter, has thicker walls, is more vascular and therefore redder, and internally its mucosa has higher and more numerous plicae circulares (circular folds) than the caudal three-fifths, the ileum. The lymph follicles in the jejunal mucosa tend to be small and scattered, unlike the larger aggregated lymph follicles found in the ileum. The jejunal blood vessels form branching arcades within the mesentery as they approach the intestine. The arcades of the jejunum tend to divide less and therefore have fewer rows of arcades than those found in the terminal ileum. There are fat-free translucent "windows" in the mesentery adjacent to the jejunum. The jejunal arcades give off long vasae rectae (straight vessels). The veins (not shown here) accompany the arteries.

B. Ileum. The ileum (from the Greek, *eileos*, twisted) is the caudal three-fifths of the mesenteric small intestine. There is no sharp demarcation between jejunum and the ileum. The ileum is characterized by blood vessels that form more rows or tiers of arcades, plus fat within its mesentery that extends up to the intestine ("encroaching fat"). Internally the ileal mucosa has lower and fewer plicae circulares that are absent at its terminal end. It also has aggregated lymph follicles that are visible to the naked eye (Peyer's patches).

C. Mesentery. The jejunum and ileum have been cut away. The mesentery is a highly folded, fan-shaped membrane that connects the jejunum and ileum to the posterior abdominal wall. It is lined on either side by a layer of peritoneum supported internally by connective tissue. It contains the superior mesenteric artery and its branches and the superior mesenteric vein and its radicles (little roots), plus lymphatic vessels, lymph nodes, sympathetic and parasympathetic nerves, and visceral afferent nerves. It may contain considerable amounts of fat. Its attachment or root on the posterior abdominal wall is only about 15 cm long (6 in). Its visceral attachment to the intestine is as long as the jejunum and ileum are, nearly 7 meters (23 ft) post mortem. However, in life its length is probably nearer to 4 meters (13 ft). (Blount and Lachman in Anson, 1966.)

A. Jejunum

1 _____
2 _____
3 _____
4 _____

B. Ileum

5 _____
6 _____
7 _____

C. Mesentry

8 _____
9 _____

Ab-27 Blood supply to the small intestine

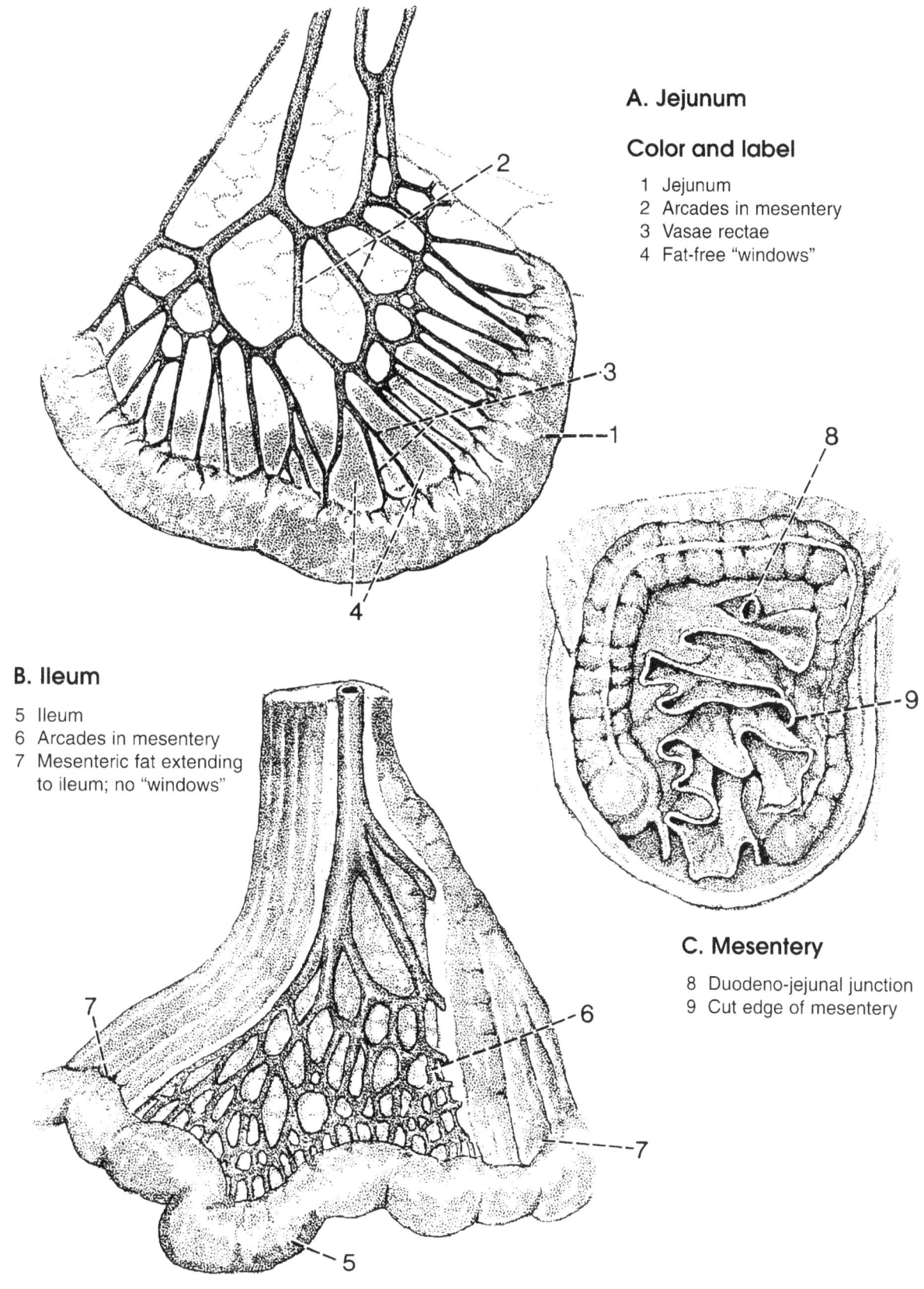

A. Jejunum

Color and label

1. Jejunum
2. Arcades in mesentery
3. Vasae rectae
4. Fat-free "windows"

B. Ileum

5. Ileum
6. Arcades in mesentery
7. Mesenteric fat extending to ileum; no "windows"

C. Mesentery

8. Duodeno-jejunal junction
9. Cut edge of mesentery

Ab-28 Mucosa of jejunum and ileum

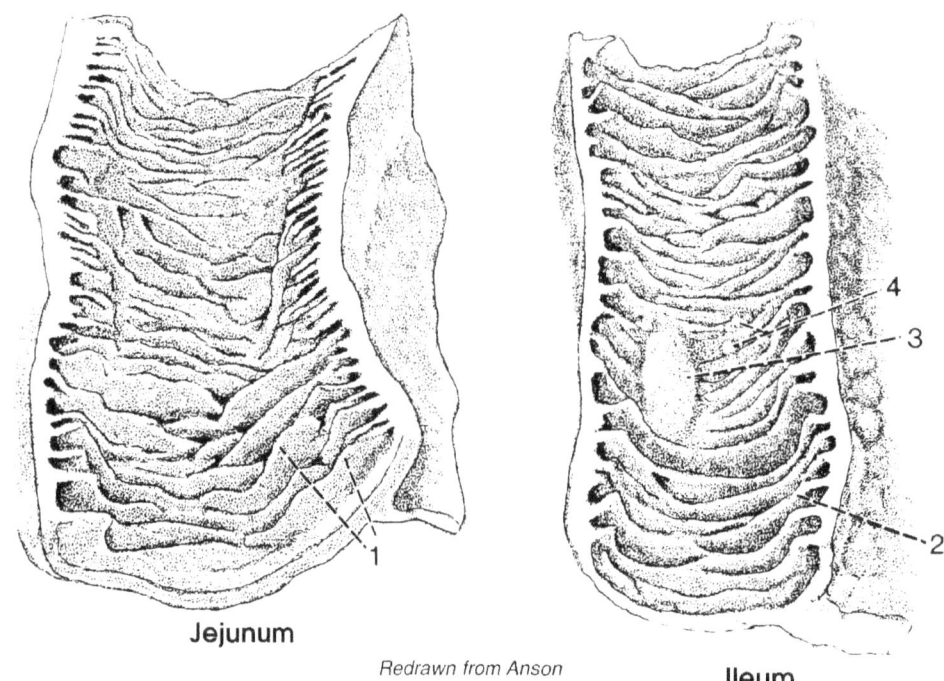

Jejunum

Redrawn from Anson

Ileum

Color and label

1. Plicae circulares (circular folds) in jejunum; tall and numerous
2. Circular folds in ileum; fewer and less prominent; absent at terminal portion of ileum
3. Aggregated lymph follicles
4. Isolated lymph follicles

Total number of plicae circulares in the adult is about 800 (Blount and Lachman in Anson, 1966).

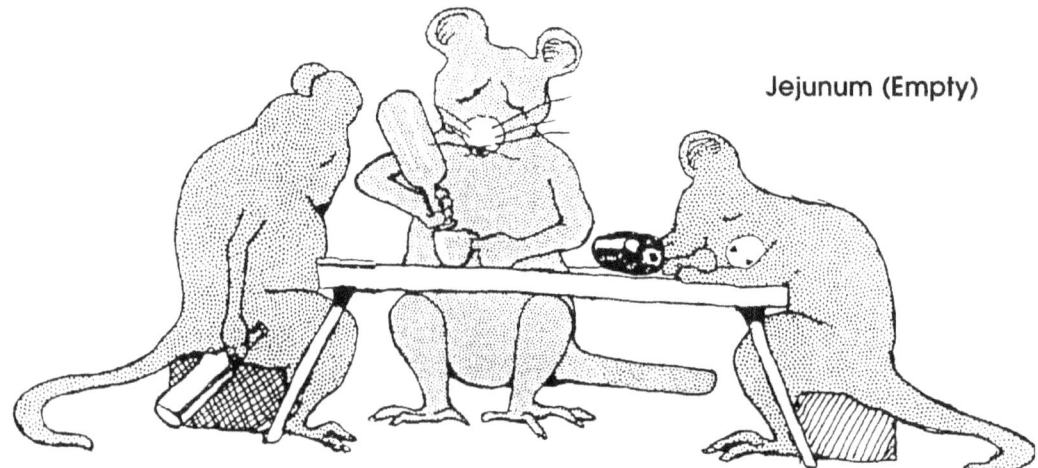

Jejunum (Empty)

The ancient anatomists named the second part of the small intestine the *jejunum*, or empty part, because after death they found it to be devoid of contents. Besides meaning "empty or wanting," jejunum also meant "hungry or fasting."

1 _____ 3 _____

2 _____ 4 _____

Ab-29 Blood supply of large intestine

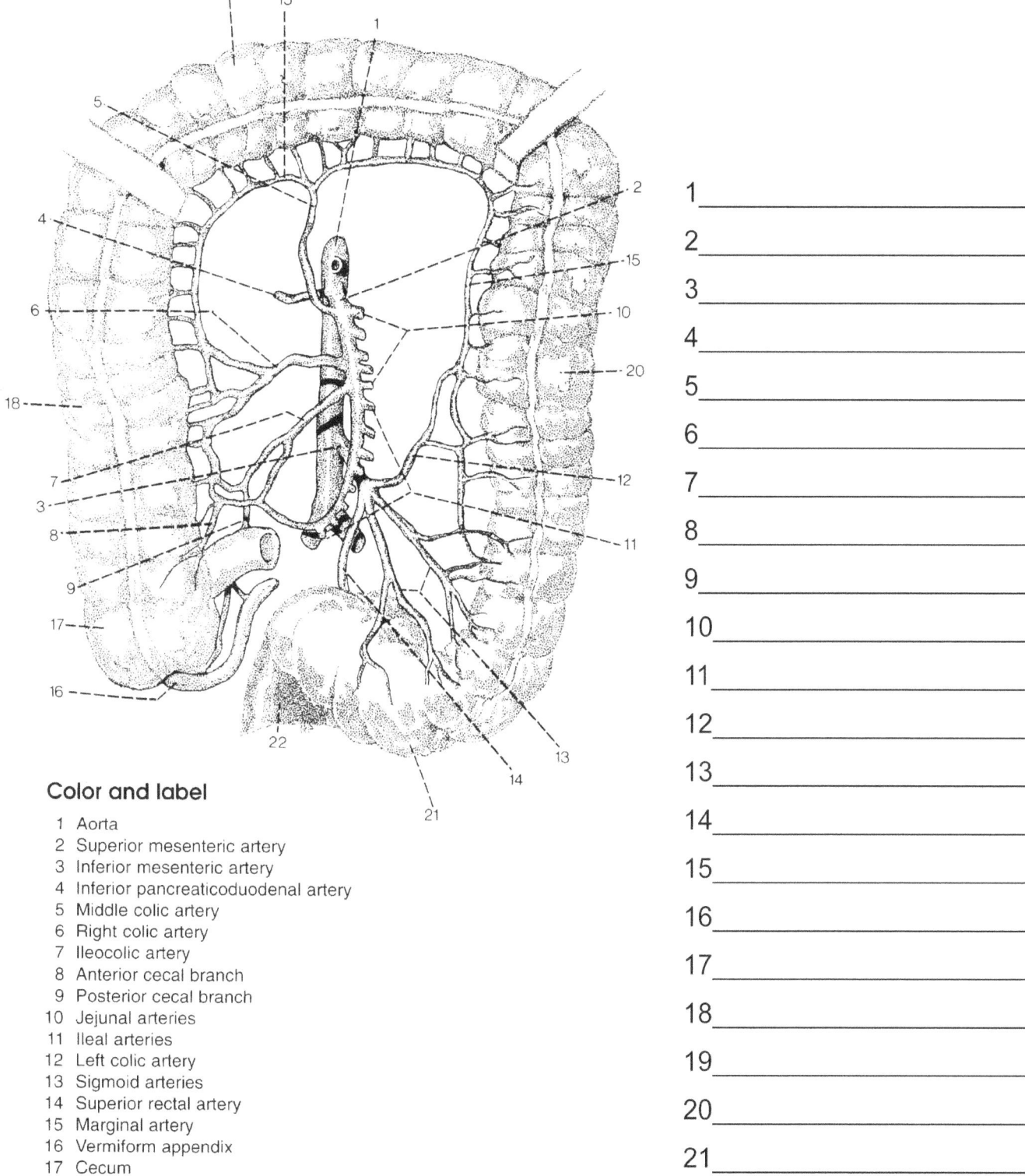

Color and label

1. Aorta
2. Superior mesenteric artery
3. Inferior mesenteric artery
4. Inferior pancreaticoduodenal artery
5. Middle colic artery
6. Right colic artery
7. Ileocolic artery
8. Anterior cecal branch
9. Posterior cecal branch
10. Jejunal arteries
11. Ileal arteries
12. Left colic artery
13. Sigmoid arteries
14. Superior rectal artery
15. Marginal artery
16. Vermiform appendix
17. Cecum
18. Ascending colon
19. Transverse colon
20. Descending colon
21. Sigmoid colon
22. Rectum

173

Ab-30 Ileocecal valve, vermiform appendix, terminal ileum, and cecum

(viewed from the front)

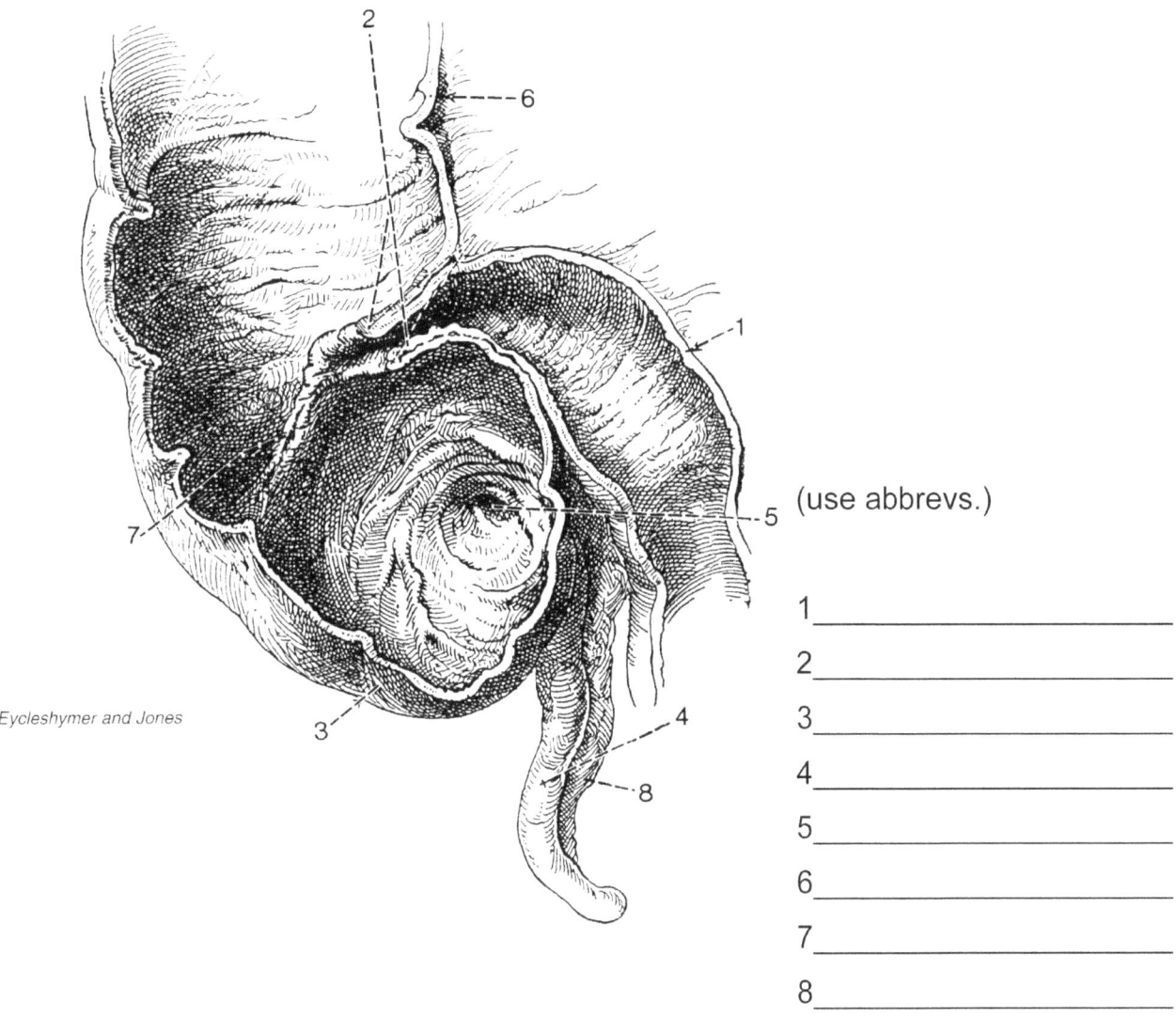

Eycleshymer and Jones

(use abbrevs.)

1 _____
2 _____
3 _____
4 _____
5 _____
6 _____
7 _____
8 _____

Color and label

1. Terminal ileum; note an absence of mucosal circular folds (plicae circulares)
2. Ileocecal valve; note that it is formed by 2 lips that project into the large intestine.
3. Cecum
4. Vermiform (*vermis*, Latin, worm) appendix. It has a small lumen that extends its entire length.
5. Orifice of vermiform appendix; occasionally guarded by a semilunar fold of mucous membrane.
6. Ascending colon
7. Frenulum of the ileocecal valve (Latin, diminutive of *frenum*, a bridle, bit, reins); a ridge that is formed by the fused lips of the the ileocecal valve. It runs downward and laterally, demarcating the cecum from the ascending colon.*
8. Flap of mesentery containing appendicular artery

*Churchill's Medical Dictionary, 1989

Ab-31 Arterial supply of vermiform appendix, terminal ileum, and cecum

Color and label (opposite page)

1. Ileocecal valve
2. Frenulum
3. Terminal ileum
4. Cecum (Latin, blind; its lumen leads nowhere). But as I used to tell my class, "cecum and ye shall find."
5. Ascending colon
6. Vermiform appendix
7. Orifice of appendix
8. Tenia (Latin, "a ribbon or tape"); the teniae coli are three prominent longitudinal bands of smooth (nonstriated) muscle positioned roughly equidistant from one another (120 degrees) in the wall of the large intestine.
9. Semilunar fold
10. Ileocolic artery
11. Anterior cecal artery
12. Posterior cecal artery
13. Appendicular artery (minus its flap of mesentery)
14. Colic branch
15. Ileal branch
16. Mesentery (cut; containing fat between its two layers of peritoneum)
17. Encroaching fat (fat next to the ileum; unlike the jejunal mesentery, which has "clear windows")
18. Arcades (an arterial formation characteristic of the ileal arteries)
19. Straight arteries (arteriae rectae); considerably shorter here than those supplying the jejunum, which tend to be long
20. Lymphatic follicles (Peyer's patches)
21. Mucosal folds. Ileum has fewer and smaller mucosal folds than those in the jejunum.

1 _____
2 _____
3 _____
4 _____
5 _____
6 _____
7 _____
8 _____
9 _____
10 _____
11 _____
12 _____
13 _____
14 _____
15 _____
16 _____
17 _____
18 _____
19 _____
20 _____
21 _____

Ab-31 Arterial supply of vermiform appendix, terminal ileum, and cecum

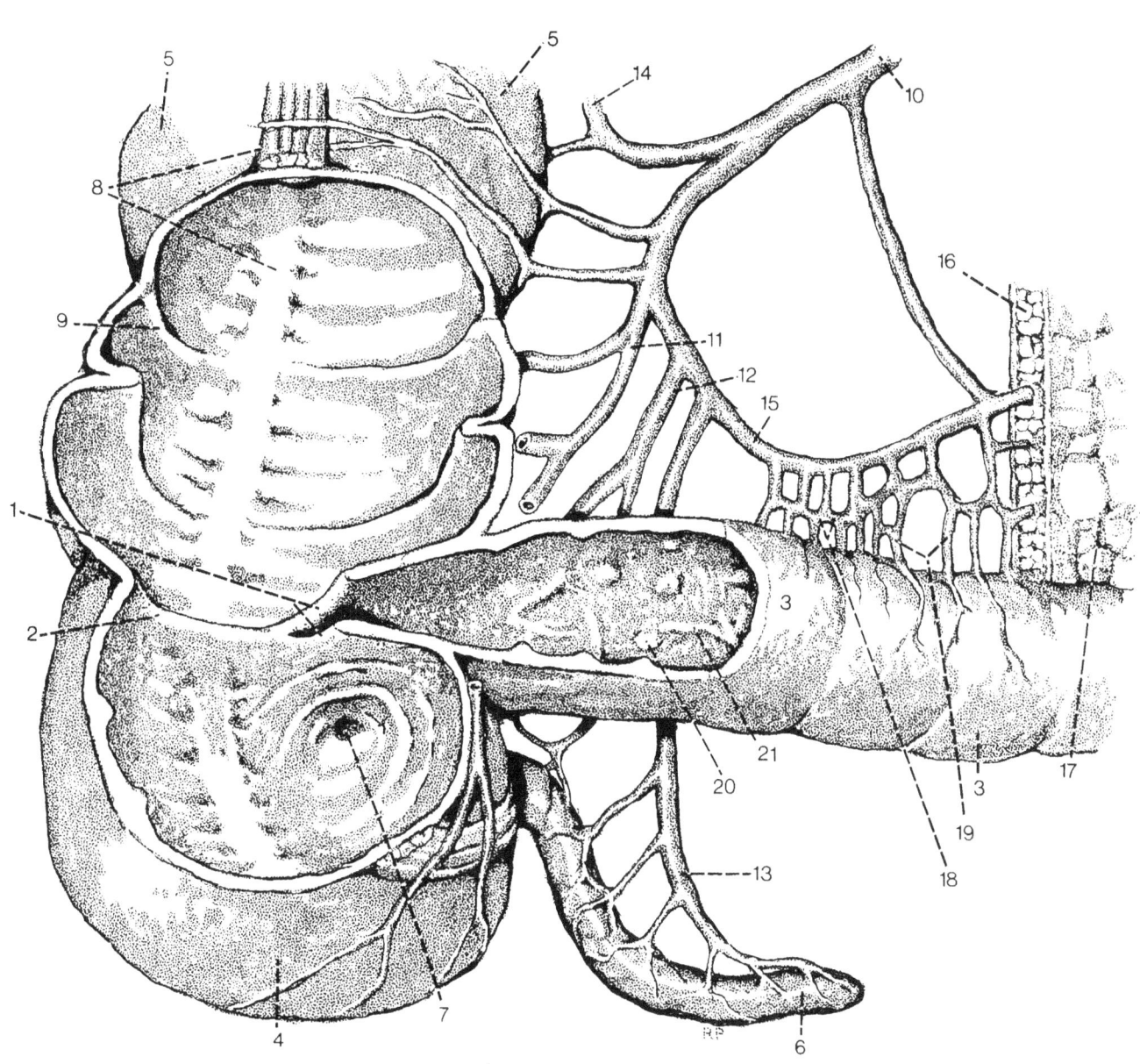

Ab-32 The hepatic portal system
(opposite page)

Color and label

1. Portal vein (also hepatic portal vein); this thick but rather short vein is formed by the convergence of the splenic vein and the superior mesenteric vein. The portal vein itself is only 7 or 8 cm long. The hepatic portal system conveys all the blood and absorbed carbohydrates and proteins from the stomach and intestines to the liver. The hepatic portal system begins with capillaries in the intestinal mucosa that feed into tiny venous tributaries or radicles. These drain into larger and larger coalescing veins that eventually end in the portal vein. However, instead of draining into the inferior vena cava, once it reaches the liver, the hepatic portal vein divides into branches inside the liver, much like an artery. The branches of the portal vein repeatedly divide into smaller and smaller branches, which end in irregular-shaped capillaries in the liver called sinusoids where the liver metabolizes the blood-borne absorbed food.
2. Superior mesenteric vein
3. Splenic vein
4. Inferior mesenteric vein. The inferior mesenteric vein usually ends in the splenic vein.
5. Left gastric vein
6. Right gastric vein
7. Superior pancreaticoduodenal vein
8. Right gastro-epiploic* vein (new name, gastro-omental vein)
9. Middle colic vein
10. Inferior pancreaticoduodenal vein
11. Right colic vein
12. Ileocolic vein
13. Appendicular vein
14. Jejunal veins
15. Ileal veins
16. Left colic vein
17. Sigmoid veins
18. Superior rectal vein
19. Dorsal pancreatic vein
20. Round ligament of the liver (obliterated umbilical vein)
21. Falciform ligament
22. Coronary ligament
23. Duodenum
24. Stomach (cut)
25. Spleen. The spleen removes old red blood cells from the circulation and sends the breakdown products to the liver via the splenic vein.
26. Right lobe of liver
27. Left gastro-epiploic (gastro-omental) vein

*Epiploic is from the Greek *epiploon*, the name used by Hippocrates for the omentum. This, in turn, came from the Greek *epipleo*, "I sail upon or float upon." The allusion, presumably, is to the omentum "floating upon" the abdominal viscera. (Haubrich, 1984)

Ab-32 The hepatic portal system

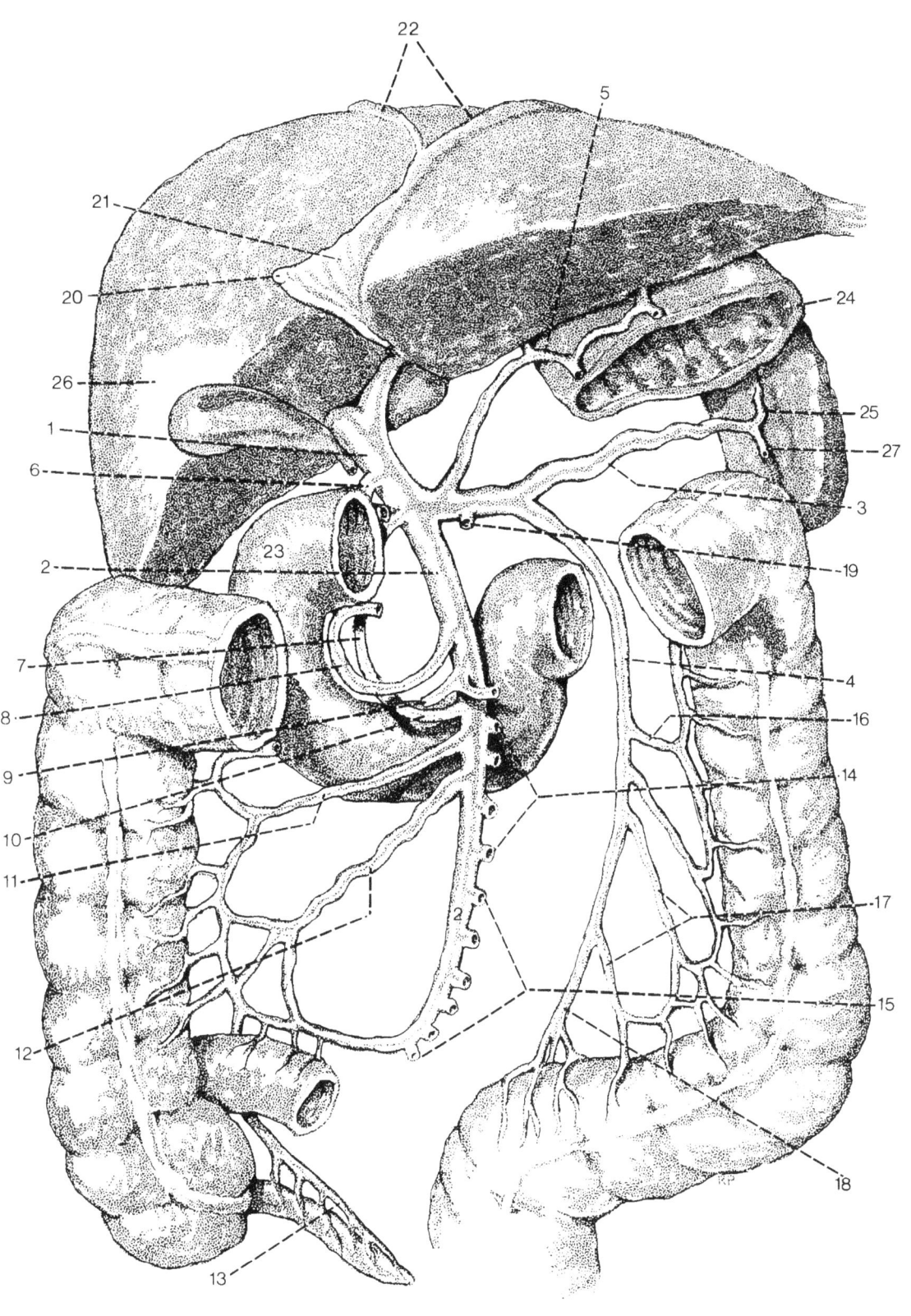

Ab-33 Posterior abdominal wall, peritoneal attachments

The stomach and liver have been removed.
(opposite page)

Color and label

1. Root of the mesentery. This is the posterior attachment of the whole jejunum and ileum. Whereas the root of the mesentery is only about about 15 cm long, its intestinal border is greatly lenghtened to about 4 meters due to its numerous folds and ruffles.
2. Site of ascending colon. During embryonic development both the ascending and descending colon as well as their mesocolons fuse to the posterior abdominal wall. This renders them relatively immobile, unlike the transverse colon and sigmoid colon, which retain their mesocolons and a fair amount of mobility.
3. Site of descending colon
4. Mesocolon of sigmoid colon
5. Transverse mesocolon
6. Greater omentum (posterior layer; the anterior layer arises from greater curvature of the stomach)
7. Ascending mesocolon, with right colic vessels, fused to posterior abdominal wall.
8. Descending mesocolon, with left colic vessels, fused to posterior abdominal wall.
9. Anterior layer (or leaf) of coronary ligament.* This anchors the liver to the diaphragm and encloses the bare area of the liver.
10. Hepatoduodenal ligament. This is part of the lesser omentum. Note the 3 cut vessels: the portal vein (posterior), the common bile duct (right), and the proper hepatic artery (left). The white arrow indicates the epiploic foramen (new name: omental foramen). It is here that the greater sac (the peritoneal cavity) communicates with the lesser sac (the omental bursa). Notice that the omental foramen lies *posterior* to the portal vein and *anterior* to the inferior vena cava.
11. Gastrosplenic ligament
12. Gastrophrenic (stomach-to-diaphragm) ligament
13. Left triangular ligament of coronary ligament
14. Superior mesenteric vein (left) and artery (right)
15. Duodenojejunal flexture
16. Area on underside of diaphragm occupied by bare area of liver
17. Hepatic veins (cut) ending in inferior vena cava
18. Inferior vena cava; this part of the inferior vena cava is firmly adherent to the liver.
19. Pancreas
20. Duodenum (first part). The 2nd, 3rd, and 4th parts of the duodenum become fused to the posterior wall, which renders the first immobile.†
21. Esophagus (thoracic part) with esophageal plexus (right and left vagus nerves).
22. Esophagus (abdominal part)
23. Posterior wall of omental bursa (lesser sac). This is a peritoneal-bound space in back of the stomach and liver. It communicates with the remainder of the peritoneal cavity by way of the omental (epiploic) foramen.
24. Rectum
25. Aorta

*Peritoneal ligaments consist of either a single layer of peritoneum (e.g., the coronary ligament) or a fused double layer (gastrosplenic ligament) reinforced with connective tissue.

†Structures such as the duodenum which lose their mesentery and become fused to the posterior abdominal wall are termed *secondarily retroperitoneal*.

(use abbrevs.)

1. _____
2. _____
3. _____
4. _____
5. _____
6. _____
7. _____
8. _____
9. _____
10. _____
11. _____
12. _____

Ab-33 Posterior abdominal wall, peritoneal attachments

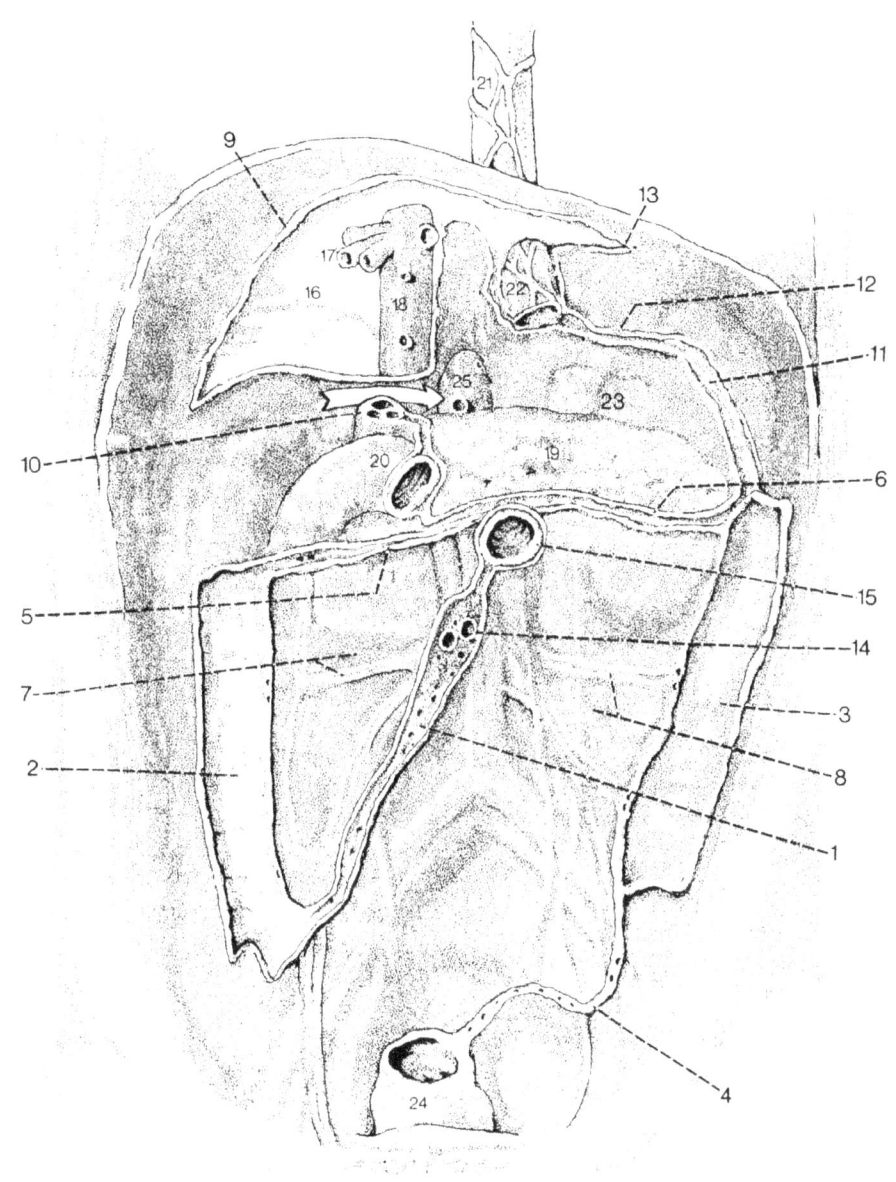

(use abbrevs.)

13 _____
14 _____
15 _____
16 _____
17 _____
18 _____
19 _____

20 _____
21 _____
22 _____
23 _____
24 _____
25 _____

Ab-34 Posterior abdominal wall, kidneys and related structures

(opposite page)

Color and label

1. Aorta
2. Inferior vena cava
3. Hepatic veins (liver has been removed)
4. Esophagus with esophageal plexus
5. Inferior phrenic artery and superior suprarenal artery
6. Middle and inferior suprarenal arteries (the latter arising from the renal artery)
7. Superior mesenteric artery
8. Left renal artery (branches)
9. Left kidney
10. Left testicular vein (ovarian in female); note that it empties into left renal vein.
11. Inferior mesenteric artery
12. Sigmoid arteries
13. Superior rectal artery
14. Left common iliac artery and vein
15. Left ureter
16. Pampiniform plexus. This plexus, which surrounds the testicular artery, is formed by the testicular vein. It absorbs heat from the testicular artery (countercurrent heat exchange), thus ensuring that the arterial blood reaching the testis will be at a temperature several degrees cooler than 98.6, thus permitting sperm production to take place.
17. Internal iliac artery
18. External iliac artery (becomes femoral artery in leg)
19. Inferior epigastric artery and vein (lateral umbilical fold)
20. Medial umbilical fold (or plica); obliterated umbilical artery
21. Rectus abdominis muscle
22. Urinary bladder (covered with peritoneum)
23. Rectum
24. Femoral nerve
25. Genital branch of genitofemoral nerve
26. Femoral branch of genitofemoral nerve
27. Lateral femoral cutaneous nerve
28. Genitofemoral nerve
29. Ilioinguinal nerve
30. Iliohypogastric nerve
31. Right testicular vein. Note it forms the pampinform plexus on the right testcular artery more caudally
32. Right testicular artery arising from the aorta
33. Subcostal nerve (nerve T12)
34. Right ureter
35. Right renal vein
36. Right kidney
37. Celiac trunk
38. Right suprarenal gland

1_____
2_____
3_____
4_____
5_____
6_____
7_____
8_____
9_____
10_____
11_____
12_____
13_____
14_____
15_____
16_____
17_____
18_____
19_____
20_____
21_____
22_____
23_____
24_____
25_____

Ab-34 Posterior abdominal wall, kidneys and related structures

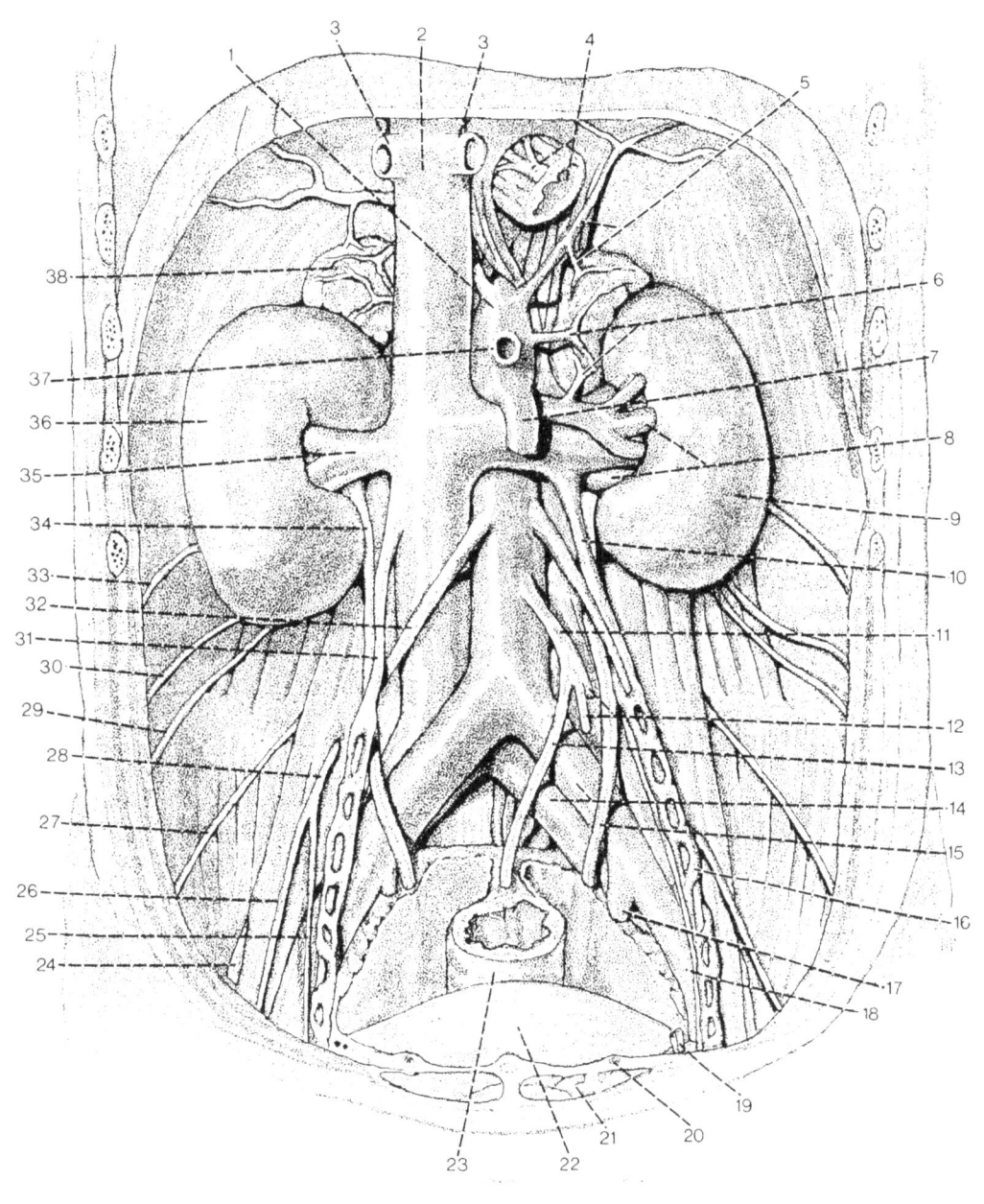

26 _____
27 _____
28 _____
29 _____
30 _____
31 _____
32 _____

33 _____
34 _____
35 _____
36 _____
37 _____
38 _____

183

Ab-35 The kidney, I
(opposite page)

Color and label

Figure A. Right kidney (anterior view)
1. Renal artery
2. Renal vein
3. Ureter

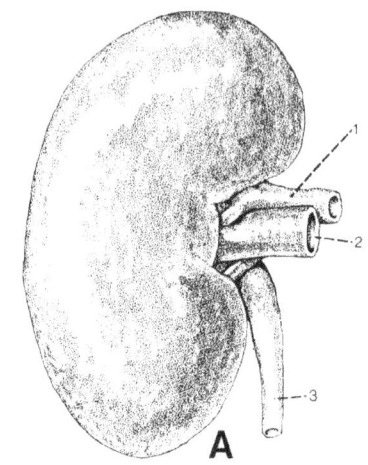

Figure B. Left kidney (partially dissected; blood vessels have been removed)

1. Ureter
2. Renal pelvis (partially opened)
3. Major renal calix (also calyx); usually 2 or 3 in number. These branch off the renal pelvis.
4. Minor renal calices. Several of these branch off of each major calix. Each minor calix has 1 to 3 expanded and indented cuplike ends that fit tightly around 1 to 3 renal papillae (7). The apices of the papillae are pierced by the openings of the collecting tubules.
5. Two minor renal calices (cut open)
6. Renal pyramids (dissected free). These are the major component of the medulla of the kidney. Note their conical shape with their apices pointing toward the renal pelvis.
7. Renal papillae. These are the prominent conical apices of the renal pyramids that project into the minor calices and are perforated by the openings of the papillary (collecting) ducts of Bellini, forming the area cribrosa (*cribrum*, Latin, a sieve or strainer). (Papilla is the diminutive of *papula*, Latin, a nipple or teat.) (Churchill's Medical Dictionary, 1989)
8. Renal papilla opening directly into a major calix.
9. Renal cortex (outer portion of the kidney)
10. Renal column. This is cortical tissue that lies in the medulla between the pyramids.
11. Renal sinus. This space actually lies outside the kidney in its medial central hollow. Blood vessels entering and leaving the kidney pass through it. Perirenal fat fills in all the interstices (small intervening spaces).

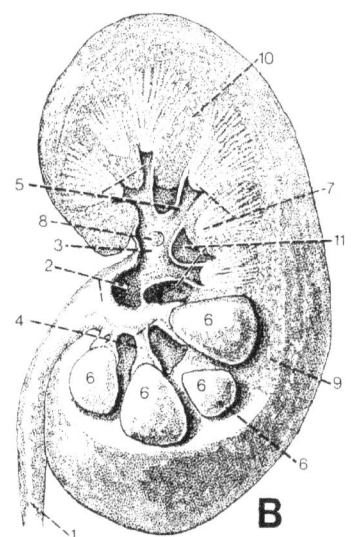

Figure C. A single pyramid
1. Base of pyramid (abuts renal cortex)
2. Apex of pyramid with papilla indenting minor calix (3)
3. Minor calix cuplike end around renal papilla
4. Plane of section (longitudinal) of figure D
5. Plane of section (transverse) of figure D

Figure D. Portion of pyramid in figure C enlarged and sectioned
1. Minor calix (expanded end surrounding papilla of pyramid)
2. Apical section of renal pyramid
3. Area cribrosa. So named because of the numerous tiny openings of the collecting ducts that give it a sievelike appearance.
4. Collecting ducts. (Also papillary ducts of Bellini)
5. Cross section of renal pyramid with collecting ducts (cut). The renal pyramid also contain the loops of Henle and the vasae rectae.

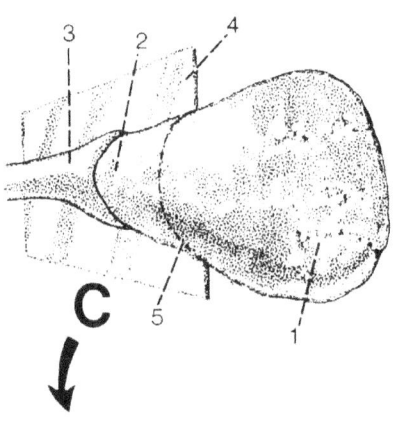

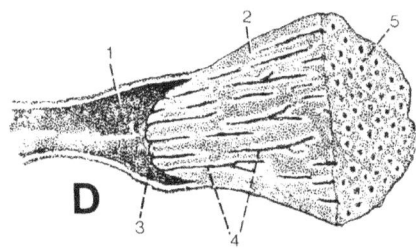

Ab-35 The kidney, I

The right kidney, anterior aspect

FIG A

1_____
2_____
3_____

FIB B (use abbrevs.)

1_____
2_____
3_____
4_____
5_____
6_____
7_____
8_____
9_____
10_____
11_____

FIG C

1_____
2_____
3_____
4_____
5_____

FIG D

1_____
2_____
3_____
4_____
5_____

Ab-36 The kidney, II
(opposite page)

Color and label

Figure A. Left kidney. Sectioned coronally
1. Ureter
2. Renal pelvis
3. Major calix
4. Minor calix
5. Renal pyramid
6. Renal papillae
7. Renal column
8. Renal cortex
9. Fat in renal sinus
10. Capsule of kidney

1. _____
2. _____
3. _____
4. _____
5. _____
6. _____
7. _____
8. _____
9. _____
10. _____

Figure B. Left kidney. Pyramids, calices, pelvis, and ureter
1. Renal pyramids
2. Minor calices
3. Major calices
4. Renal pelvis
5. Ureter
6. Opening of minor calix pyramid removed)

1. _____
2. _____
3. _____
4. _____
5. _____
6. _____

Figure C. Detail of calix and papilla
1. Minor calix enclosing papilla
2. Minor calix with papilla missing
3. Minor calix cut open to expose papilla with openings of papillary ducts into minor calix
4. Cribriform area containing openings of papillary ducts. The latter are formed by the coalescing of the collecting tubules.
5. Renal papilla
6. Renal pyramid

1. _____
2. _____
3. _____
4. _____
5. _____
6. _____

Ab-36 The kidney, II

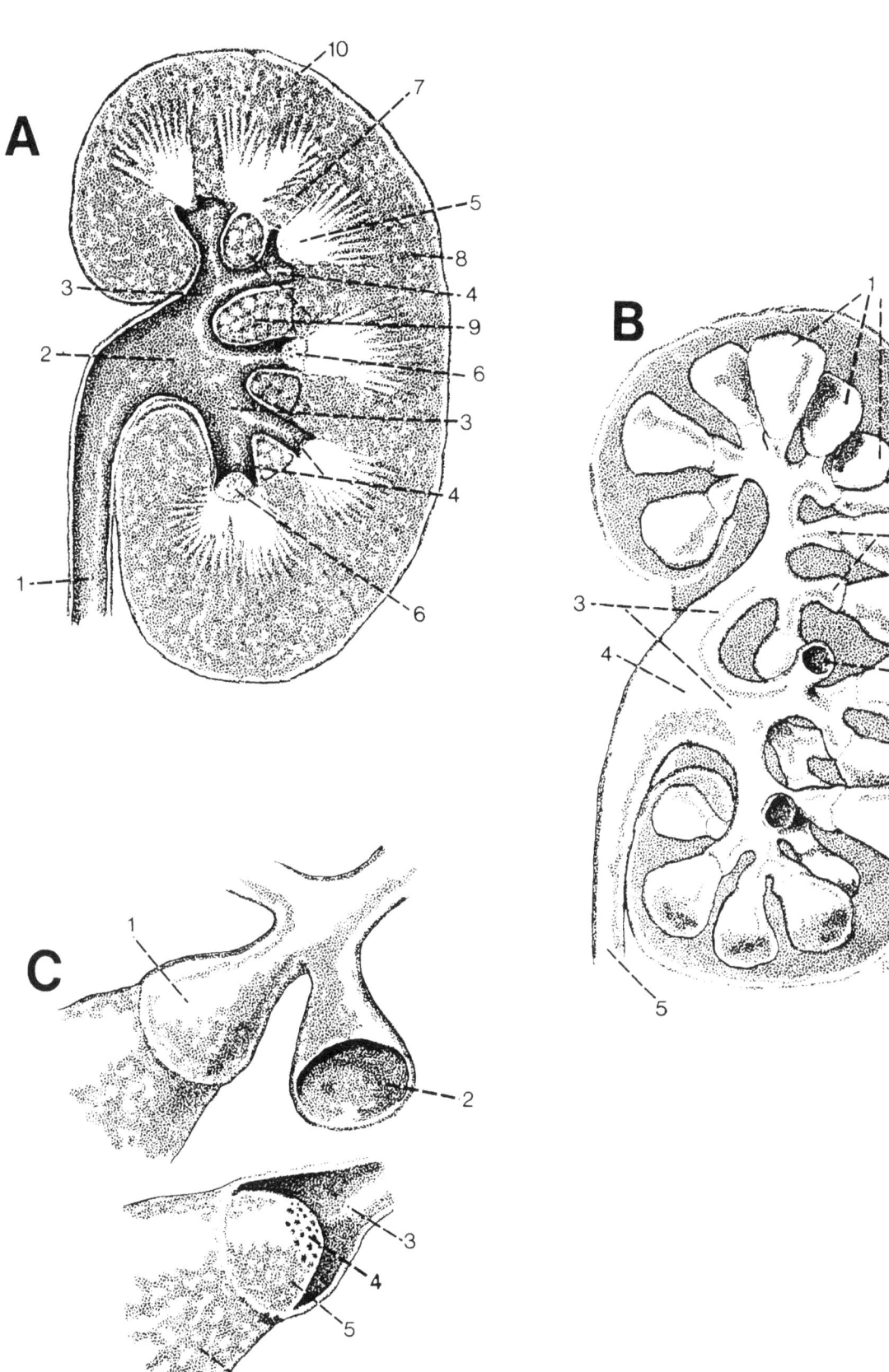

Ab-37 Posterior abdominal wall, showing principal muscles and nerves
(opposite page)

Color and label

1. Aortic hiatus and median (central) arcuate ligament. Note that the aorta passes posterior to the diaphragm so that, unlike the inferior vena cava which passes through the central tendon of the diaphragm, the aorta will be least affected by the contraction and relaxation of the diaphragm.
2. Inferior vena cava with hepatic veins
3. Esophagus
4. Diaphragm (muscular part)
5. Left crus of diaphragm
6. Subcostal nerve (nerve T12)
7. Transversus abdominis muscle
8. Iliohypogastric nerve
9. Iliacus muscle. The iliacus inserts on the tendon of the psoas major muscle. Together, as the iliopsoas muscle, they insert on the lesser trochanter of the femur where they act as a powerful flexor of the thigh upon the pelvis.
10. Genitofemoral nerve. Note that it emerges from the anterior surface of the psoas major muscle and splits into a genital branch and a femoral branch (labels 14 and 15 on the right side).
11. Tendon of psoas minor muscle. This thin shiny tendon is easily mistaken for a nerve.
12. Bladder (urinary bladder)
13. Rectum
14. Genital branch of genitofemoral nerve. The genital branch traverses the inguinal canal and supplies the cremaster muscle and the skin of the scrotum in males or the labium majus in females.
15. Femoral branch of genitofemoral nerve. The femoral branch passes into the thigh beneath the inguinal ligament, supplying the skin of the middle and upper anterior part of the thigh.
16. Femoral nerve. This large mixed (sensorimotor) nerve supplies the skin and muscles of the anterior thigh and the skin on the medial lower leg.
17. Lateral femoral cutaneous nerve. Supplies skin of lateral thigh.
18. Psoas major muscle. A major flexor of the thigh.
19. Ilioinguinal nerve. A mixed nerve supplying the lower anterolateral abdominal muscles. It accompanies the spermatic cord through the superficial inguinal ring and distibutes cutaneous fibers to the skin of the proximal and medial part of the thigh, the root of the penis, and the scrotum in males, or the mons pubis and labium majus in the female.
20. Iliohypogastric nerve. A mixed nerve supplying the skin of the gluteal region and lower anterior abdomen and motor fibers to the lower transversus abdominis, internal oblique, and external oblique muscles
21. Quadratus lumborum muscle
22. Psoas minor muscle
23. Medial and lateral arcuate ligaments. Anatomists agree that these are not ligaments in the true sense of the word, but the names will have to do until better ones come along.
24. Aorta and right crus of diaphragm

(use abbrevs.)

Ab-37 Posterior abdominal wall, showing principal muscles and nerves

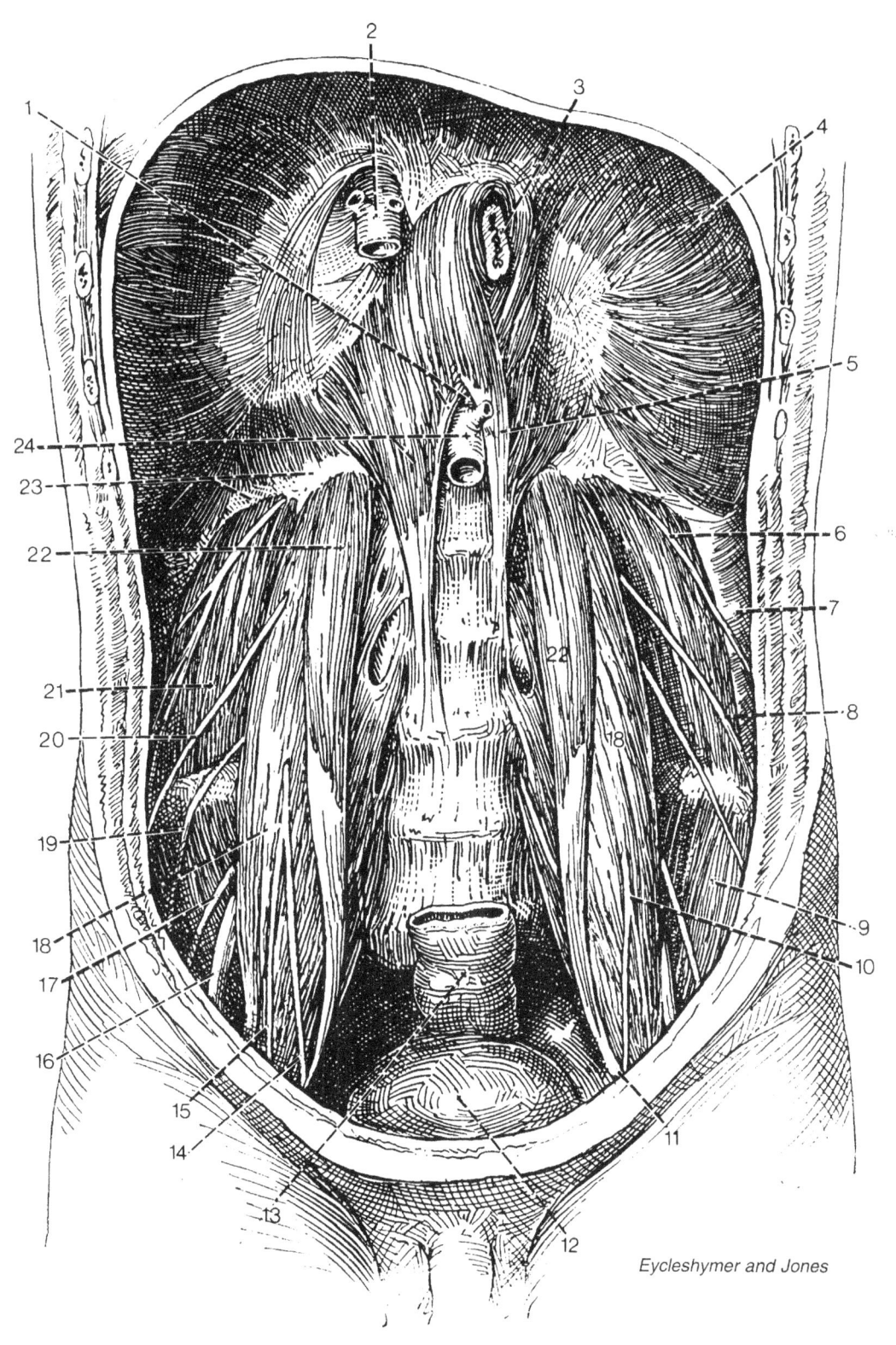

Eycleshymer and Jones

Part III: Pelvis and Perineum

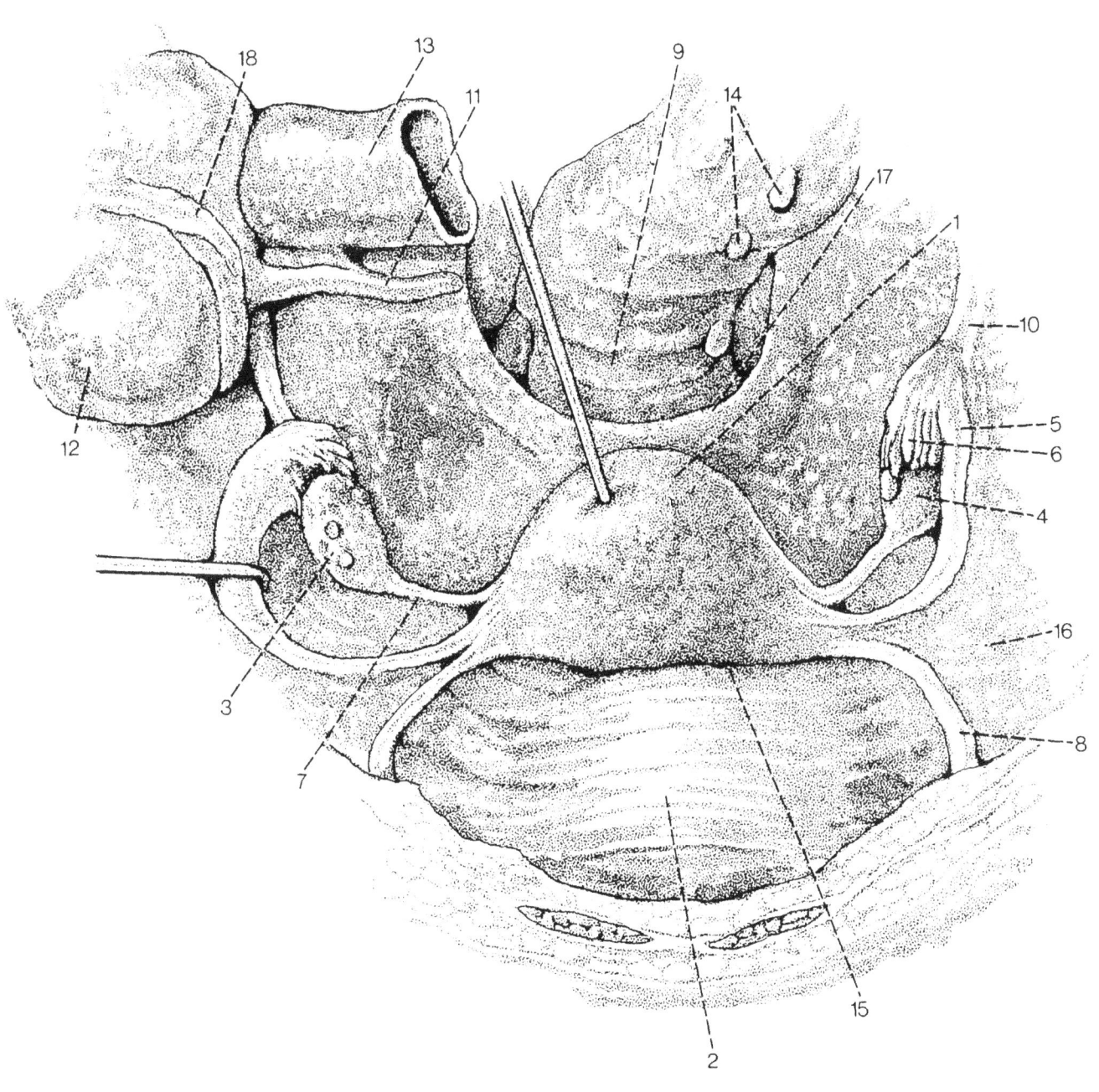

P-1 Hip (coxal) bone

Right hip bone, lateral aspect

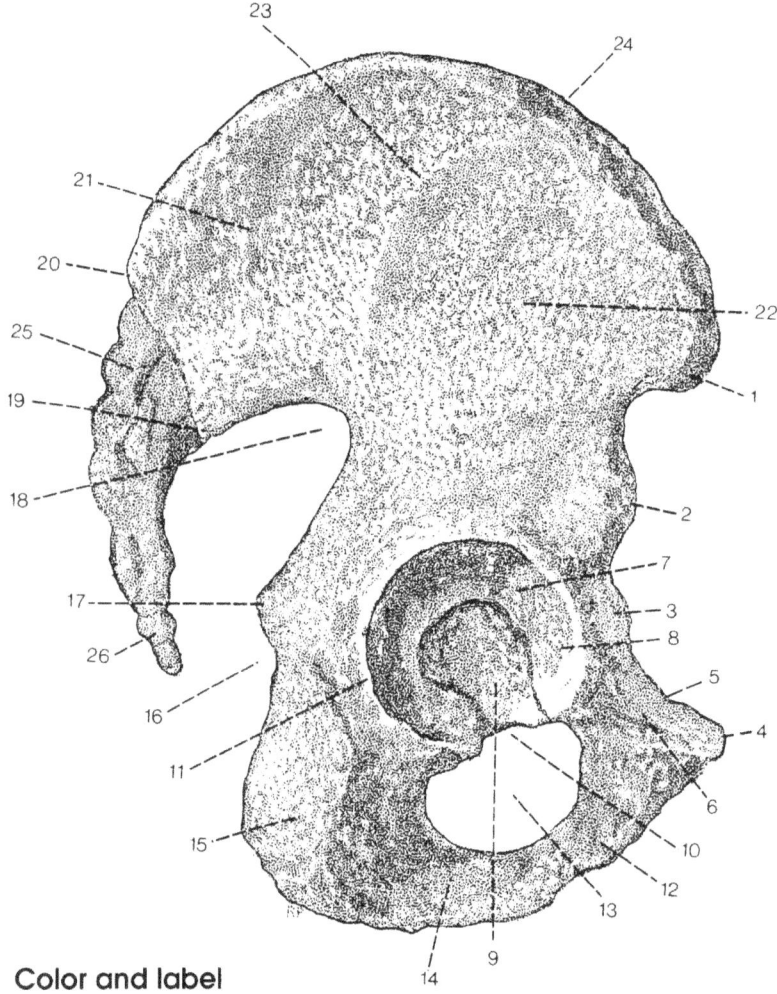

Color and label

1. Anterior superior iliac spine
2. Anterior inferior iliac spine
3. Iliopectineal (iliopubic) eminence
4. Pubic tubercle
5. Pecten (Latin, comb) of pubic bone
6. Superior ramus of pubis
7. Acetabulum (Latin, vinegar cup) socket for head of the femur
8. Lunate surface of acetabulum; covered with articular cartilage
9. Acetabular fossa; the depressed area in the floor of the acetabulum above the acetabular notch.
10. Acetabular notch
11. Border (limbus) of acetabulum
12. Inferior ramus of pubis; this fuses with the ramus of the ischium to form the ischiopubic ramus.
13. Obturator foramen (Latin, *obturo*, to stop up or block)
14. Ramus of ischium
15. Ischial tuberosity
16. Lesser sciatic notch
17. Ischial spine
18. Greater sciatic notch
19. Posterior inferior iliac spine
20. Posterior superior iliac spine
21. Posterior gluteal line
22. Ala (Latin, wing) of ilium
23. Anterior gluteal line
24. Iliac crest
25. Sacrum
26. Coccyx

P-2 Hip bone

Right hip bone, medial aspect

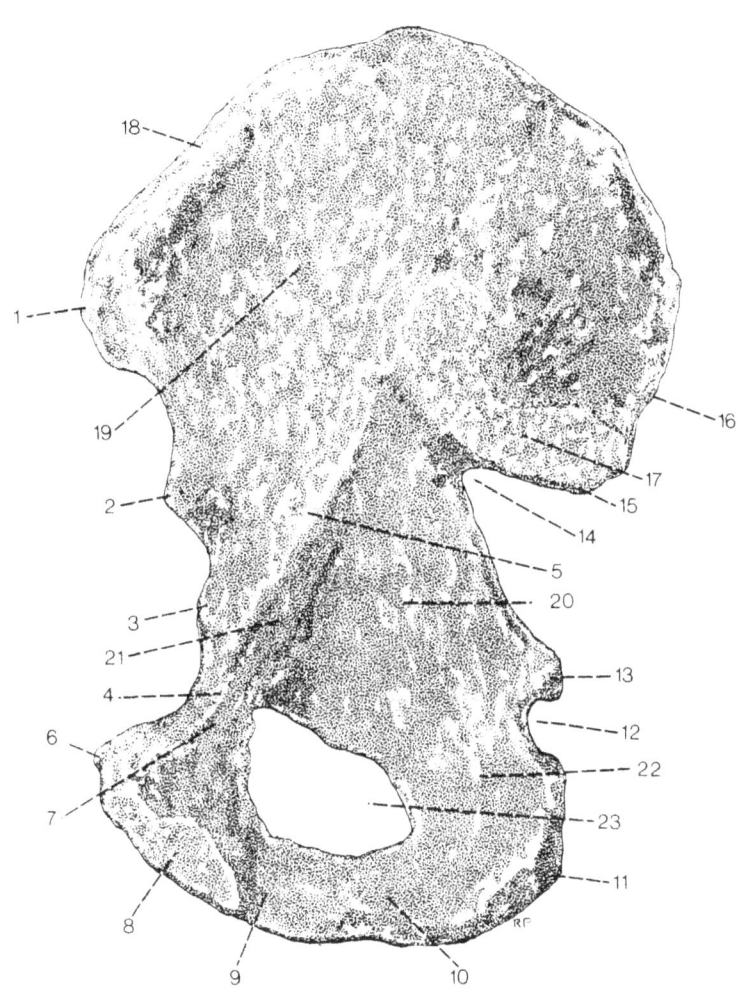

Color and label

1. Anterior superior iliac spine
2. Anterior inferior iliac spine
3. Iliopectineal eminence
4. Pecten of pubis
5. Arcuate line
6. Pubic tubercle
7. Superior ramus of pubic bone
8. Symphysis surface
9. Inferior ramus of pubic bone
10. Ramus of ischium; fusion of 9+10 = ischiopubic ramus.
11. Ischial tuberosity
12. Lesser sciatic notch
13. Ischial spine
14. Greater sciatic notch
15. Posterior inferior iliac spine
16. Posterior superior iliac spine
17. Auricular surface for sacroiliac joint
18. Iliac crest
19. Iliac fossa
20. Body of ilium
21. Body of pubis
22. Body of ischium
23. Obturator foramen

1 _____
2 _____
3 _____
4 _____
5 _____
6 _____
7 _____
8 _____
9 _____
10 _____
11 _____
12 _____
13 _____
14 _____
15 _____
16 _____
17 _____
18 _____
19 _____
20 _____
21 _____
22 _____
23 _____

P-3 Hip bone lines of fusion

Color and label
1. Ilium
2. Ischium
3. Pubis
4. Acetabulum (fuses at 15 years)
5. Iliac crest (appears at 16 years; fuses at 25 years)
6. Anterior inferior iliac spine (appears at 16 years; fuses at 25)
7. Pubic tubercle (appears at 16; fuses at 25)
8. Ischial tuberosity (appears at 16; fuses at 25 years)
9. Sacrum

1 _____
2 _____
3 _____
4 _____
5 _____
6 _____
7 _____
8 _____
9 _____

The hip bone consists of the ilium, ischium, and pubis. At birth these bones are separated and joined to one another by cartilage. They do not coalesce into the bony hip bone until the age of 15. Notice how the socket-like acetabulum is formed by each of the three bones. Peripheral parts of the hip bone such as the iliac crest, anterior inferior iliac spine, pubic tubercle, and ischial tuberosity remain as cartilage longer. Bone formation in these peripheral parts first appears at 16 years and fuses with the main bone mass at 25-30 years. The presence of cartilage between the three main bones and the extent of bone fusion are useful clues in estimating the age of the skeleton.

P-4 Male pelvis dissection
(opposite page)

Color and label

1. Skin
2. Superficial (fatty) layer of superficial fascia (Camper's)
3. Deep (membranous) layer of superficial fascia (Scarpa's)
4. Skin of scrotum
5. Dartos tunic; the layer of subcutaneous areolar connective tissues of the scrotum that contains fibers of smooth muscle (dartos muscle, responsible for the deep wrinkles in the skin of the scrotum).
6. Tunica vaginalis (parietal layer). This thin, moist layer which covers most of the testis is reflected posteriorly to form a surrounding parietal layer. The tunica vaginalis is derived in the embryo from a tubular extension of peritoneum (processus vaginalis) that descended with the testis into the developing scrotum. It is usually closed off at the deep inguinal ring at birth.
7. Testis; covered with tunica vaginalis (visceral layer)
8. Epididymis (head); this contains the beginning of the convoluted ductus epididymis that conveys the spermatozoa from the testis to the ductus (vas) deferens which carries them, within the spermatic cord, into the abdomen to the prostate gland where they enter the prostatic urethra.
9. Pampiniform plexus (cut); formed by the intertwining radicles of the testicular vein that surround the testicular artery. This plexus of vine-like venules absorbs heat from the testicular artery so that the arterial blood reaching the testis has cooled enough for spermatogenesis to take place. Undescended testes that remain in the abdomen will not produce viable sperm.
10. Ductus deferens (vas deferens)
11. Superior ramus of pubic bone (cut)
12. Ramus of ischium (cut); this has fused with the more medial inferior ramus of pubis to form the ischiopubic ramus.
13. Colles' fascia (superficial perineal fascia continuous with Scarpa's fascia)
14. Testicular artery (cut)
15. Levator ani muscle
16. Rectum
17. Peritoneum (cut); on superior surface of bladder
18. Prostate gland
19. Bladder (urinary bladder)
20. Seminal vesicle
21. Ureter
22. Superficial fascia of penis (loose areolar connective tissue)
23. Corpus cavernosus penis
24. Corpus spongiosum penis
25. Prepuce of penis (foreskin)
26. Glans of penis
27. External anal sphincter

(use abbrevs.)

1. _____
2. _____
3. _____
4. _____
5. _____
6. _____
7. _____
8. _____
9. _____
10. _____
11. _____
12. _____
13. _____
14. _____
15. _____
16. _____
17. _____
18. _____
19. _____
20. _____
21. _____
22. _____
23. _____
24. _____
25. _____
26. _____
27. _____

P-4 Male pelvis dissection

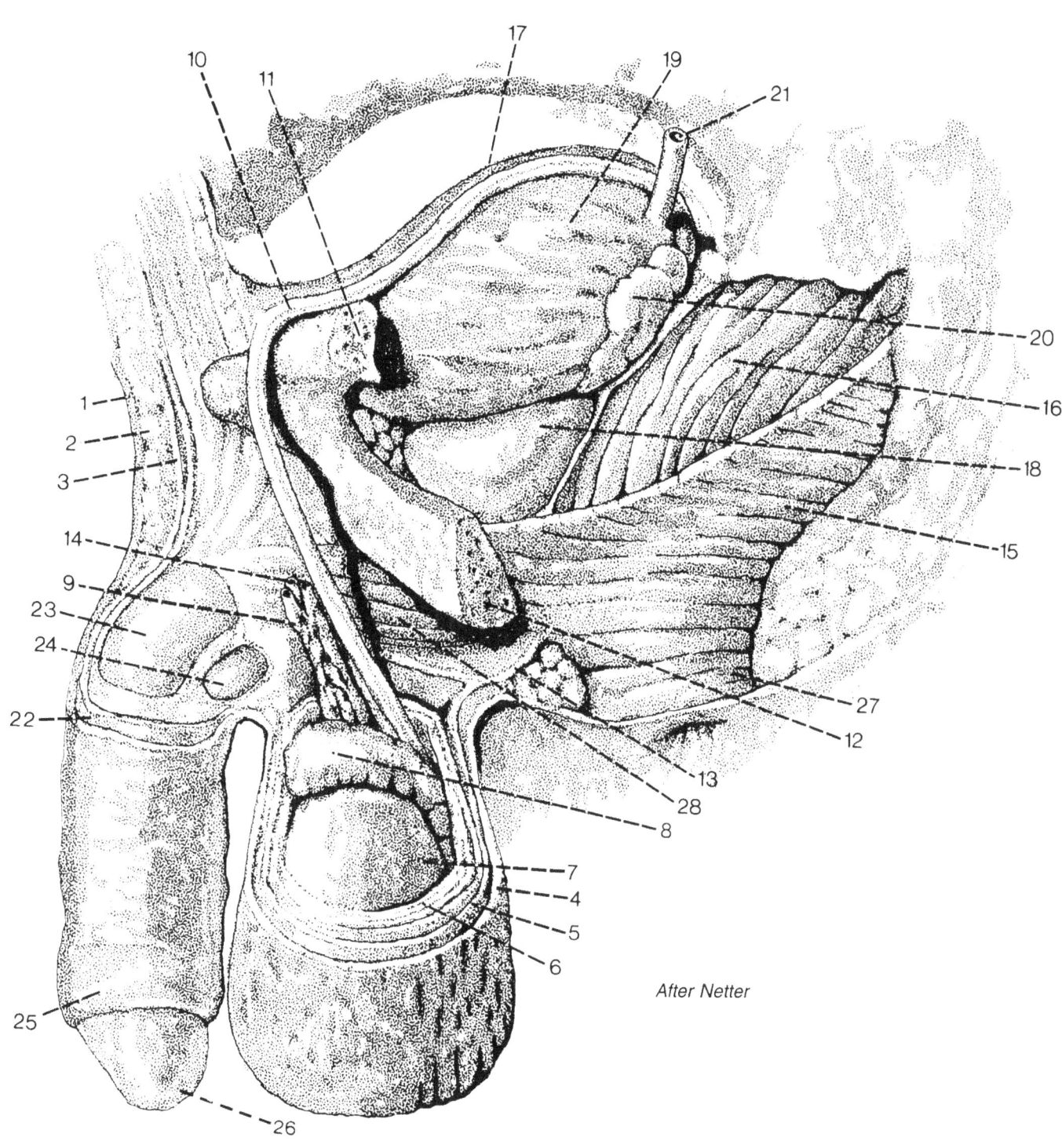

After Netter

P-5 Male pelvis median section
(opposite page)

Color and label

1. Pubic symphysis
2. Bladder
3. Peritoneum on superior surface of bladder; its vertical displacement will depend upon the fullness of the bladder.
4. Suspensory ligament of penis
5. Prostate gland; it surrounds the proximal (upper) portion of the male urethra; its secretion contributes to the seminal fluid.
6. Ejaculatory duct; this receives both the semen from the testis as well as the seminal vesicle secretion, both of which it conveys through the prostate gland to the urethra. The 2 ducts actually lie obliquely on either side of the median plane so that a median section would most likely not pass totally through either of them as pictured here passing through the right ejaculatory duct.
7. Vas (ductus) deferens (terminal portion)
8. Urethra; note that the urethra passes first through the prostate gland, then the urethral sphincter muscle, and then through the length of the corpus spongiosum of the penis; recent investigations list many more subdivisions and parts of the male urethra.*
9. Corpus cavernosum penis
10. Corpus spongiosum penis; it contains the penile (spongy) urethra
11. Bulbospongiosus muscle
12. Urethral sphincter muscle; note that it is more vertical than horizontal as sometimes described. It extends from the bladder to the perineal membrane.†
13. Seminal vesicle; this convoluted tubular structure joins the vas deferens to form the ejaculatory duct. It produces part of the seminal fluid.
14. Perineal membrane
15. Bulbo-urethral gland and duct (left)
16. Superficial perineal fascia (Colles' fascia)
17. Deep fascia of penis (Buck's fascia)
18. Dartos tunic (membranous/smooth muscle layer of superficial fascia of testes; devoid of fat)
19. Septum of scrotum
20. Glans penis; this is the expanded end of the corpus spongiosum penis.
21. Prepuce of penis (foreskin); a fold of skin that covers the glans; removed in circumcision.
22. Navicular fossa of the urethra
23. External anal sphincter
24. Rectum

*The Terminologia Anatomica lists 31 successive parts of the male urethra.
† Oelrich, American Journal of Anatomy, Vol. 158, 1980.

P-5 Male pelvis median section

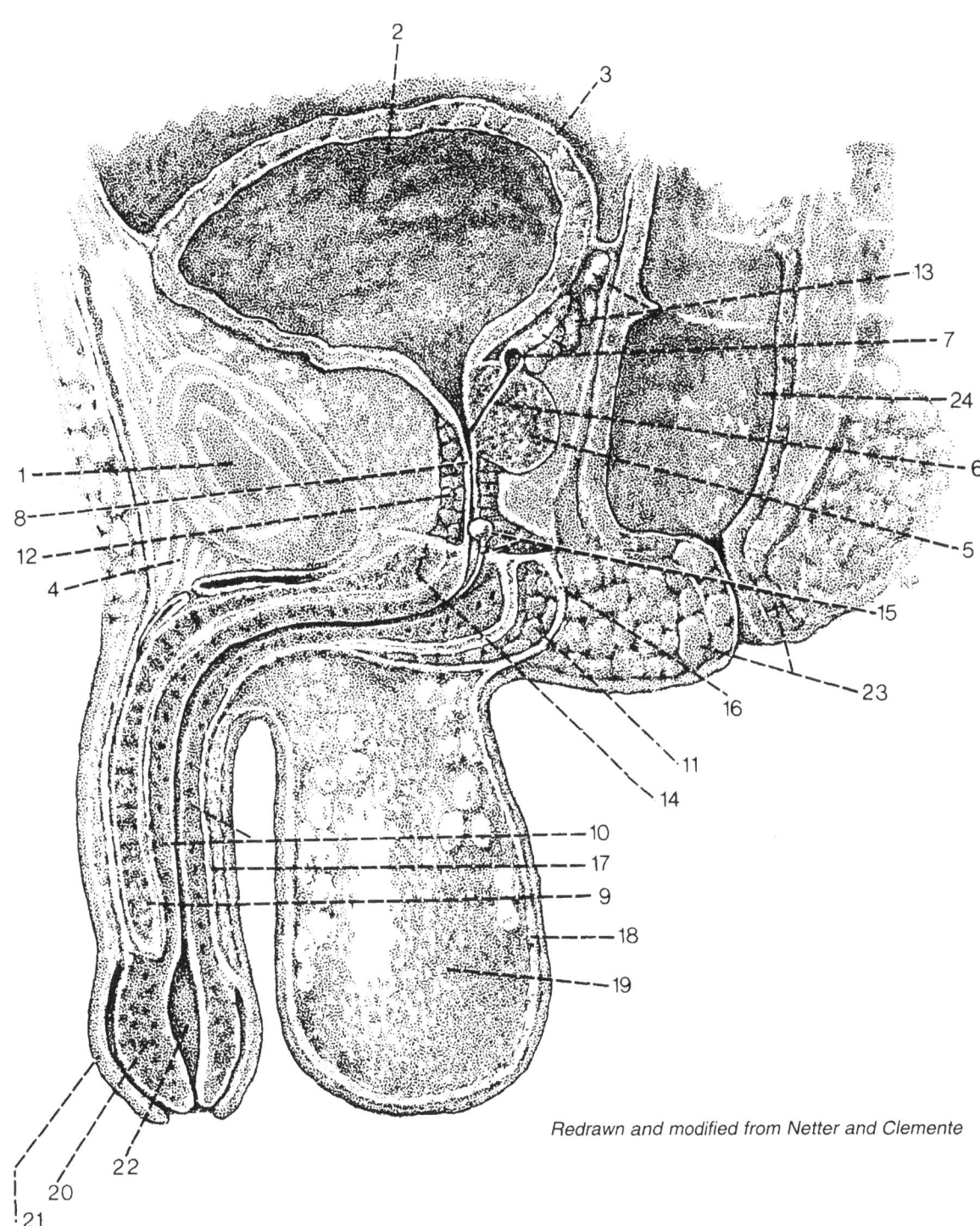

Redrawn and modified from Netter and Clemente

P-6 Male reproductive organs

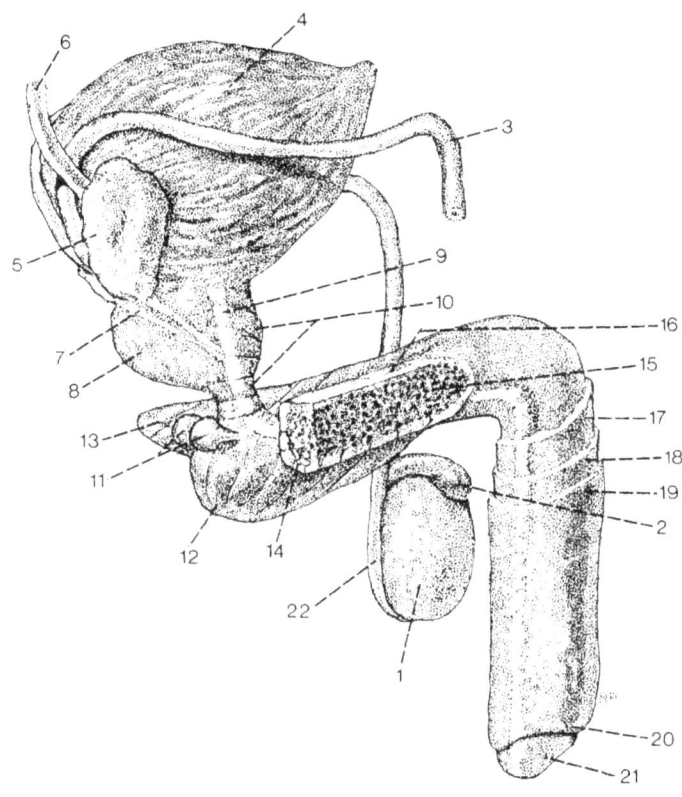

Color and label

1. Left testis
2. Epididymis
3. Ductus deferens (right; cut)
4. Bladder
5. Seminal vesicle (right)
6. Right ureter
7. Ejaculatory duct; this receives the semen from the testis plus the secretion from the seminal vesicle and conveys them through the prostate to the urethra.
8. Prostate gland
9. Prostatic urethra
10. Urethral sphincter muscle; its individual muscle fibers are smaller than those in associated muscles and are embedded in connective tissue, which obscures the visibility of the whole muscle (Oelrich, 1980).
11. Bulbourethral glands; these lie within the basal posterolateral portions of the urethral sphincter muscle (not shown); this portion corresponds to the deep transverse perineus muscle in the male.
12. Bulb of penis and bulbospongiosus muscle
13. Left crus of penis and ischiocavernosus muscle
14. Right crus of penis; cut both on superior surface (16) and lateral surface (15).
15. Site of attachment to ischiopubic ramus
16. Site of attachment to overlying perineal membrane (not shown)
17. Deep fascia of penis
18. Superficial fascia of penis
19. Skin of penis
20. Prepuce (foreskin)
21. Glans
22. Left ductus deferens

1_____
2_____
3_____
4_____
5_____
6_____
7_____
8_____
9_____
10_____
11_____
12_____
13_____
14_____
15_____
16_____
17_____
18_____
19_____
20_____
21_____
22_____

P-7 The penis

Anterior aspect

Color and label

Figure A. Three erectile bodies

The skin, superficial fascia, and attached muscles (ischiocavernosus and bulbospongiosus) have been removed.

1. Corpus spongiosum penis; contains the penile (spongy) urethra. Proximally its enlarged bulb is firmly attached to the underside of the perineal membrane.
2. Glans of penis. This is the expanded, acorn-shaped end of the corpus spongiosum (whence its name). The glans and distal corpus spongiosum have been separated from the two corpora cavernosa. (Glans is Latin for acorn)
3. Corpus cavernosum penis. Proximally the two crura of the corpora cavernosa are firmly attached to the perineal membrane and the ischiopubic ramus. The two overlying ischiocavernosus muscles have been removed. The conical end of the two united corpora fit into the concavity of the glans
4. Bulb of the penis; the overlying bulbospongiosus muscle has been removed.
5. Crus of penis; the two immobile crura and the bulb comprise the root of the penis. The pendulous free portion is the body of the penis.
6. Perineal membrane (formerly called inferior fascial layer of the urogenital diaphragm; there is no urogenital diaphragm as such).

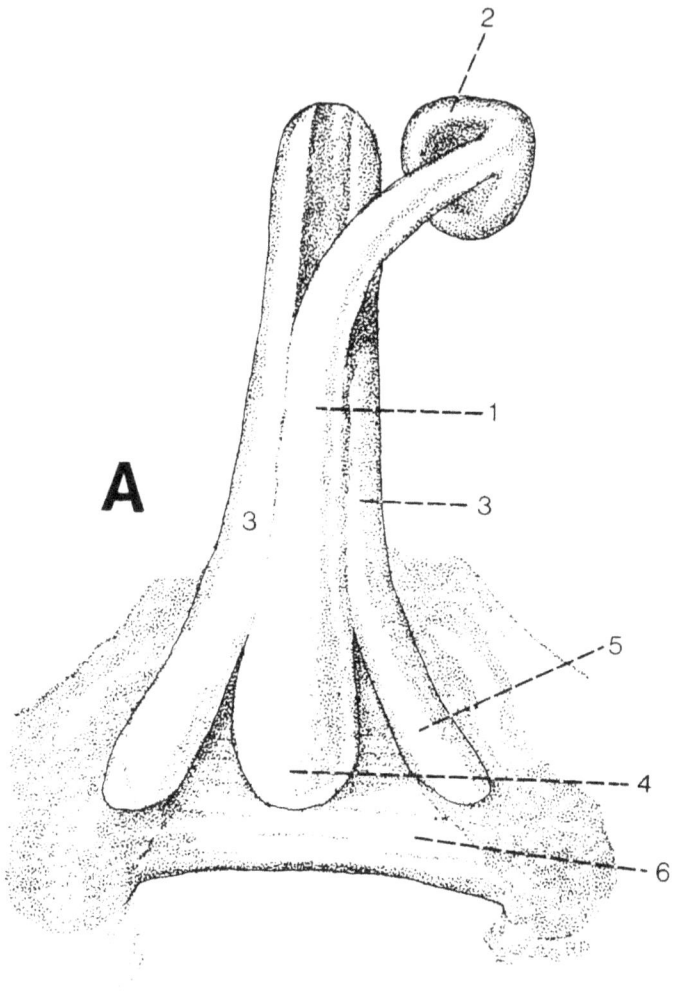

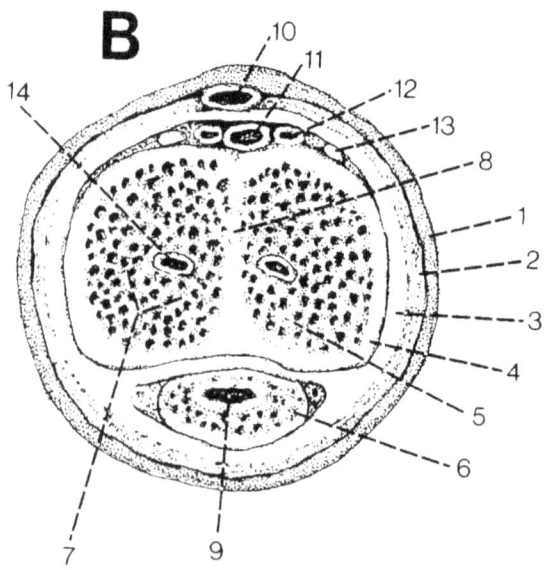

Figure B. Body of penis in cross section

1. Skin
2. Loose connective tissue (superficial fascia)
3. Deep fascia of penis (Buck's fascia)
4. Tunica albuginea
5. Corpus cavernosum penis
6. Corpus spongiosum penis
7. Erectile tissue with cavernous spaces
8. Septum of penis
9. Spongy (penile) part of urethra
10. Superficial dorsal vein of penis
11. Deep dorsal vein of penis
12. Dorsal artery of penis
13. Dorsal nerve of penis
14. Deep artery of penis

The penis becomes erect and enlarged by blood filling the cavernous spaces in the erectile tissue.

P-7 The penis

Anterior aspect
(opposite page)

FIG A

1. _____
2. _____
3. _____
4. _____
5. _____
6. _____

FIG B

1. _____
2. _____
3. _____
4. _____
5. _____
6. _____
7. _____
8. _____
9. _____
10. _____
11. _____
12. _____
13. _____
14. _____

P-8 Scrotum and spermatic cord

(opposite page)

Color and label

1. Spermatic cord
2. Ductus (vas) deferens; this is the only structure in the spermatic cord solid enough be identified by palpation.
3. Epididymis (head); the Greek *didymos* actually meant "double, twofold, or twins" but was also used to refer to the paired testes and ovaries.*
4. Pampiniform plexus; this intertwining plexus of small veins which surrounds the testicular artery drains into the testicular vein. It acts as a countercurrent heat exchanger with the testicular artery, thus cooling the arterial blood and allowing the testes to maintain a temperature several degrees below body temperature.
5. Testicular artery
6. Ductus deferens artery; this lies on the ductus deferens. It arises from the patent (open) part of the umbilical artery.
7. Testis; covered with the visceral layer of the tunica vaginalis
8. Superficial inguinal ring; opening in the aponeurosis of the external abdominal oblique muscle
9. Ilioinguinal nerve; this is the major continuation of the first lumbar nerve; in the abdomen this nerve supplies the abdominal muscles and the skin over the pubic symphysis; it then passes through the deep inguinal ring and spermatic cord to supply the skin of the anterior scrotum in the male and anterior labia in the female.
10. Genitofemoral nerve; this nerve derived mainly from nerves L1 and L2 divides into a femoral branch, which supplies the skin of the medial thigh, and a genital branch, which enters the deep inguinal ring and supplies the cremaster muscle. Scratching of the medial thigh will cause the cremaster muscle to contract and the testis to rise (cremasteric reflex).
11. Tunica vaginalis (parietal layer)
12. External spermatic fascia; a tubular layer of fibrous tissue that forms the outermost covering of the spermatic cord and testis; it extends downward from the margins of the superficial inguinal ring.
13. Cremasteric fascia and cremaster muscle
14. Internal spermatic fascia; innermost sheath surrounding the spermatic cord and the testis; it is a tubular prolongation of the transversalis fascia at the deep inguinal ring.
15. Epididymis (Greek, "upon the testis"); shown here isolated with efferent ductules; it receives the immature spermatozoa from the efferent ductules; its elongated coiled duct provides for the storage, transit, and maturation of spermatozoa and is continuous with the ductus deferens at the inferior pole of the testis. It consists of a head, body, and tail.
16. Testis; sectioned with lobules visible; each lobule contains a convoluted seminiferous tubule from whose lining the spermatozoa develop.
17. Skin of scrotum; the underlying smooth muscle (dartos tunic) gives the skin the characteristic corrugated appearance.
18. Dartos tunic
19. Septum of scrotum

1_____
2_____
3_____
4_____
5_____
6_____
7_____
8_____
9_____
10_____
11_____
12_____
13_____
14_____
15_____
16_____
17_____
18_____
19_____

*Haubrich, Medical Meanings, 1984.

P-8 Scrotum and spermatic cord

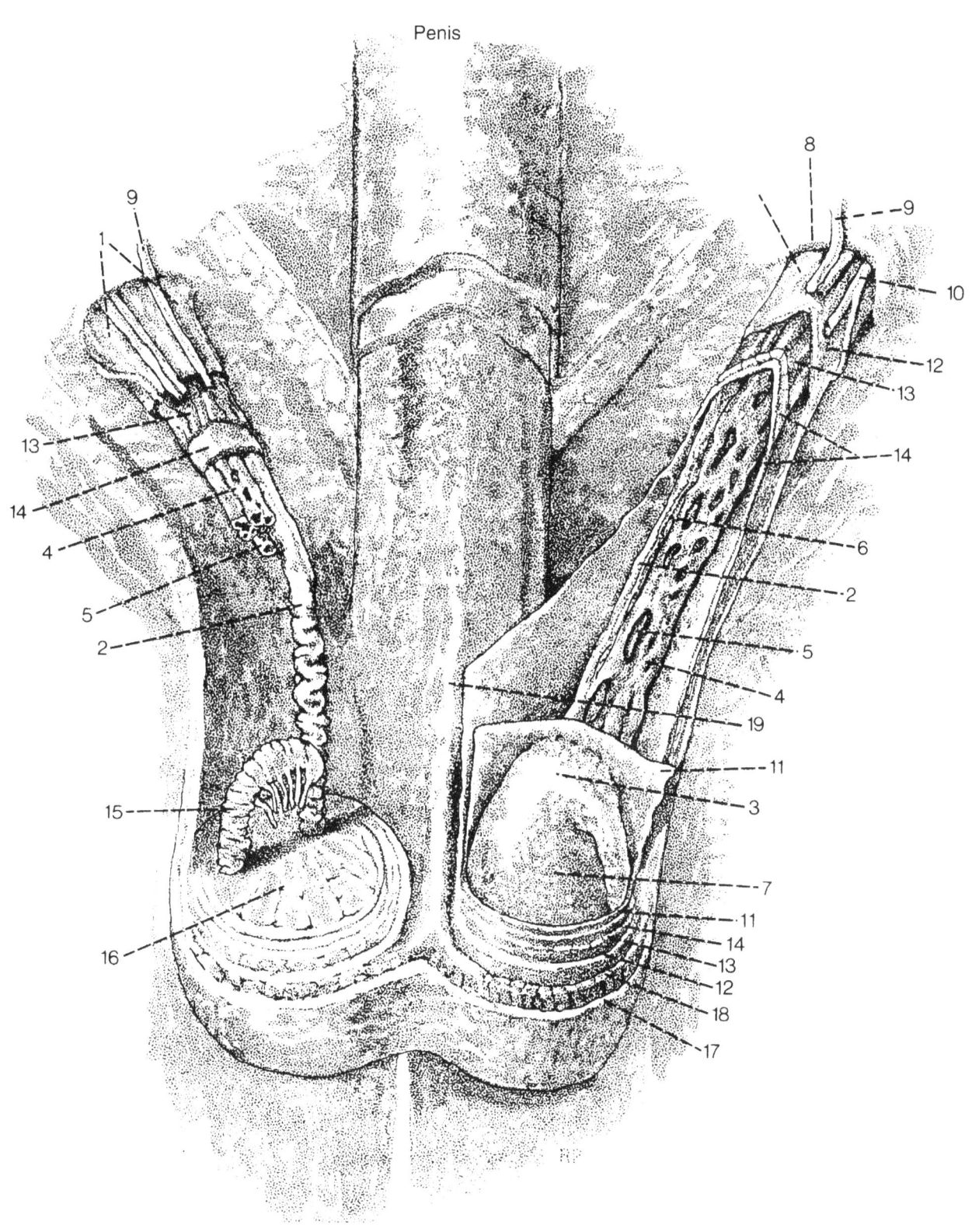

P-9 The testis

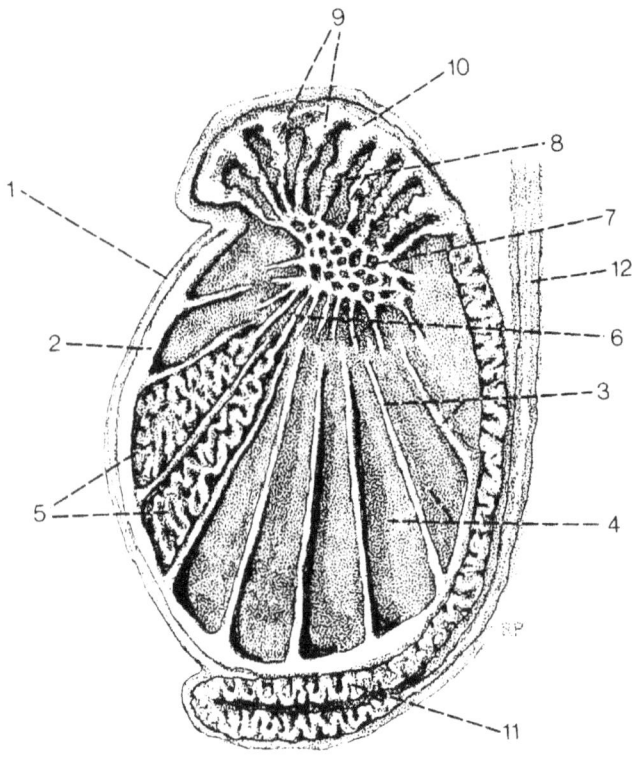

Color and label

1. Tunica vaginalis (visceral layer); derived from the peritoneum during development
2. Tunica albuginea; dense, bluish-white covering consisting of collagen fibers
3. Septula (septums); these divide the testis into wedge-shaped lobules.
4. Lobules of testis; these number 200-300 in each testis. Each contains 1-3 seminiferous tubules Only two lobules are shown here containing seminiferous tubules.
5. Seminiferous tubules (convoluted part); these are highly contorted closed loops that open at both ends into straight tubules (tubuli recti). There are an estimated 400-600 seminiferous tubules in each testis. Each seminiferous tubule is about 70-80 cm long.
6. Seminiferous tubules (tubuli recti, straight part)
7. Rete testis; network of channels formed by the straight seminiferous tubules, traversing the mediastinum testis and draining into the efferent ductules.
8. Efferent ductules of testis; these number between 12 and 20. They become the conical lobules of the epididymis.
9. Lobules of epididymis; each contains a highly contorted efferent ductule. Together they comprise the head of the epididymis.
10. Head of epididymis
11. Tail of epididymis; the epididymis is extremely coiled; unraveled, its total length is about 3 meters.

Bannister and Dyson in Gray's Anatomy, 1995.

P-10 Urethral sphincter in the male

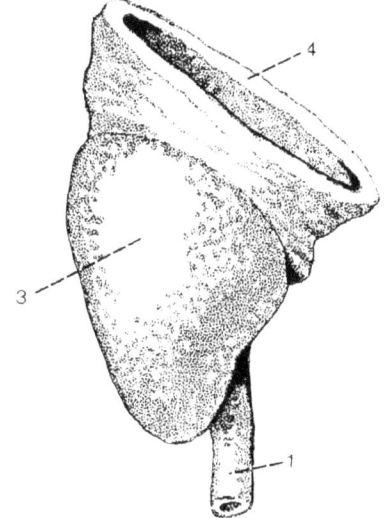

Lateral view with urethral sphincter muscle removed

Color and label
1. Urethra (membranous part)
2. Urethral sphincter muscle
3. Prostate gland
4. Bladder (lower part)
5. Lateral part of urethral sphincter muscle (this part corresponds to deep transverse perineus muscle)

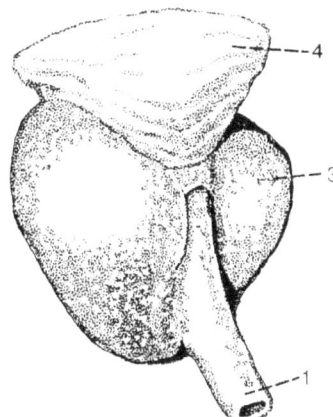

Oblique view with urethral sphincter muscle removed

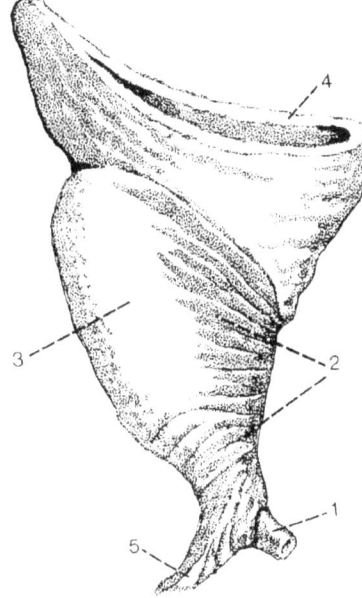

Lateral view from the right

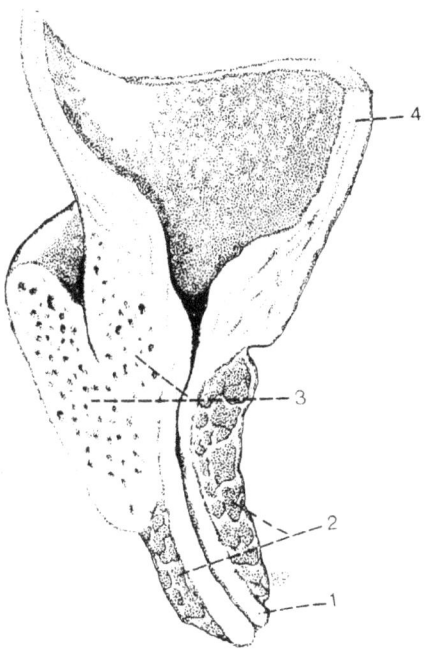

Median section showing extent of contact between urethra and urethral sphincter muscle

There is no distinct superior fascia of the so-called urogenital diaphragm separating the sphincter muscle from the prostate. The fascia of the sphincter muscle is inseparable from the prostatic sheath, is oriented vertically, and passes through the urogenital hiatus to unite with the fascia of the pudendal canals at the ischiopubic rami. Thus the sphincter muscle is a component of the bladder-urethra-prostate-shincter unit which lies within the pelvis, in the urogenital hiatus, and rests upon the perineal membrane. The concept of a urogenital diaphragm is not borne out by this study (Oelrich, 1980, Am J Anat 158).

1_____
2_____
3_____
4_____
5_____

P-11 Male pelvis, frontal section I

Viewed from behind

Color and label

1 Ductus deferens
2 Ampulla* of ductus deferens
3 Seminal vesicle
4 Ejaculatory duct
5 Urethra (prostatic part)
6 Prostate gland (a wedge has been cut out)
7 Urethral sphincter muscle
8 Bulbourethral glands (also called Cowper's glands); these two small glands lie in the urethral sphincter; their small ducts discharge a mucoid secretion into the spongy (penile) urethra.
9 Urethral sphincter muscle (lateral part)
10 Bladder
11 Pudendal canal; containing pudendal nerve and internal pudendal artery and vein.
12 Ischiopubic ramus
13 Perineal membrane
14 Levator ani muscle
15 Obturator internus muscle
16 Obturator membrane
17 Ischiocavernosus muscle covering crus of penis
18 Bulbospongiosus muscle
19 Superficial perineal fascia (Colles' fascia)
20 Fascia lata (deep fascia of thigh)
21 Superficial perineal pouch
22 Ureter

*A saccular dilation of a canal or duct.

Redrawn from Oelrich

P-12 Male pelvis, frontal section II

Posterior aspect - viewed from behind

Color and label

1. Perineal membrane
2. Urethra (membranous part)
3. Urethral sphincter muscle
4. Deep transverse perineus muscle
5. Prostate gland
6. Ductus deferens
7. Seminal vesicle
8. Levator ani muscle; note the thickening of its inferior border
9. Obturator internus muscle
10. Inferior pubic ramus
11. Corpus cavernosus penis
12. Ischiocavernosus muscle
13. Corpus spongiosus penis
14. Bulbospongiosus muscle
15. Superficial perineal fascia (Colles')
16. Deep fascia of penis (Buck's)
17. Obturator membrane
18. Pudendal canal with internal pudendal artery, vein, and pudendal nerve
19. Fascia lata (deep fascia of thigh)
20. Ilium
21. Sheath of prostate
22. Transversalis fascia
23. Puboprostatic ligament
24. Ejaculatory duct

1. Plane of section
2. Bladder
3. Ductus deferens
4. Seminal vesicle
5. Epididymis
6. Testis
7. Bulb of penis
8. Corpus cavernosus penis
9. Corpus spongiosus penis
10. Urethra
11. Perineal membrane
12. Urethral sphincter muscle

P-13 Pelvis and perineum

Viewed from below

The perineum is a diamond-shaped area defined by four landmarks that border the pelvic outlet. These are the pubic symphysis, the two ischial tuberosities, and the coccyx. It is divided into two regions or triangles: the anterior **urogenital triangle** (UGT) and the posterior **anal triangle** (AT). The anterior urogenital triangle is outlined by lines drawn from the pubic symphysis to each ischial tuberosity, and by a third line connecting the tuberosities. The posterior anal triangle is defined anteriorly by the same line between the two ischial tuberosities and two lines connecting them posteriorly to the coccyx. The term perineum also includes all the structures superficial to (below) the diamond shape shown here; these include the bulb of the penis and anus in the male, and the lower vagina, external genital organs, and anus in the female. In obstetrics and gynecology the term perineum is usually restricted to the region between the anal and vaginal orifices. More loosely, the term refers to that part of the lower trunk that lies between the thighs.

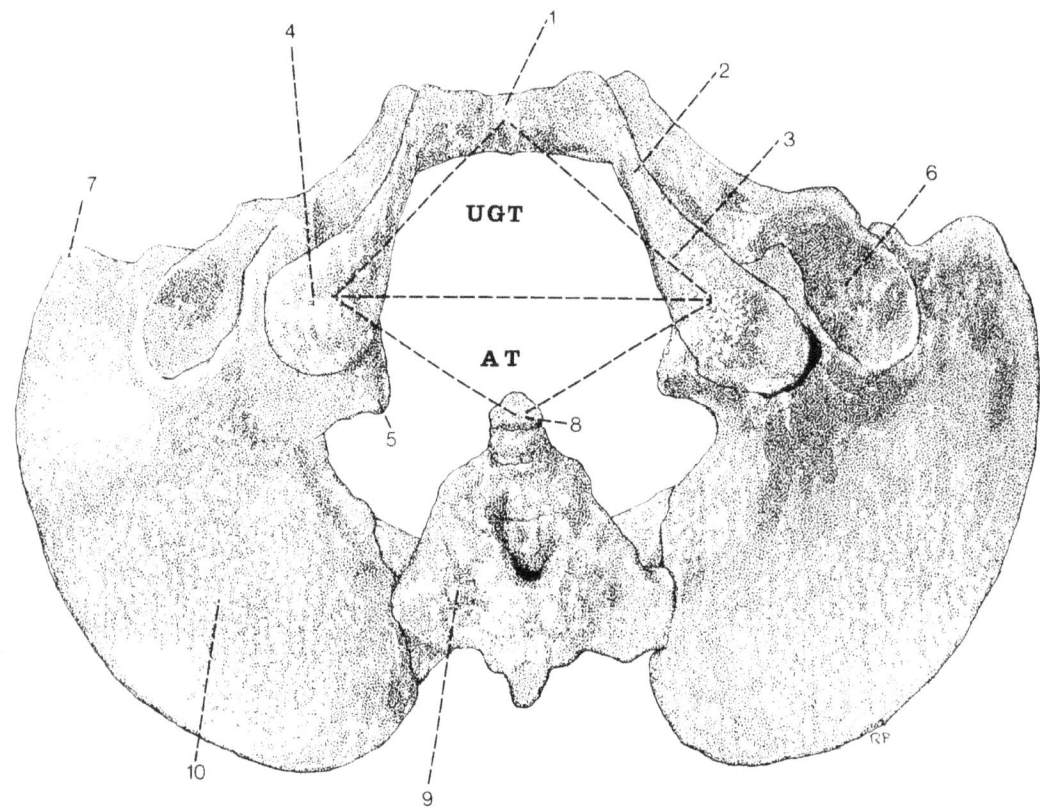

Color and label
UGT Urogenital triangle, AT Anal triangle

1. Pubic symphysis
2. Inferior ramus of the pubic bone
3. Ramus of the ischial bone; this fuses with the inferior pubic ramus by the 3rd decade, forming the ischiopubic ramus
4. Ischial tuberosity
5. Ischial spine
6. Acetabulum
7. Anterior superior iliac spine
8. Coccyx
9. Ala of sacrum
10. Ala of ilium

P-14 Muscles of male perineum

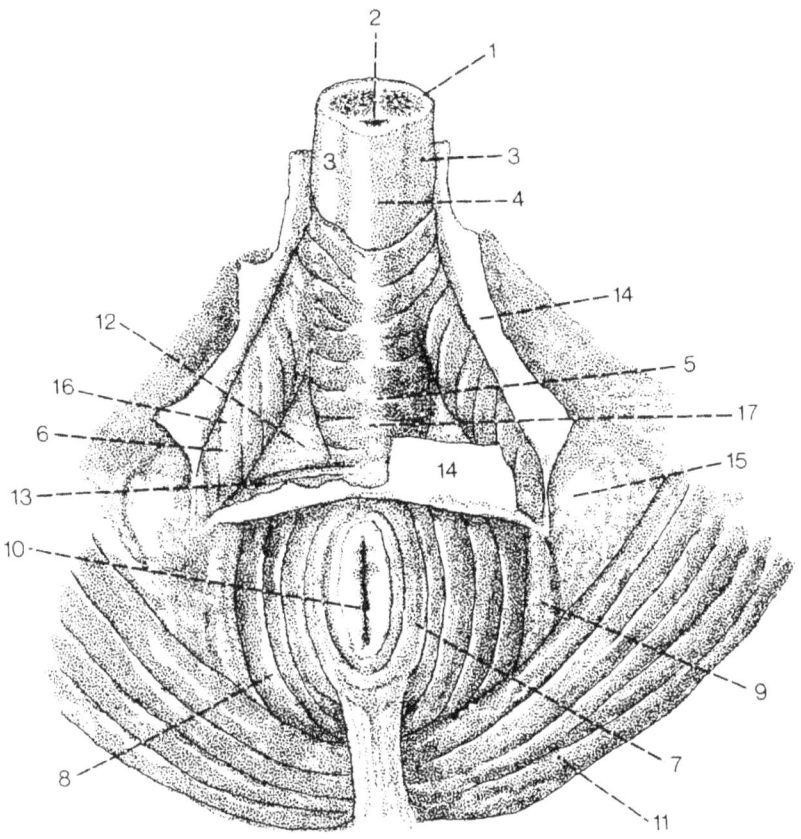

Color and label

1. Penis (cut)
2. Urethra
3. Corpus cavernosum penis; these separate posteriorly and form the two crura.
4. Corpus spongiosum penis; posteriorly this expands into the bulb of the penis.
5. Bulbospongiosus muscle; this covers the bulb of the penis
6. Ischiocavernosus muscle; this covers the crus and anchors it to the ischiopubic ramus and the perineal membrane.
7. External anal sphincter
8. Levator ani muscle; this funnel-shaped muscle is surrounded externally by a wedge of fat that fills the space, the ischiorectal fossa; here shown empty.
9. Pudendal canal
10. Anus
11. Gluteus maximus muscle
12. Perineal membrane
13. Superficial transverse perineus muscle
14. Superficial perineal fascia (Colles', cut and partially reflected)
15. Ischial tuberosity
16. Crus of penis (covered by ischiocavernosus muscle)
17. Bulb of penis (enlarged proximal part; covered by bulbospongiosus muscle)

1_____
2_____
3_____
4_____
5_____
6_____
7_____
8_____
9_____
10_____
11_____
12_____
13_____
14_____
15_____
16_____
17_____

P-15 Nerves and arteries of the male perineum

(opposite page)

Color and label

1. Pudendal canal; this conveys the internal pudendal artery and vein, and pudendal nerve (the veins are not shown).
2. Inferior rectal artery (branch of internal pudendal); fat has been removed from the ischiorectal fossa.
3. Perineal artery (branch of internal pudendal artery)
4. Branch to superficial transverse perineus muscle
5. Perineal artery in superficial perineal space; this space lies between the deep perineal membrane and the superficial Colles' fascia.
6. Dorsal artery of the penis; this gives off a medial branch to the bulb of the penis and a lateral deep artery of the penis that supplies each corpus cavernosum; here it courses deep to the perineal membrane within the substance of the deep transverse perineus muscle and sphincter urethra muscle.
7. Posterior scrotal branches; these are terminal branches of the perineal artery.
8. Pudendal nerve within pudendal canal; derived from sacral nerves S2, S3, S4.
9. Inferior rectal nerves; these supply the external anal sphincter and skin of the anal region
10. Dorsal nerve of the penis; this supplies the glans and prepuce of the penis; here it travels deep to the perineal membrane within the substance of the sphincter urethra and deep transverse perineus muscles.*
11. Perineal nerve; this supplies the muscles in the superficial perineal space (or pouch) (bulbospongiosus, ischiocavernosus, and superficial transverse perineus muscles).
12. Perineal membrane (partially removed)
13. Perineal nerve on left crus of penis.
14. Posterior scrotal nerves (terminal branches of perineal nerve)
15. Left superficial transverse perineus muscle (cut and reflected)
16. Ischiocavernosus muscle on left crus of penis (pulled laterally)
17. Right crus of penis (covered with ischiocavernosus muscle)
18. Bulb of penis (covered by bulbospongiosus muscle)
19. Penis (corpus spongiosum with urethra)
20. Testes
21. Central perineal tendon (or perineal body)
22. Anus
23. Anococcygeal ligament
24. Coccyx
25. External anal sphincter
26. Levator ani muscle (pelvic diaphragm); this marks the superior extent of the perineum; structures inferior to this muscle are considered within the perineum.
27. Gluteus maximus muscle
28. Colles' fascia (membranous layer of superficial perineal fascia; external or inferior layer of superficial perineal space)

* These muscles and enclosing fascial membranes were formerly believed to form a flat "urogenital diaphragm." The space occupied by the two muscles was called the "deep perineal pouch"; however, because the sphincter urethra in the male appears to be more cylindrical than flat and extends from the perineal membrane to the bladder with no intervening superior fascial layer, the use of the term "urogenital diaphragm" remains questionable.

P-15 Nerves and arteries of the male perineum

Inferior aspect; nerves on the left; arteries on the right

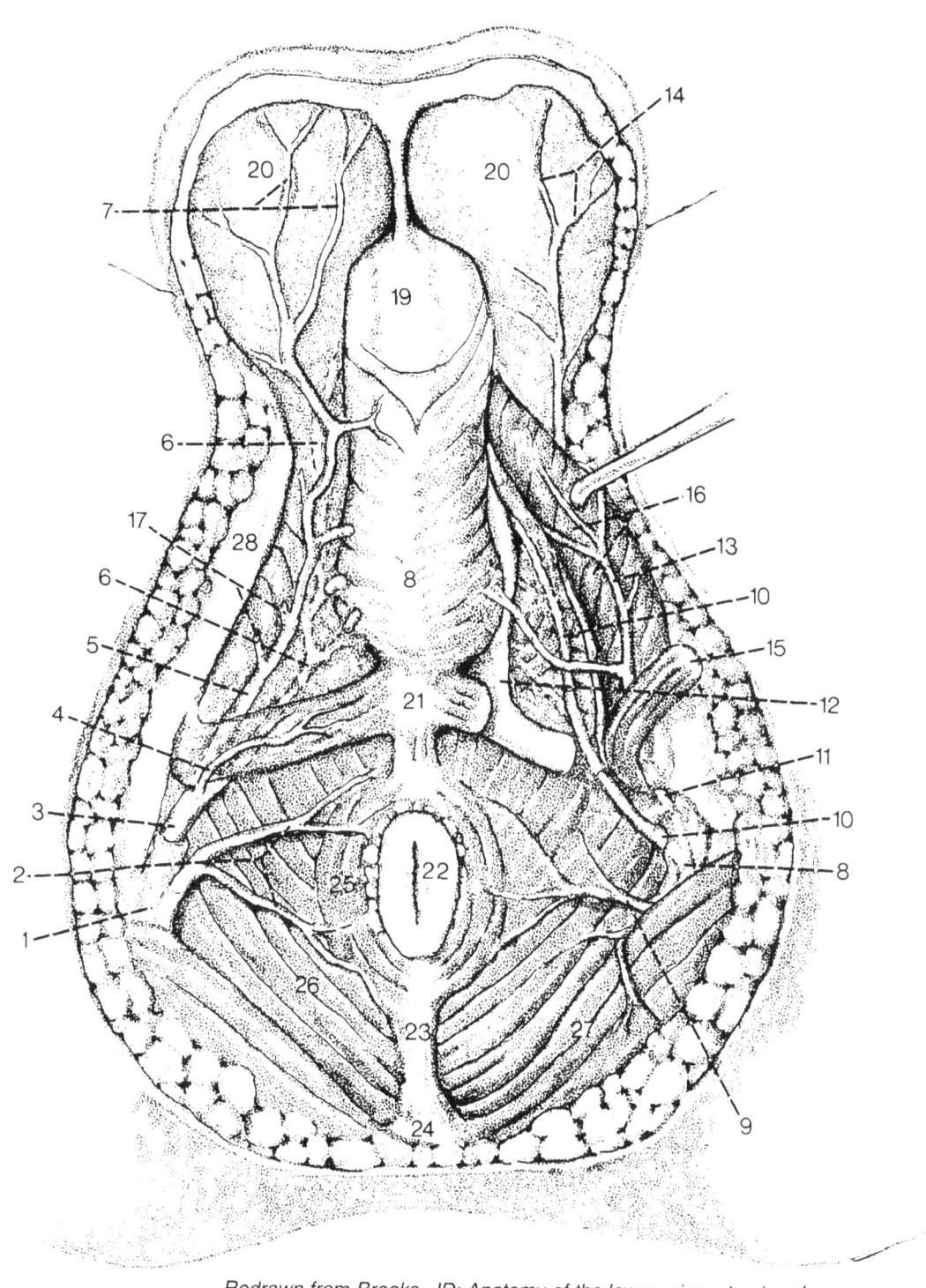

Redrawn from Brooks, JD: Anatomy of the lower urinary tract and male genitalia. In Campbell's Urology, 7th ed., Philadelphia, W.B. Saunders, 1998.

P-16 Male pelvis and perineal muscles

Viewed from the left; sectioned sagittally to the left of the rectum and penis

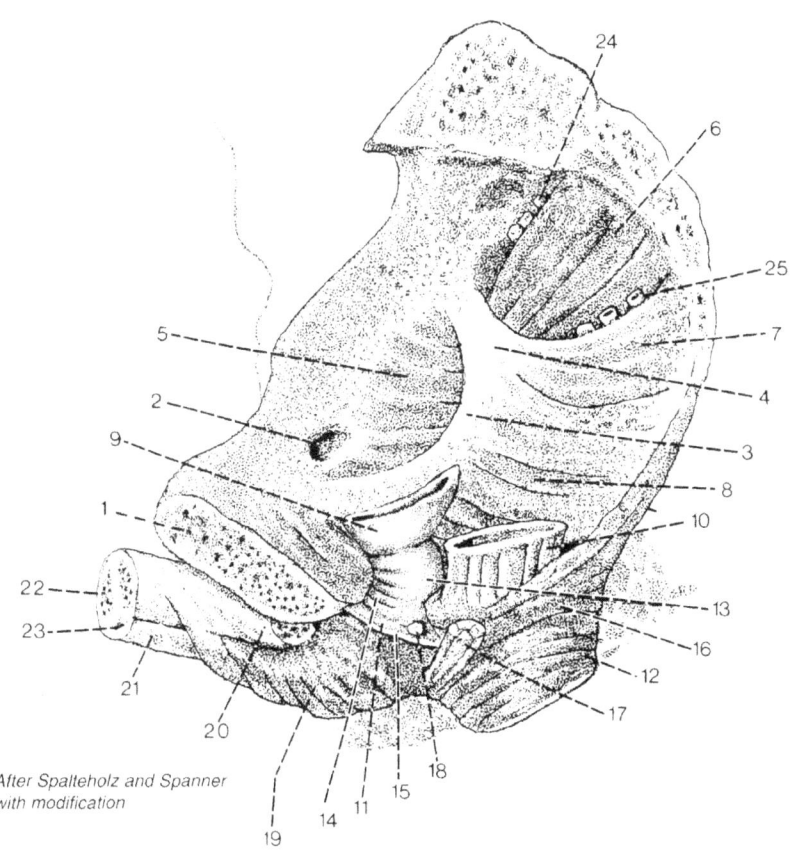

After Spalteholz and Spanner with modification

Color and label

1. Pubic bone (sectioned)
2. Obturator canal
3. Tendinous arch of levator ani muscle
4. Ischial spine
5. Obturator internus muscle
6. Piriformis muscle
7. Coccygeus muscle
8. Levator ani muscle
9. Bladder (cut, lower portion)
10. Rectum (cut)
11. Deep transverse perineus muscle
12. External anal sphincter
13. Prostate gland
14. Urethral sphincter muscle (sphincter urethrae)
15. Perineal membrane
16. Puborectalis muscle (part of the levator ani muscle)
17. Superficial transverse perineus muscle
18. Bulbo-urethral gland
19. Bulbospongiosus muscle
20. Ischiocavernosus muscle (left, covering the left crus of penis)
21. Penis (cut)
22. Urethra (spongy, in corpus spongiosum penis)
23. Superior gluteal artery, vein, and nerve
24. Inferior gluteal artery, vein, and nerve

1 _____
2 _____
3 _____
4 _____
5 _____
6 _____
7 _____
8 _____
9 _____
10 _____
11 _____
12 _____
13 _____
14 _____
15 _____
16 _____
17 _____
18 _____
19 _____
20 _____
21 _____
22 _____
23 _____
24 _____

P-17 Arterial supply of male pelvis

Mainly arteries on right side
(opposite page)

Color and label

1. Abdominal aorta; note that it divides (or bifurcates) into a right and a left common iliac artery.
2. Left common iliac artery and vein (both cut)
3. Inferior mesenteric artery; this supplies the lower (distal) half of the large intestine (or colon) and the upper two-thirds of the rectum.
4. Right common iliac artery
5. Right external iliac artery and vein; below the inguinal ligament they become the femoral artery and vein.
6. Inferior epigastric artery; this supplies the lower half of the rectus abdominis muscle. It anastomoses with the superior epigastric artery at approximately the level of the umbilicus.
7. Deep circumflex artery
8. Right internal iliac artery
9. Anterior trunk of internal iliac artery
10. Posterior trunk of internal iliac artery; this division of the internal iliac artery into two trunks is often not present; rather its terminal branches may arise directly from the internal iliac artery.
11. Umbilical artery; after birth only its proximal section and its branch to the bladder (superior vesical artery) remain open or patent; the remainder becomes the obliterated cord-like medial umbilical ligament.
12. Right superior vesical artery; the left superior vesical artery has been cut.
13. Obturator artery; this frequently arises from the external iliac artery.
14. Inferior vesical artery (right; left cut); *vesica* is Latin for the urinary bladder.
15. Middle rectal artery
16. Inferior gluteal artery
17. Internal pudendal artery
18. Iliolumbar artery
19. Lateral sacral artery
20. Superior gluteal artery
21. Middle sacral artery
22. Inferior rectal artery
23. Perineal artery
24. Dorsal artery of penis
25. Deep artery of penis
26. Obturator nerve
27. Lumbosacral trunk; this supplies nerve fibers from lumbar nerves L4 and L5 to the sacral plexus, which supplies the leg.
28. First sacral nerve S1
29. Obturator internus muscle
30. Coccygeus muscle
31. Ductus (vas) deferens (right; left cut and unlabelled)
32. Bladder
33. Prostate gland
34. Ureter (right; left cut and unlabelled)

After Spalteholz and Spanner with modification.

1_____
2_____
3_____
4_____
5_____
6_____
7_____
8_____
9_____
10_____
11_____
12_____
13_____
14_____
15_____
16_____
17_____
18_____
19_____
20_____
21_____
22_____
23_____
24_____
25_____
26_____
27_____
28_____
29_____
30_____
31_____
32_____
33_____
34_____

P-17 Arterial supply of male pelvis

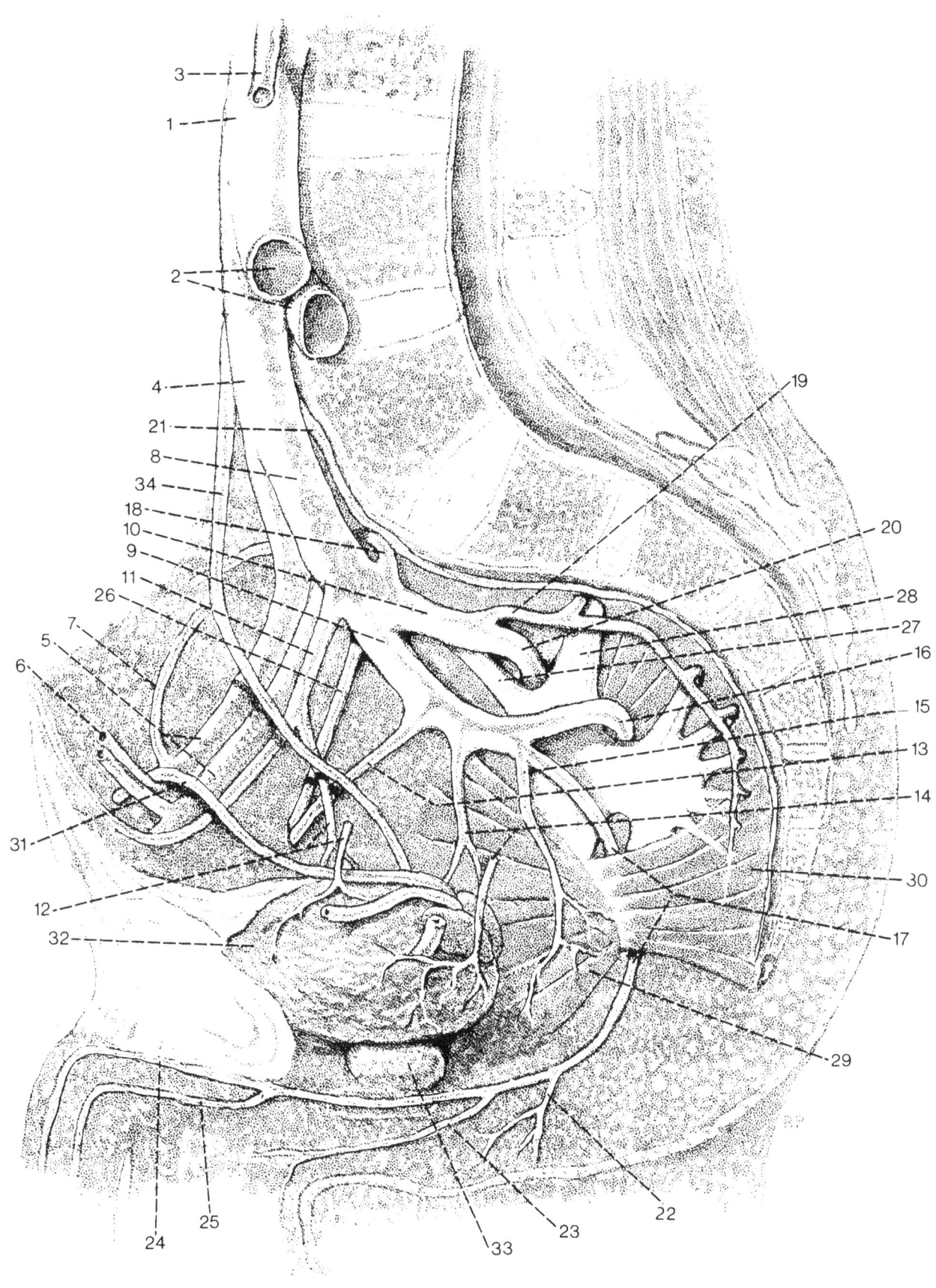

P-18 Male urogenital tract

**Bladder, prostate, and penis have been cut open ventrally
Viewed from the front**

1. _____
2. _____
3. _____
4. _____
5. _____
6. _____
7. _____
8. _____
9. _____
10. _____
11. _____
12. _____
13. _____
14. _____
15. _____
16. _____
17. _____
18. _____
19. _____
20. _____
21. _____
22. _____
23. _____
24. _____
25. _____
26. _____
27. _____

P-18 Male urogenital tract

Bladder, prostate, and penis have been cut open ventrally
Viewed from the front

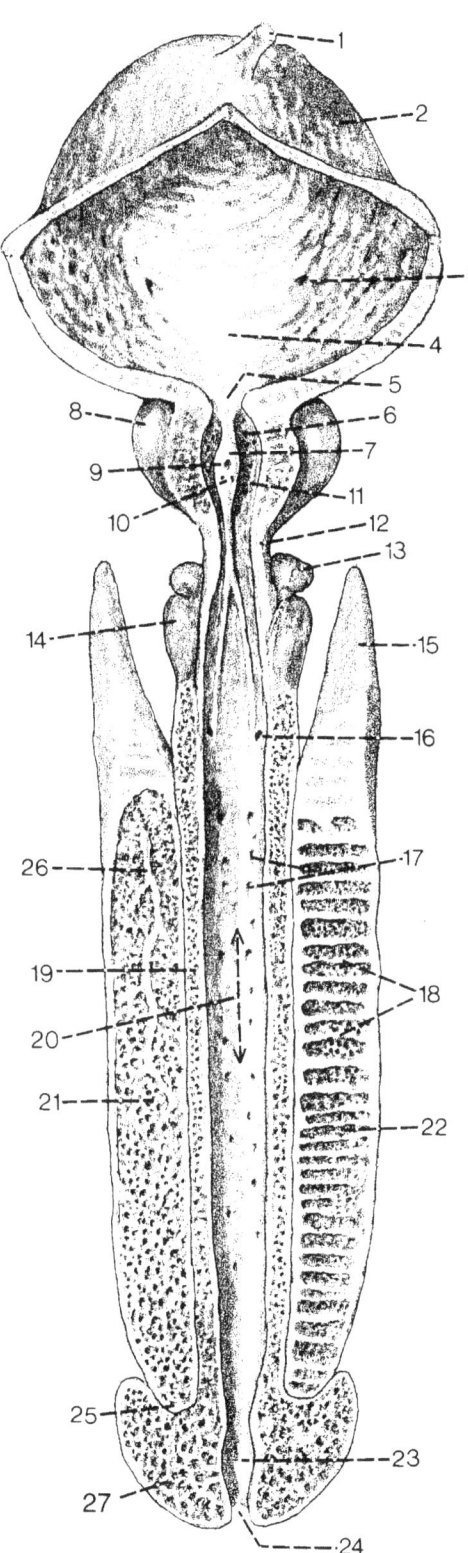

Color and label

1 Urachal cord or ligament; remnant of the the fetal urachus; it persists as a midline fibrous cord between the apex of the bladder and the umbilicus; it forms the median umbilical fold (or plica).
2 Urinary bladder
3 Opening (ostium) of the left ureter into the bladder
4 Trigone of bladder (trigonum vesicae)
5 Internal urethral opening (ostium)
6 Openings of prostatic ductules
7 Seminal colliculus
8 Prostate gland
9 Prostatic utricle; a minute saccular depression in the seminal colliculus; it is the remnant of the embryonic paramesonephric (Mullerian) ducts, which in the male largely disappear; in the female the lower parts form the uterus and upper vagina.
10 Openings of right and left ejaculatory ducts
11 Prostatic sinus
12 Membranous part of urethra; narrowest part of urethra; here the urethra is surrounded by striated muscle.
13 Bulbo-urethral gland
14 Bulb of penis
15 Left crus of penis; the two crura of the penis are firmly attached to the two ischiopubic rami.
16 Opening of bulbourethral glands
17 Urethral lacunae; small recesses in the urethral wall into which the ducts of the urethral glands empty
18 Septum of penis; the penis is divided here slightly to the right of the midline septum, thus causing the midline septa to lie with the left corpus cavernosum.
19 Corpus spongiosum; note that the urethra passes through the corpus spongiosum
20 Penile (spongy) portion of urethra
21 Erectile tissue in right corpus cavernosum
22 Erectile tissue in left corpus cavernosum
23 Navicular fossa
24 External urethral opening
25 Apex of right corpus cavernosum
26 Deep artery of penis
27 Glans of penis

Redrawn from Pernkopf

P-19 Autonomic ganglia and nerves in the male abdomen and pelvis

Viewed from the left
(opposite page)

Color and label

1. Diaphragm (a small portion arising from the posterior wall)
2. 12th thoracic nerve (subcostal nerve)
3. Lesser (or minor) splanchnic nerve; arises from the last two thoracic ganglia and passes to the aorticorenal ganglion. It carries preganglionic sympathetic fibers.
4. Greater splanchnic nerve: contains preganglionic sympathetic nerves from thoracic sympathetic ganglia T5 to T9, which end in the celiac ganglion, celiac plexus, and adrenal medulla.
5. Second lumbar sympathetic ganglion with communicating rami
6. Iliohypogastric nerve; notice its origin from 1st lumbar nerve.
7. Ilioinguinal nerve; it also contains nerve fibers from lumbar nerve L1.
8. Obturator nerve; it carries fibers from lumbar nerves L2, L3, L4.
9. Fifth lumbar nerve (L5)
10. Femoral nerve; notice its fibers also come from lumbar nerves L2, L3, L4.
11. Sacral nerve S2; notice its communicating rami.
12. Communicating ramus from sacral nerves S2, S3, and S4; named pelvic nerve (also *nervus erigens*, because of its reported role in penile erection).
13. Pelvic plexus
14. Vesical (bladder) plexus
15. Prostatic plexus on the side of prostate gland; this plexus contains largely microscopic nerves destined for the corpus spongiosum, the dorsal, deep, and urethral arteries. The nerves destined for the corpora cavernosa of the penis (cavernous nerves) are responsible for erection of the penis. As these nerves pass downward and forward they intermingle with the extensive prostatic venous plexus and form a neurovascular bundle (not shown here) (Lepor et al, J Urol, 133, 1985). The terminal branches of these nerves innervate the helicine arteries and the erectile tissue within the corpora cavernosa. (Lue et al, J Urol, 131, 1984).
16. Aortic plexus
17. Celiac gangion (left); note its relation to the celiac arterial trunk and the latter's three branches, the common hepatic artery, the left gastric artery, and the splenic artery. It contains sympathetic neurons whose unmyelinated postganglionic axons* innervate the stomach, liver, gallbladder, spleen, kidney, small intestine, and ascending and transverse colon.
18. Aorticorenal ganglion. It innervates the vasculature of the kidney.
19. Superior mesenteric plexus on superior mesenteric artery
20. Renal plexus on left renal artery
21. Abdominal aortic plexus
22. Inferior aortic plexus
23. Inferior mesenteric artery
24. External iliac plexus on right common iliac artery; left common iliac artery has been cut.
25. Hypogastric plexus
26. Branches of vesical plexus on side of bladder
27. Dorsal nerve of penis; this is the deep terminal branch of the pudendal nerve. It supplies the skin of the penis, the prepuce, and the glans.

g, sympathetic chain ganglia; B, urinary bladder; ur, ureter; A, abdominal aorta; dd, ductus deferens.

* Preganglionic (myelinated) fibers exit the spinal cord with spinal nerves that they then leave by way of *white communicating rami*. Postganglionic (unmyelinated) axons travel within *gray communicating rami*. The distinction between white and gray is attributed to the presence or absence of myelin. However, in the dissecting laboratory it is impossible to distinguish between the two types of fibers, white or gray, with the naked eye.

Redrawn from Francis and Voneida in Morris' Anatomy, 1966.

P-19 Autonomic ganglia and nerves in the male abdomen and pelvis

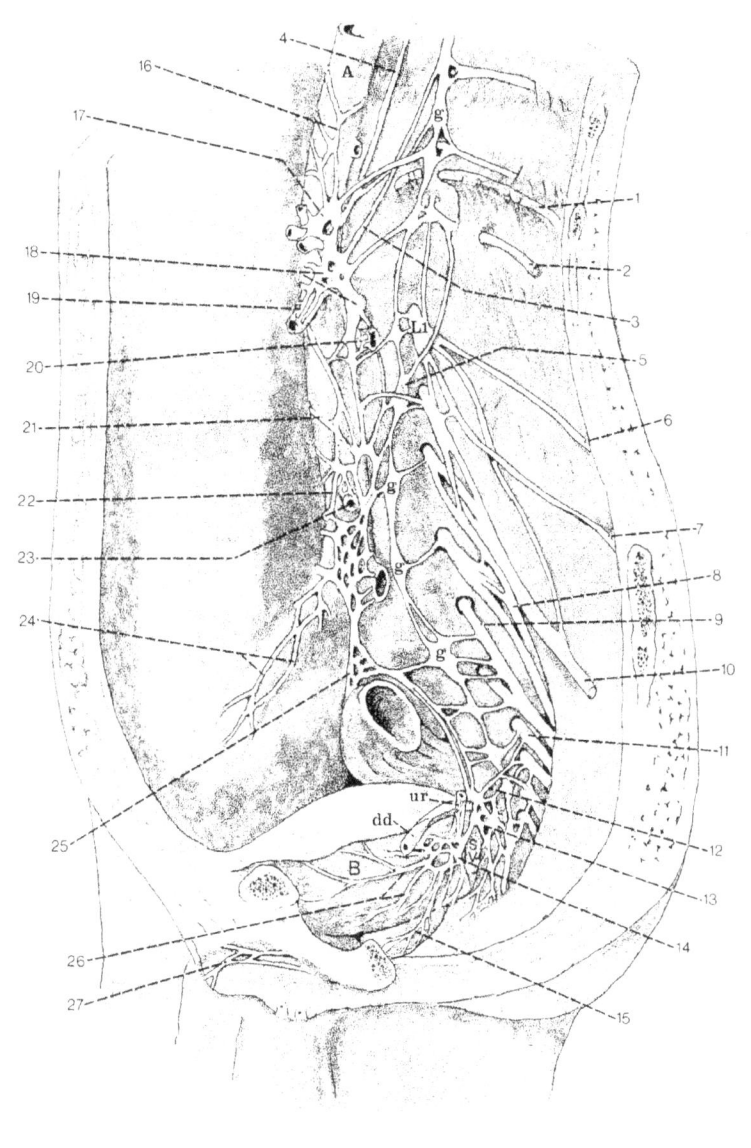

1_____
2_____
3_____
4_____
5_____
6_____
7_____
8_____

9_____
10_____
11_____
12_____
13_____
14_____
15_____
16_____
17_____
18_____
19_____
20_____
21_____
22_____
23_____
24_____
25_____
26_____
27_____

P-20 Female perineum

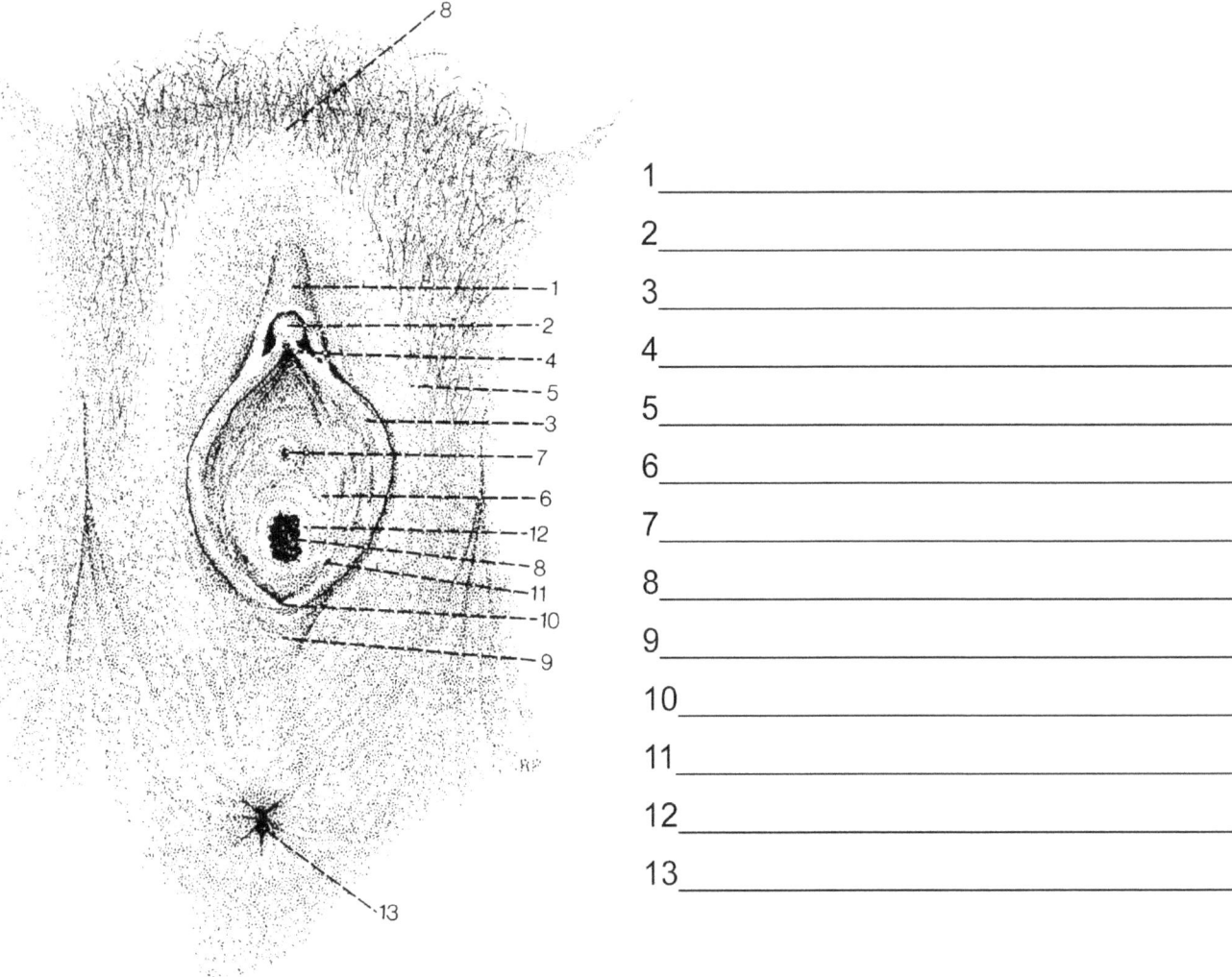

1 _____
2 _____
3 _____
4 _____
5 _____
6 _____
7 _____
8 _____
9 _____
10 _____
11 _____
12 _____
13 _____

Color and label

1 Prepuce of clitoris; a fold of skin that covers the body of the clitoris; formed by the anterior union of the labia minora.
2 Glans of clitoris; erectile tissue at the end of the clitoris; richly supplied with nerve endings making it extremely sensitive.
3 Labium minus (singular; plural is *labia minora*, minor lips); a fold of skin bordering the vestibule of the vagina. Anteriorly the two labia minora split into a medial and lateral fold; the lateral folds unite anteriorly over the clitoris and form its prepuce; the medial folds insert on the deep surface of the clitoris and form the frenulum of the clitoris.
4 Frenulum of clitoris (Latin *frenum*, rein); attached to the under surface of the clitoris; formed by the insertion of the two medial folds of the labia minora.
5 Labium majus (singular; plural is *labia majora*, major lips)
6 Vestibule of vagina; almond-shaped space opening between the labia minora containing the openings of the vagina, urethra, and the two ducts of the greater vestibular glands.
7 External urethral opening
8 Mons pubis; the rounded fleshy prominence over the pubic symphysis
9 Posterior labial commissure; a slight fold uniting the labia majora posteriorly in front of the anus
10 Frenulum of labia minora; posterior union of the labia minora (also called the fourchette, French, diminutive of *fourche*, pitchfork).
11 Opening (left) of greater vestibular gland
12 Hymen (remains of); the membranous fold that partially or wholly occludes the external opening of the vagina.
13 Anus

P-21 Female erectile tissue

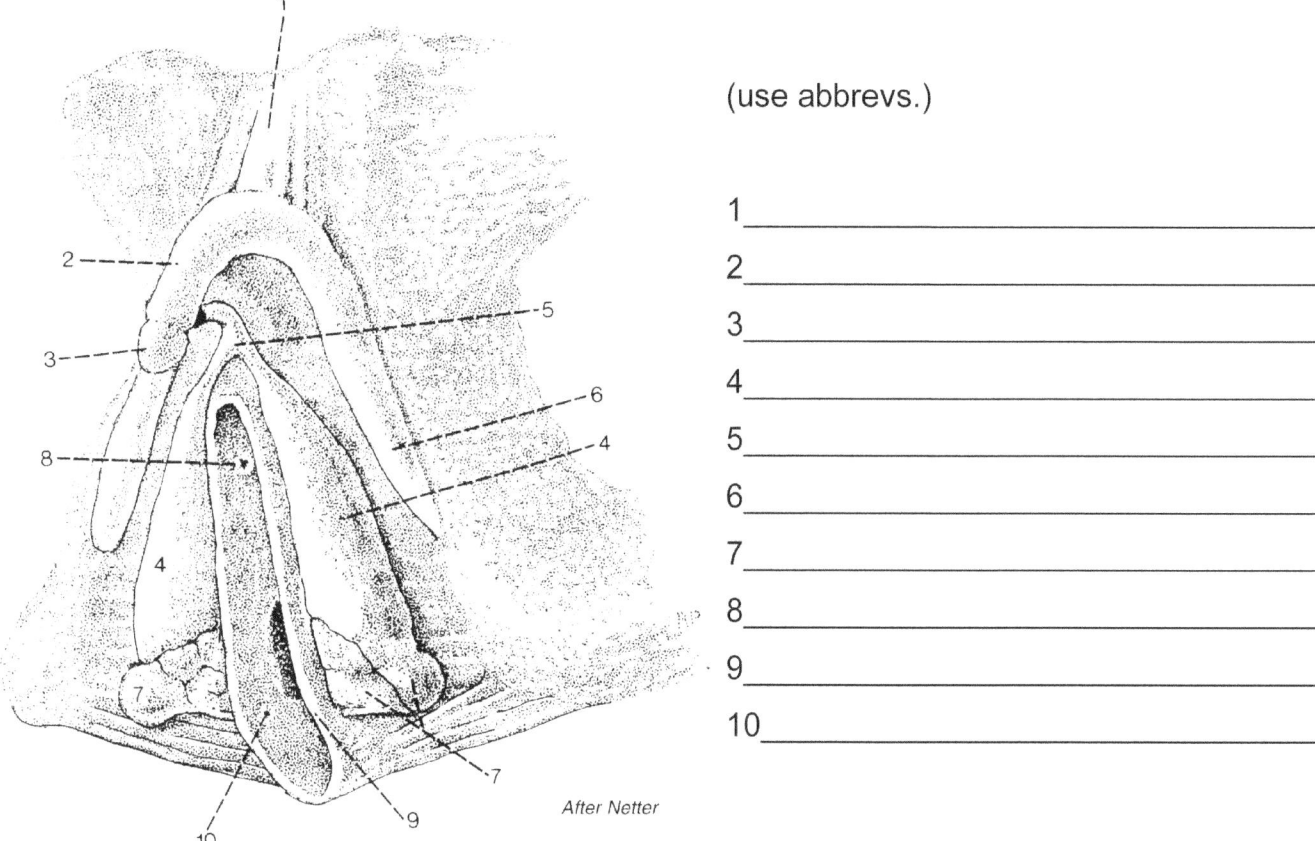

After Netter

(use abbrevs.)

1_____
2_____
3_____
4_____
5_____
6_____
7_____
8_____
9_____
10_____

Color and label

1. Suspensory ligament of clitoris; this suspends the body of the clitoris from the pubic symphysis.
2. Body of the clitoris. The clitoris is homologous to the male penis. Like the penis, it is an erectile organ. It consists of a body, two crura, and a glans. The body, about 2 cm (1 inch) long, consists of two fused corpora cavernosa. It is covered by the prepuce of the clitoris.
3. Glans of clitoris; the glans is a small rounded tubercle located at the free distal end of the body. It is partly covered by the hood-like prepuce of the clitoris. It is highly sensitive.
4. Vestibular bulb; these are two oval masses of erectile tissue on either side of the opening of the vagina. They are situated on the inferior surface of the perineal membrane and each is covered by the bulbospongiosus muscle (not shown).They are homologous to the corpus spongiosus of the male penis. They differ from the male, however, in that they are not fused but remain separate and do not contain the urethra, as does the male corpus spongiosum. Each is connected to the other anteriorly by a narrow pars intermedia bulborum, which together form the commissure of the vestibular bulb. The commissure is also continuous with the glans of the clitoris by a short narrow extension.
5. Commissure of vestibular bulb; formed by the joining of the two pars intermedia bulborum (two intermediate parts of the bulbs).
6. Left crus of clitoris; The two crura are continuous with the corpora cavernosa and serve to attach them to the inferior rami of the pubic bone. They are both covered by the ischiocavernosa muscles (not shown here).
7. Greater vestibular gland and duct (also called Bartholin's gland); these lie posterior to the bulb of the vestibule and discharge their mucoid secretion into the vestibule of the vagina. They correspond to the bulbo-urethral glands in the male.
8. External urethral orifice
9. Labium minus
10. Orifice of duct of greater vestibular gland

P-22 Clitoris and vestibular bulb

After injection of resin through the veins
Labia minora and majora cut and removed

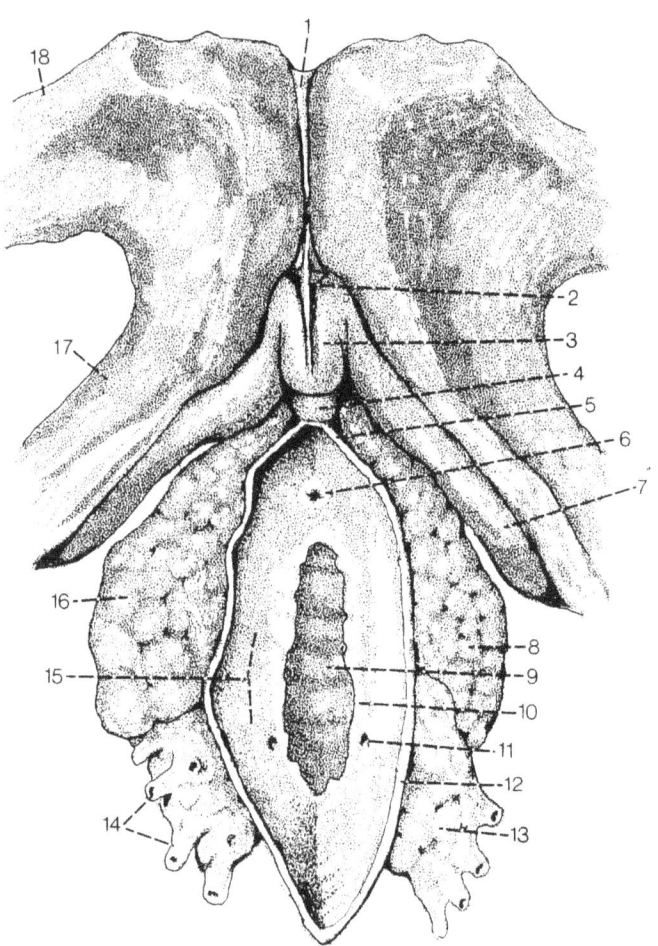

Color and label

1. Pubic symphysis
2. Suspensory ligament of clitoris
3. Body of clitoris
4. Glans of clitoris
5. Frenulum of clitoris
6. Urethral external orifice
7. Crus (left) of clitoris
8. Vestibular bulb (left)
9. Vagina
10. Opening of vagina (vaginal orifice)
11. Opening of duct of greater vestibular gland
12. Line of excision of labia minora
13. Greater vestibular gland
14. Venous plexus
15. Vestibule of the vagina
16. Right vestibular bulb
17. Inferior ramus of pubis
18. Superior ramus of pubis

Redrawn from Toldt

1 _____
2 _____
3 _____
4 _____
5 _____
6 _____
7 _____
8 _____
9 _____
10 _____
11 _____
12 _____
13 _____
14 _____
15 _____
16 _____
17 _____
18 _____

P-23 Female pelvis, median section

Ileum and colon removed except for terminal portion of large intestine

Color and label

1. Uterus (body)
2. Cervix of uterus
3. Fundus of uterus
4. Ovary
5. Bladder
6. Urethra
7. Vagina
8. Anus
9. Rectum
10. Uterine tube (also oviduct, fallopian tube, salpinx)
11. Ampulla (dilation) of oviduct
12. Infundibulum (funnel-like) of fallopian tube
13. Fimbria (Latin, fringe) of fallopian tube
14. Proper ovarian ligament
15. Ovarian suspensory ligament
16. Rectouterine pouch
17. Posterior lip of cervix
18. Glans and prepuce of clitoris
19. Pubic symphysis
20. Posterior part of fornix of vagina
21. Vesicouterine pouch
22. Peritoneum on the uterus forming the tunica serosa (serosal coat) or perimetrium. Trace the peritoneum as it covers the uterus and bladder and forms the deep folds of the vesicouterine and rectouterine pouches.

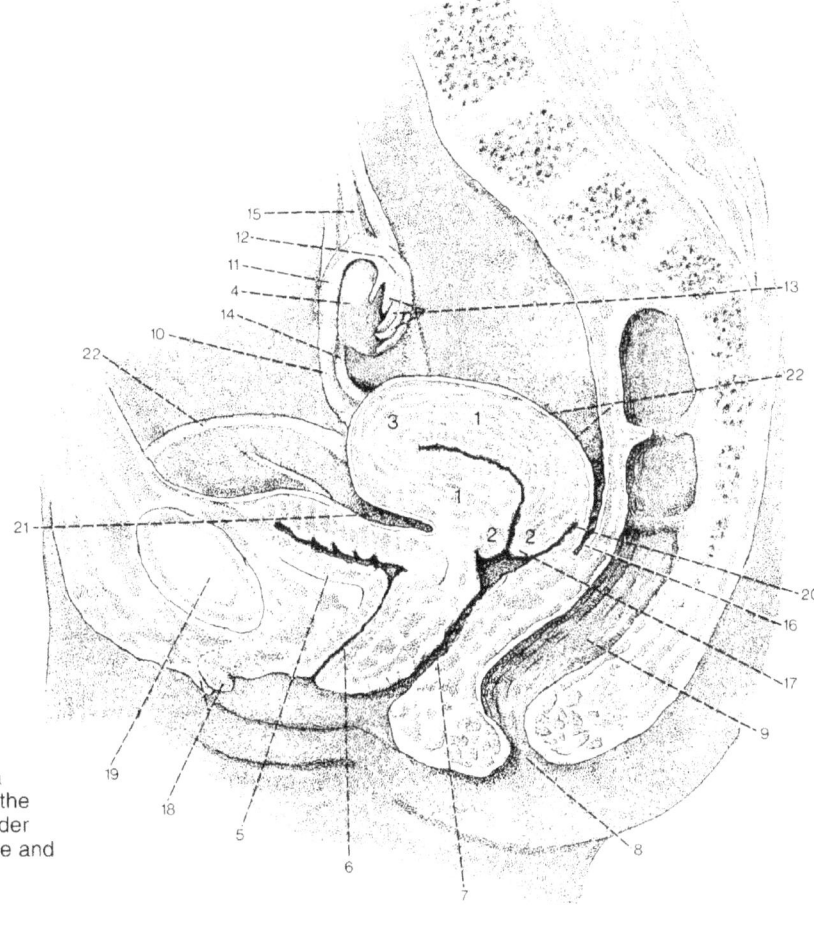

1_____ 12_____
2_____ 13_____
3_____ 14_____
4_____ 15_____
5_____ 16_____
6_____ 17_____
7_____ 18_____
8_____ 19_____
9_____ 20_____
10_____ 21_____
11_____ 22_____

P-24 Female superficial perineal muscles

Color and label

1. Suspensory ligament of clitoris
2. Prepuce covering body of clitoris
3. Bulbospongiosus muscle* (covering bulb of vestibule and greater vestibular gland)
4. Ischiocavernosus muscle* (covering the left crus of the clitoris)
5. Glans of the clitoris
6. External urethral opening (orifice)
7. Vagina
8. Labium minus (cut)
9. Perineal membrane
10. Superficial transverse perineus muscle
11. Levator ani muscle
12. External anal sphincter muscle
13. Anus
14. Gluteus maximus muscle

*These muscles are thinner and more delicate than those in the male.

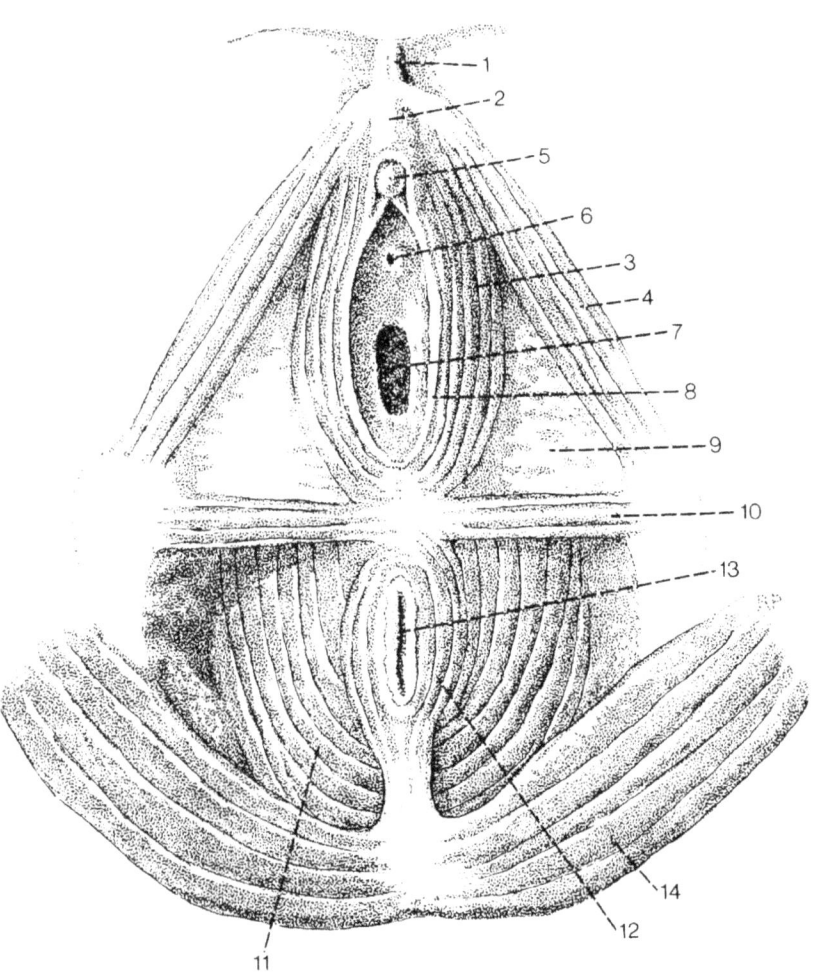

P-25 Nerves of the female perineum

Color and label

1. Clitoris (prepuce removed)
2. Vestibule of vagina
3. Anus
4. Superficial transverse perineus muscle (cut on left side)
5. Gluteus maximus muscle
6. Labium majus pudendi (major pudendal lip) (cut)
7. Perineal nerve; this is a branch of the pudendal nerve; it gives off the posterior labial nerves and supplies the bulbospongiosus and ischiocavernosus muscles and the vestibular bulb.
8. Posterior labial nerves
9. Inferior rectal nerves
10. Dorsal nerve of clitoris; note that it becomes more superficial by penetrating the perineal membrane
11. Posterior femoral cutaneous nerve
12. Perineal branch of posterior femoral cutaneous nerve
13. Inferior clunial nerve
14. Perineal membrane

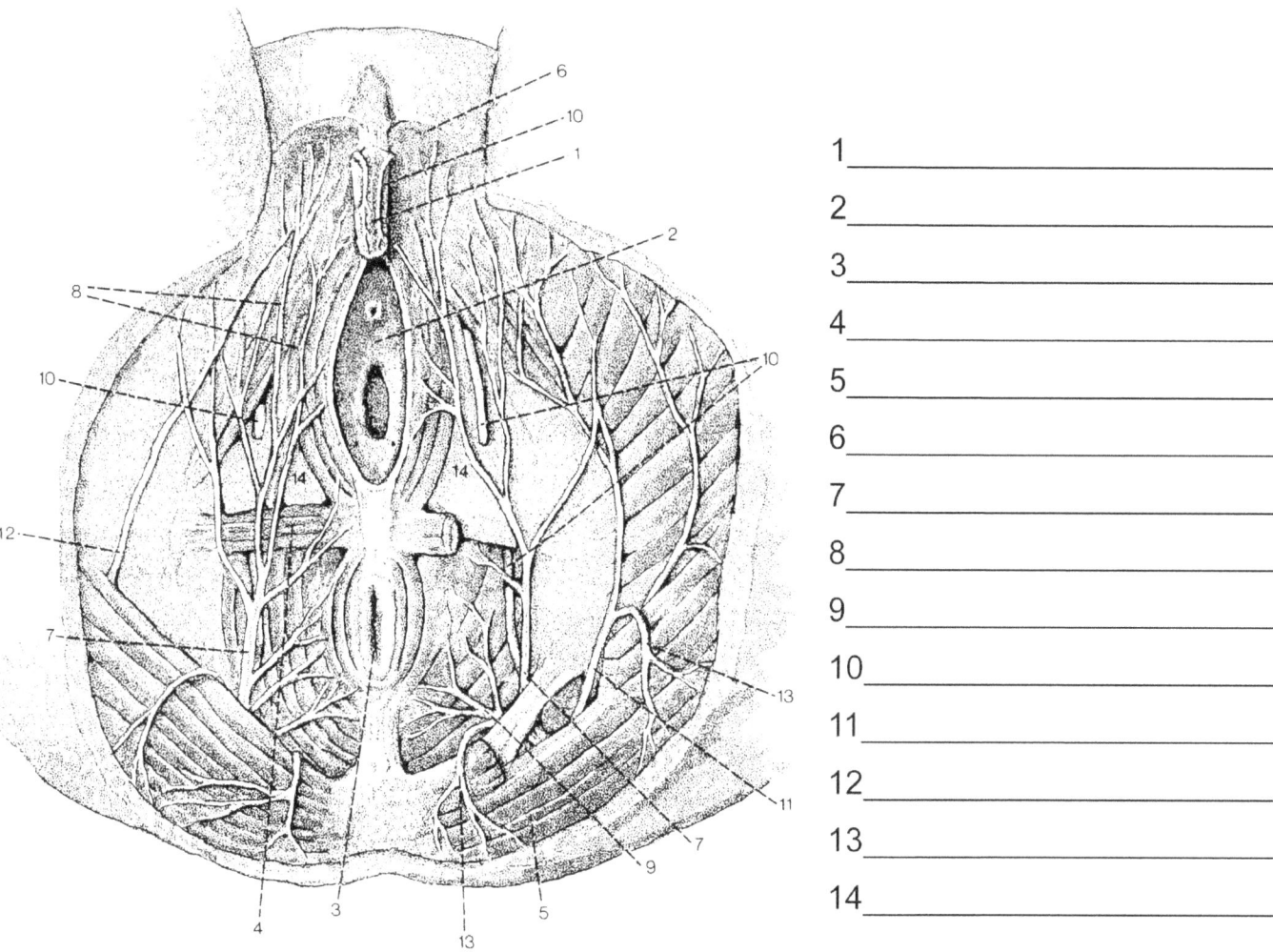

P-26 Arteries of female perineum

Veins (not shown) would accompany arteries

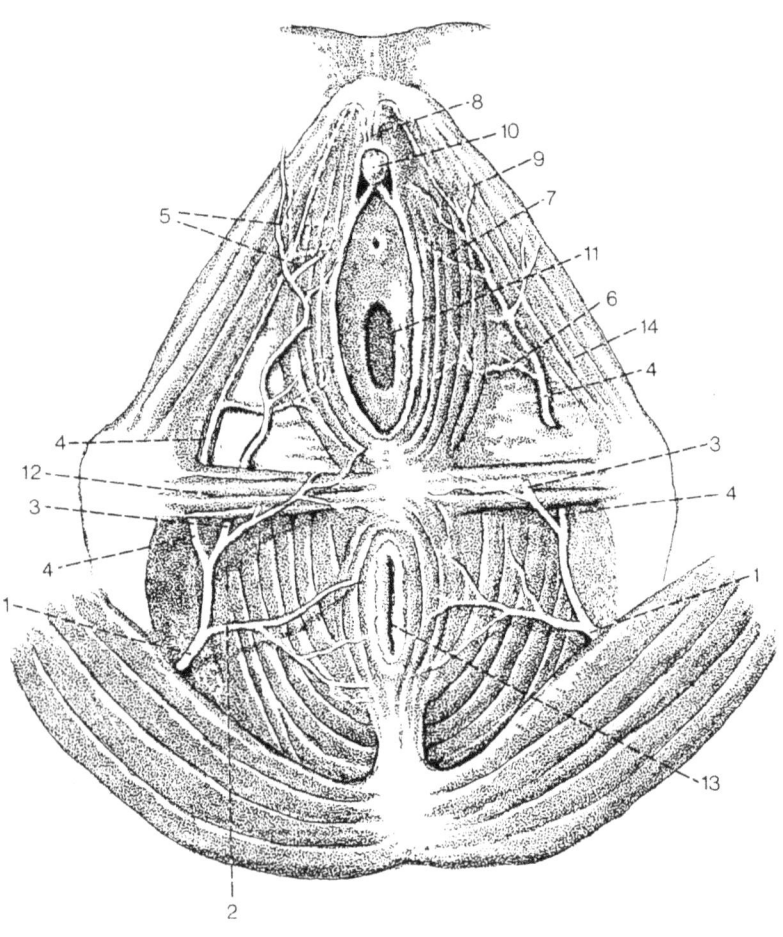

Color and label

1 Internal pudendal artery
2 Inferior rectal artery and branches
3 Perineal artery (cut on left)
4 Artery of clitoris
5 Posterior labial arteries;
    terminal branches of perineal artery
6 Artery of vestibular bulb; off clitoral artery
7 Urethral artery
8 Dorsal artery of clitoris
9 Deep artery of clitoris; to crus of clitoris
10 Glans of clitoris
11 Vagina
12 Superficial transverse perineus muscle
14 Ischiocavernosus muscle

P-27 The uterus
Viewed from the left
Parasagittal section to the left of the uterus

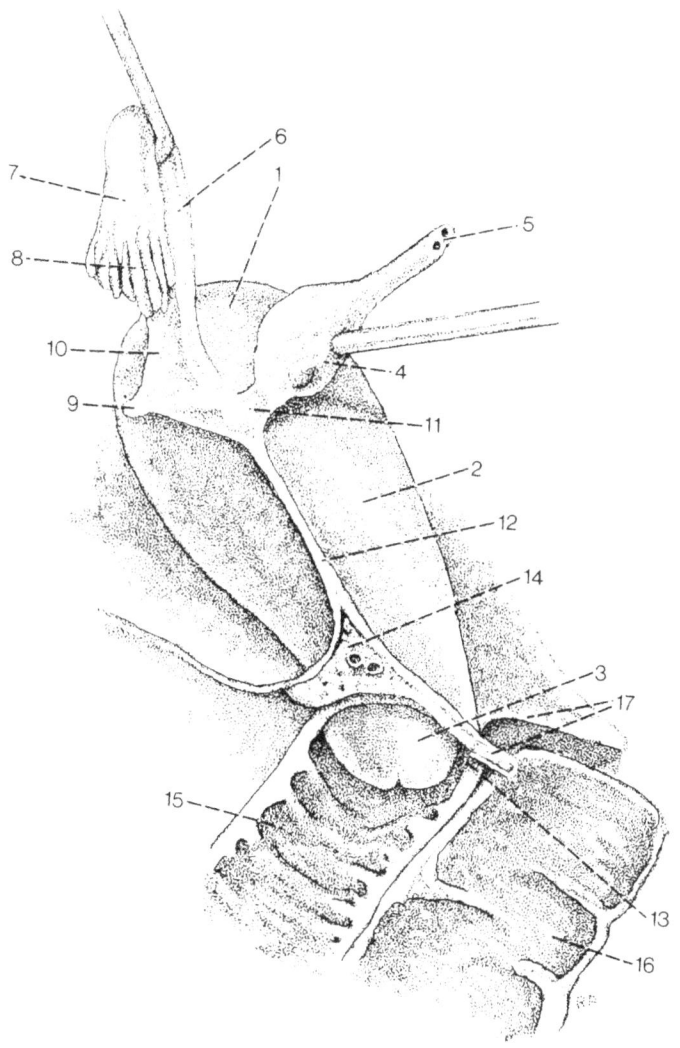

1 ___
2 ___
3 ___
4 ___
5 ___
6 ___
7 ___
8 ___
9 ___
10 ___
11 ___
12 ___
13 ___
14 ___
15 ___
16 ___
17 ___

Color and label

1 Fundus of uterus
2 Body of uterus
3 Cervix of uterus (intravaginal part)
4 Ovary
5 Suspensory ligament of ovary with ovarian artery and vein (cut)
6 Uterine tube (oviduct)
7 Infundibulum of uterine tube
8 Fimbria of uterine tube
9 Round ligament of uterus (cut)
10 Mesosalpinx; fold of broad ligament attached to uterine tube (*salpinx* is Greek for trumpet or tube)
11 Mesovarium; fold of broad ligament attached to ovary
12 Mesometrium; major part of broad ligament; attached to sides of uterus
13 Posterior fornix of vagina; the vaginal fornix is actually a circular cleft around the intravaginal cervix; for descriptive purposes it is divided into an anterior part, right and left lateral parts, and a posterior part.
14 Lateral cervical ligament with uterine artery and vein(s)
15 Vagina (cut midsagittally)
16 Rectum (midsagittal cut)
17 Uterosacral ligament and fold

P-28 Female pelvic diaphragm and related structures (viewed from below and from the right) (opposite page)

The fat in the **ischiorectal fossa** (the wedge-shaped space between the obturator internus muscle and the pelvic diaphragm) has been removed.

The **pelvic diaphragm** consists of two paired muscles, the **levator ani** and the **coccygeus**, which meet in the midline and together form the hammock-like muscle. The pelvic diaphragm forms the floor of the pelvis. It supports the pelvic viscera and raises the pelvic floor. It resists increased intra-abdominal pressure and constricts the anorectal junction and the vagina. It is pierced by the anal canal, the urethra, and the vagina. Each levator ani consists of three muscles: the pubococcygeus, the puborectalis, and the iliococcygeus. The puborectalis lies internal to the pubococcygeus and cannot be seen from below. In addition to the three muscles named above, two additional muscles are sometimes considered part of the levator ani: the levator prostate in the male and the pubovaginalis in the female (not shown here).

Color and label

1. Anus
2. External anal sphincter (superficial layer)
3. Pubococcygeus muscle.
4. Iliococcygeus muscle. This forms the lateral and posterior part of the levator ani muscle.
5. Coccygeus muscle. This forms the posterior superior part of the pelvic diaphragm. The levator ani and the coccygeus together form the pelvic diaphragm.
6. Coccyx (the tail bone)
7. Anococcygeal ligament. This is a fibromuscular band extending from the external anal sphincter to the coccyx. Some of the fibers from the two sides of the levator ani interdigitate across this ligament while other fibers terminate on the ligament.
8. Obturator internus muscle. This leg muscle along with the obturator membrane and the obturator externus muscle largely block off the obturator foramen.
9. Superficial transverse perineal muscle
10. Perineal body (also central tendon of perineum). A fibromuscular mass between the anus and bulb of the penis in the male, and between the vagina and anus in the female. It serves as an anchor and attachment for the muscles in the region.
11. Perineal membrane (formerly called inferior fascia of urogenital membrane)
12. Greater vestibular gland and its opening in the vestibule of the vagina
13. Vestibular bulb. This is female erectile tissue. It is homologous to the corpus spongiosus penis in the male.
14. Vagina
15. Bulbospongiosus muscle. This thin, delicate muscle overlies the vestibular bulb in the female. It is partly removed on the left side.
16. Glans and prepuce of the clitoris
17. Obturator (Latin, *obturare*, to stop up) membrane. This membrane and the obturator internus and obturator externus muscles almost completely seal off the obturator foramen.
18. Ischiocavernosus muscle. This delicate muscle covers the crus of the clitoris in the female.
19. Obturator nerve, artery, and vein. These exit the pelvis through a small opening in the obturator membrane and supply the medial thigh muscles and medial skin of the thigh.
20. Acetabulum. This cup-shaped socket fits over the head of the femur. Together they form the hip joint.
21. Sacrotuberous ligament (extends from sacrum to ischial tuberosity). This strong ligament along with the deeper sacrospinous ligament (not seen here) convert the two sciatic notches into two foramina, the greater and lesser sciatic foramina.
22. Ischial tuberosity (right and left)
23. Anterior superior iliac spine
24. Right obturator internus. This leg muscle arises mainly from the internal surface of the obturator membrane. It leaves the pelvis through the lesser sciatic foramen and inserts on the greater trochanter of the femur.
25. Sciatic nerve. This is the largest nerve in the body. It is actually a double nerve that divides lower in the thigh into its two component parts: the common peroneal nerve and the tibial nerve.
26. Pudendal nerve and internal pudendal artery and vein. These exit the pelvis through the greater sciatic foramen and re-enter the pelvis through the lesser sciatic foramen. They supply the anus and external genitalia.
27. Piriformis muscle. This leg muscle leaves the pelvis through the greater sciatic foramen, which it largely fills, and inserts on the greater trochanter of the femur.
28. Supraspinal ligament

P-28 Female pelvic diaphragm and related structures

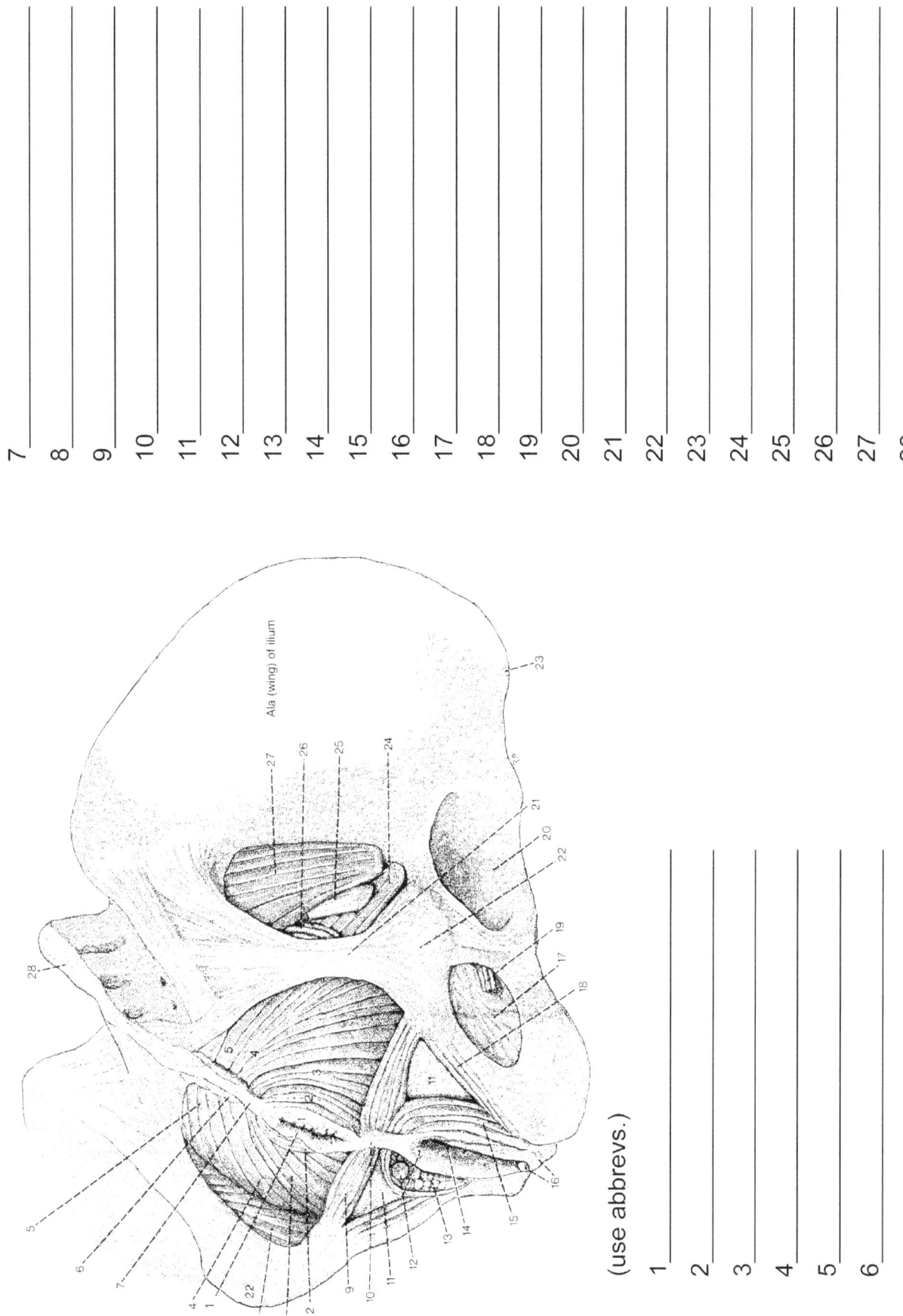

1. _____
2. _____
3. _____
4. _____
5. _____
6. _____
7. _____
8. _____
9. _____
10. _____
11. _____
12. _____
13. _____
14. _____
15. _____
16. _____
17. _____
18. _____
19. _____
20. _____
21. _____
22. _____
23. _____
24. _____
25. _____
26. _____
27. _____
28. _____

(use abbrevs.)

P-29 Female pelvis from the front and above
(opposite page)

Color and label

1. Fundus of uterus
2. Bladder (superior surface covered by peritoneum); all the intraperitoneal pelvic and abdominal organs are covered on their external surface by peritoneum, which forms the outer tunica serosa or serosal layer.
3. Right ovary; with developing follicles
4. Left ovary; with developing follicles. These rupture at ovulation and release their eggs into the oviduct. Only about 300 follicles mature and rupture at ovulation during a woman's reproductive life.
5. Uterine tube (also called fallopian tube, oviduct). Salpingitis is inflammation of the fallopian tube (salpingo- is the combining form from *salpinx,* Greek for a trumpet or tube)
6. Fimbriae (L. fringe, thread, fiber) of the uterine tube. They are finger-like processes extending from the circumference of the distal expanded end (infundibulum) of the uterine tube.
7. Proper ovarian ligament
8. Round ligament of the uterus. This is a narrow fibrous band that extends from the uterus to the deep inguinal ring where it passes through the inguinal canal to end in the labium majus.
9. Rectum
10. Suspensory ligament of the ovary with the ovarian artery and vein
11. Vermiform appendix (worm-like, L. *vermis*, worm)
12. Cecum of large intestine; this is the beginning of the large intestine. "Cecum and ye shall find."
13. Ileum (terminal portion)
14. Appendices epiploica (fatty appendages). These small globules of fat are found only on the large intestine and are an aid in distinguishing an empty, constricted colon from a full, small intestine.
15. Vesicouterine pouch; the peritoneal-lined space or recess between the bladder and uterus.
16. Broad ligament
17. Rectouterine fold; a crescentric fold of peritoneum extending from the rectum to the base of the broad ligament.
18. Tenia coli; there are three of these thickened, tapelike bands of smooth muscle arranged longitudinally on the surface of the large intestine. They are responsible for the bulging haustra of the large intestine.

1 _____
2 _____
3 _____
4 _____
5 _____
6 _____
7 _____
8 _____
9 _____
10 _____
11 _____
12 _____
13 _____
14 _____
15 _____
16 _____
17 _____
18 _____

P-29 Female pelvis from the front and above

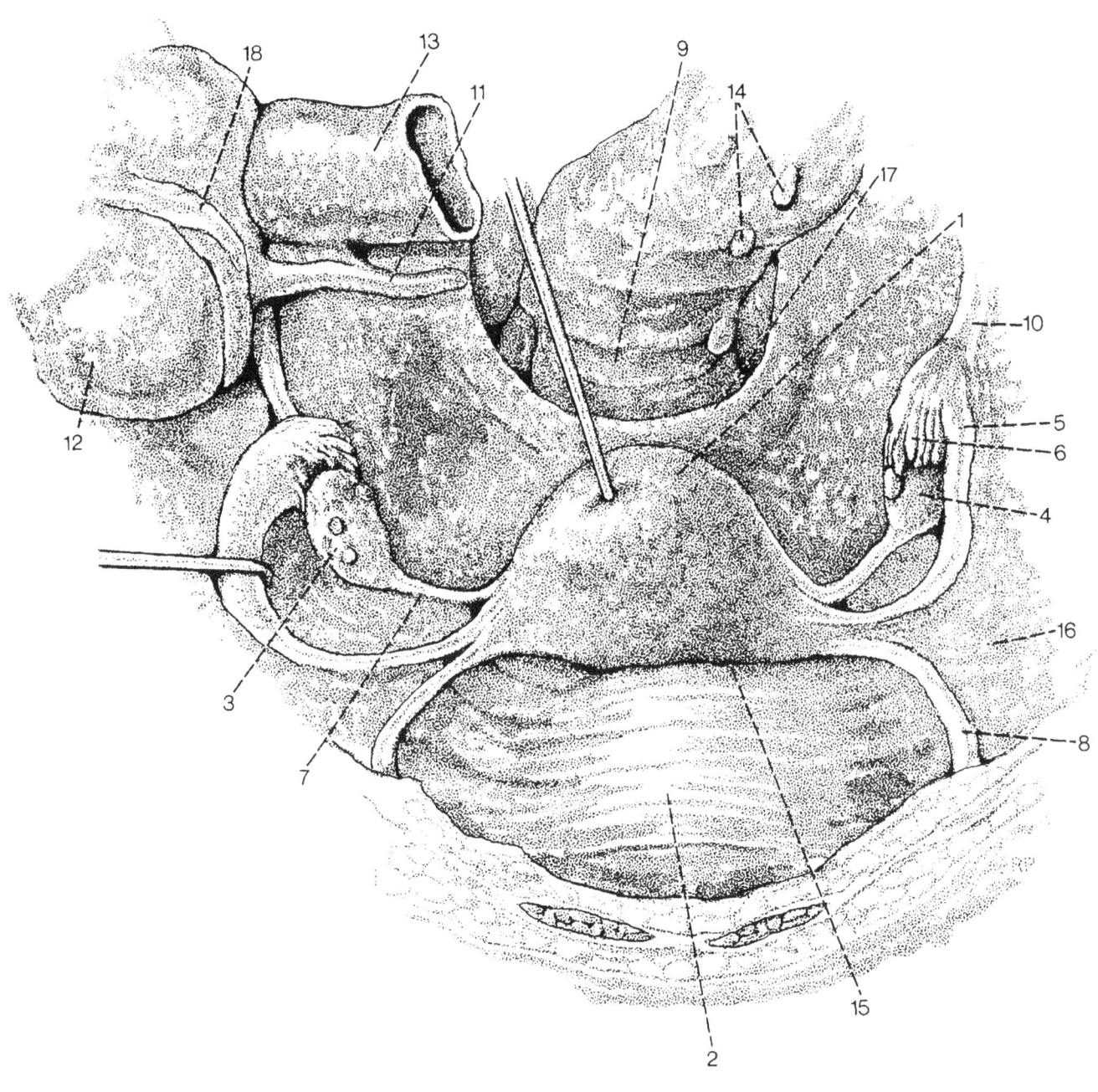

P-30 Uterus and related structures

Viewed from behind
(opposite page)

Color and label

1. Fundus of uterus (the word *uterus* is probably derived from the Greek *hystera*, womb). Hysterectomy is surgical excision of the uterus. Hysteria was originally thought to be caused by the internal movements of an unrestrained uterus that had broken free of its moorings.
2. Cavity of uterus
3. Body of uterus (a segment of the uterus has been removed to expose its cavity and the layers of its wall)
4. Cervix of uterus (supravaginal part; that portion above the vagina; *cervix*, Latin, neck)
5. Cervix of uterus (vaginal part; that portion projecting into the vagina)
6. Cervical canal
7. Vagina (anterior wall)
8. Opening of the uterus (ostium uteri)
9. Anterior lip of the cervix
10. Lateral fornices of vagina (left and right); actually the vaginal fornix is a circular cleft between the intravaginal cervix and the superior wall of the vagina; for descriptive purposes, it is divided into right, left, anterior, and posterior fornix.
11. Isthmus of uterus (narrow portion)
12. Endometrium (mucosal lining); this is lost and restored each month during the menstrual cycle.
13. Myometrium (muscular layer, consisting of nonstriated or smooth muscle); this becomes greatly enlarged and thickened in pregnancy.
14. Perimetrium (outer covering of peritoneum, also tunica serosa)
15. Mesometrium of broad ligament (that part attached to the sides of the uterus)
16. Mesovarium of broad ligament (that part attached to the ovary)
17. Mesovarium of broad ligament (part attached to the uterine tube)
18. Uterine tube (opened on the left side) eggs released from the ovary travel down the uterine tube into the uterus. Fertilization of the egg by a spermatozoon usually occurs within the uterine tube.
19. Infundibulum of uterine tube (expanded end)
20. Ampulla of uterine tube (dilation of tube)
21. Fimbria of uterine tube
22. Ureter
23. Uterine artery; it connects with both the artery of the vagina and the ovarian artery.
24. Recto-uterine ligament with smooth muscle
25. Lateral cervical ligament (cardinal ligament, Mackenrodt's ligament)
26. Ovary (cut open on left); mature follicle on right ovary
27. Proper ovarian ligament
28. Ovarian artery and vein within suspensory ligament of the ovary
29. Corpus albicans; remnant of the ovarian corpus luteum weeks after ovulation.
30. Corpus luteum (yellow body of the ovary). The yellow progesterone-secreting body formed in the ovary at the site of a ruptured ovarian follicle.
31. Artery of the vagina

P-30 Uterus and related structures
Viewed from behind

P-31 Female pelvic diaphragm from above

Color and label
1. Urethra
2. Vagina
3. Rectum
4. Puborectalis muscle (part of levator ani)
5. Pubococcygeus muscle (part of levator ani)
6. Iliococcygeus muscle (part of levator ani)
7. Coccygeus muscle (part of pelvic diaphragm)
   (coccygeus + levator ani = pelvic diaphragm)
8. Obturator internus muscle
9. Tendinous arch of levator ani
10. Pubovaginalis (part of levator ani)
11. Ischial spine
12. Obturator canal
13. Dorsal vein of clitoris
14. Pubic symphysis
15. Piriformis muscle

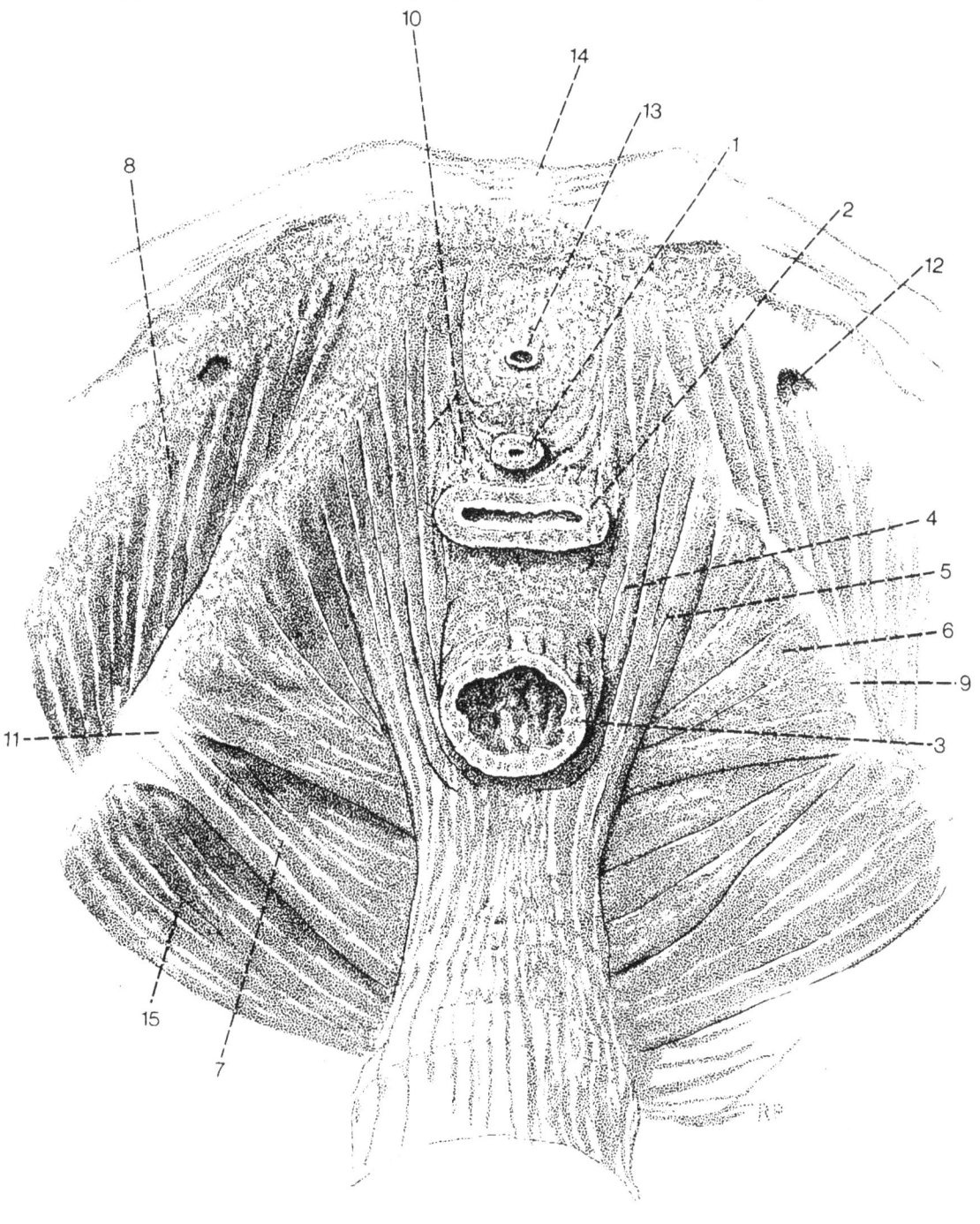

P-32 Arterial supply of the female pelvis

Viewed from the left; part of the left hip bone has been removed; veins (not shown) accompany artery
(opposite page)

Color and label

1. Aorta; the aorta bifurcates (divides) into the right and left common iliac arteries
2. Inferior mesenteric artery; this artery supplies the lower one half of the colon
3. Right common iliac artery; the common iliac artery divides into an external iliac artery and an internal iliac artery.
4. Right external iliac artery and vein; these continue into the leg as the femoral artery and vein.
5. Left common iliac artery and vein (vein is cut)
6. Left external iliac artery and vein (both cut)
7. Internal iliac artery (old name, hypogastric artery)
8. Superior gluteal artery
9. Inferior gluteal artery
10. Internal pudendal artery; this exits the greater sciatic foramen and reenters the lesser sciatic foramen (accompanied with the vein and pudendal nerve)
11. Inferior rectal artery
12. Obturator artery; this usually arises from the internal iliac artery, but it may arise from the external iliac artery and complicate exploratory surgery in this area.
13. Umbilical artery; the proximal portion of this artery (that part to the bladder) remains patent (open), whereas after birth the distal portion up to the umbilicus becomes obliterated and forms the medial umbilical plica
14. Superior vesical (*vesica* Latin, bladder, blister) artery; supplies the superior portion of the bladder.
15. Obliterated part of umbilical artery (median umbilical plica or fold)
16. Uterine artery; note that it anastomoses with both the ovarian artery and the vaginal artery.
17. Vaginal artery
18. Piriformis muscle; note that the superior gluteal artery (and vein and nerve) comes out of the greater sciatic foramen **above** the piriformis, whereas the inferior gluteal vessels and nerve exit the same foramen **below** the piriformis muscle.
19. Coccygeus muscle (part of the pelvic diaphragm)
20. Levator ani muscle
21. Obturator internus muscle
22. External anal sphincter
23. Labia minora
24. Glans of clitoris
25. Left ureter
26. Fundus of uterus
27. Bladder
28. Inferior vena cava
29. Branch of uterine artery to ovarian artery

1 _____
2 _____
3 _____
4 _____
5 _____
6 _____
7 _____
8 _____
9 _____
10 _____
11 _____
12 _____
13 _____
14 _____
15 _____
16 _____
17 _____
18 _____
19 _____
20 _____
21 _____
22 _____
23 _____
24 _____
25 _____
26 _____
27 _____
28 _____
29 _____

P-32 Arterial supply of the female pelvis

Viewed from the left; part of the left hip bone has been removed; veins (not shown) accompany artery

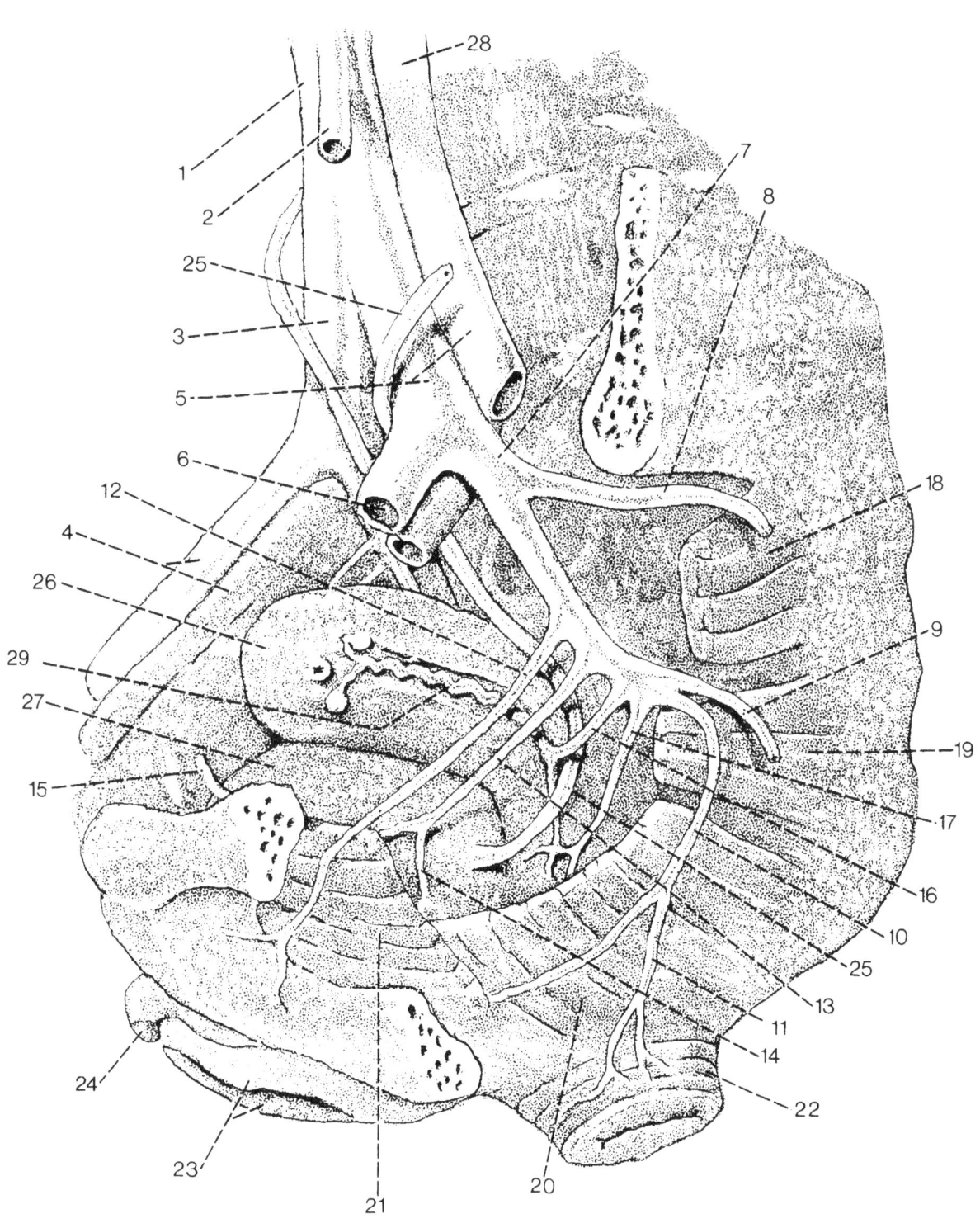

239

P-33 Muscles on medial surface of pelvis

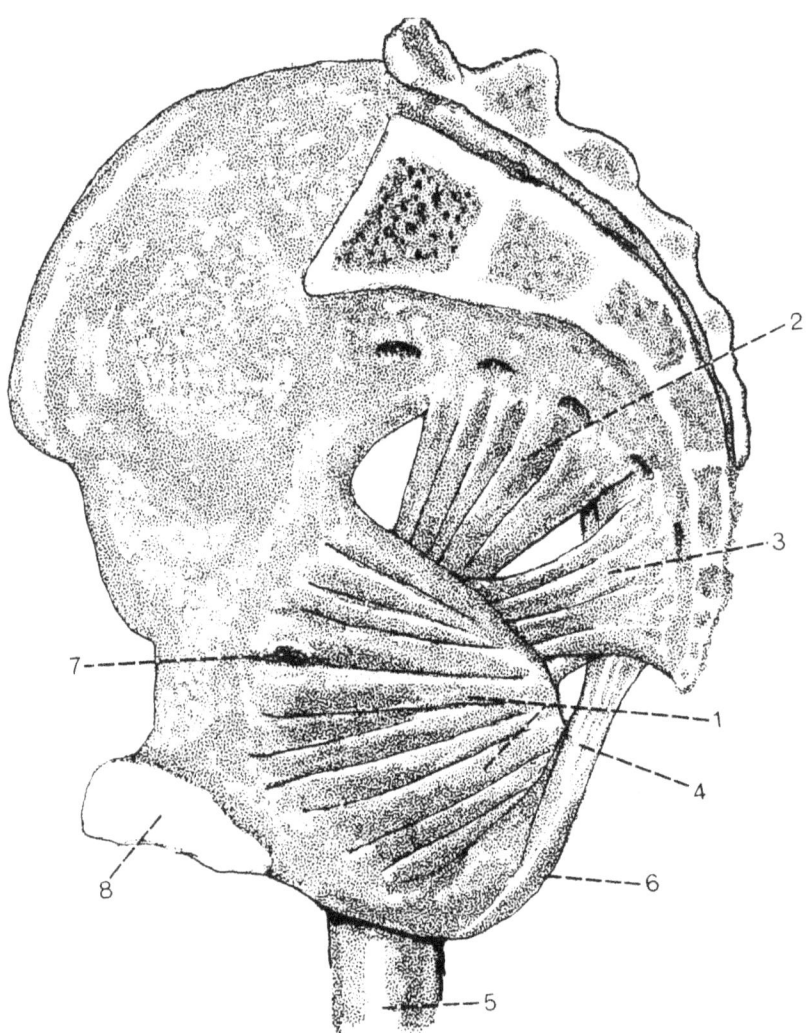

Color and label

1. Obturator internus muscle; note how it covers the obturator foramen internally; it exits the pelvis through the lesser sciatic foramen and inserts on the femur.
2. Piriformis muscle. This muscle exits the pelvis via, the greater sciatic foramen, which it largely fills; it also inserts on the femur.
3. Coccygeus muscle; in tailed mammals this muscle pulls the tail between the legs.
4. Sacrotuberous ligament; this extends from the sacrum to the ischial tuberosity.
5. Femur
6. Ischial tuberosity
7. Obturator canal; this small opening transmits the obturator nerve, artery, and vein.
8. Pubic symphysis

1 _____
2 _____
3 _____
4 _____
5 _____
6 _____
7 _____
8 _____

P-34 Female urogenital sphincter I
Viewed from below

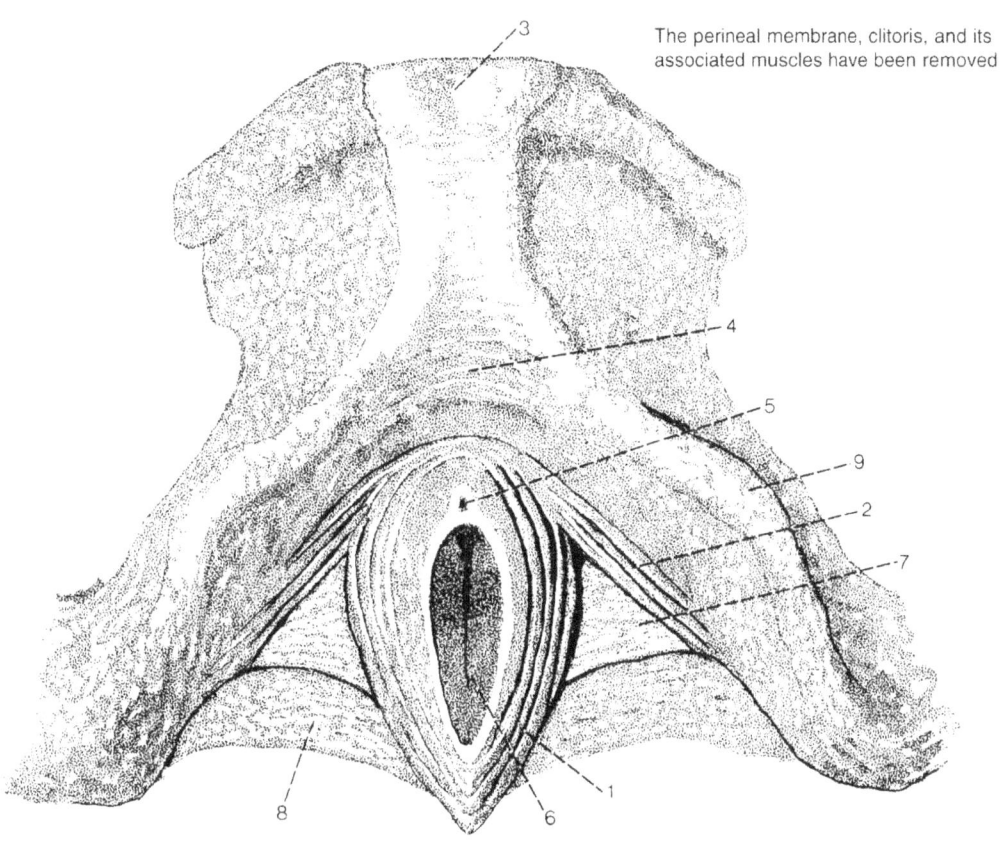

The perineal membrane, clitoris, and its associated muscles have been removed

The striated urogenital sphincter muscle of the female consists of:
  The **urethrovaginal sphincter** surrounding the urethra and the vaginal vestibule (1)
  The **compressor of the urethra** arching across the ventral side of the urethra (2)
  The **sphincter** surrounding the middle third of the urethra (see figure P-35)

Color and label

1 Urethrovaginal sphincter muscle
2 Urethral compressor muscle: this arches across the ventral side of the uretha
3 Pubic symphysis
4 Arcuate pubic ligament
5 Urethra
6 Vagina
7 Transverse vaginal muscle; this is a variable striated muscle
8 Smooth muscle of urethrovaginal compartment
9 Ischiopubic ramus

After Oelrich T, Anat Rec 205:223, 1983.

1_____ 6_____
2_____ 7_____
3_____ 8_____
4_____ 9_____
5_____

P-35 Female striated urethral sphincter II

(opposite page)

The body and crura of the clitoris and the vestibular bulb with the associated muscles plus the perineal membrane have been removed. The three striated muscles (5,6,7 below) that comprise the striated urethral sphincter in the female lie above (deep to or cephalic to) the perineal membrane.

Color and label

1. Bladder; cephalic portion has been removed
2. Vagina
3. Urethra; the urethra is not a straight tube but is concave forward.
4. Vaginal wall
5. **Urethral sphincter muscle**; this lies in the pelvic cavity. It surrounds the middle third of the urethra for approximately 1.5 cm. Caudally it is continuous with the compressor urethrae muscle, which lies in the perineum. In the adult the sphincter muscle is thickest ventrally and thins as it passes dorsally.
6. **Compressor urethrae muscle**; this muscle lies in the perineum. It begins at a point anterior to the ischial tuberosity. It extends forward and medially to the anterior surface of the urethra where it forms a thick bundle around the anterior urethra and then becomes continuous with corresponding fibers from the opposite side of the body, thus forming a broad arching muscle. Its superior fibers on the urethra are continuous with the inferior fibers of the urethral sphincter. Because it approaches the urethra at an angle of 130 degrees, it appears to have the action of pulling the urethral meatus caudally, thus elongating the urethra, which may be important in providing continence (along with elevation of the bladder by the pelvic diaphragm).
7. **Urethrovaginal sphincter**; this muscle also lies in the perineum and is continuous ventrally with the compressor urethra. It surrounds both the vagina and urethra. It begins ventral to the urethra and passes dorsally deep to the vestibular bulb (removed) along the sides of the vagina until it reaches its posterior point where its fibers interdigitate with corresponding fibers of the opposite side.
8. Transverse vaginal muscle; this very thin, fan-shaped muscle attaches to the anterior portion of the lateral wall of the vagina. It varies in both size and extent. It seldom attaches to the posterior half of the vagina.
9. Smooth muscle of the urethrovaginal compartment. The amount and density of smooth muscle and connective tissue tend to increase with age, making the identification of striated muscle more difficult in the adult. The smooth muscle is extensive throughout the perineal region from the ischiopubic rami to the lateral wall of the urethra.
10. Ischiopubic ramus (pubic symphysis and medial portion removed)
11. Uterus (cephalic portion removed)

After Oelrich: The striated urogenital sphincter in the female. Anat Rec 205:223-232, 1983.

Recent work has shown the striated muscle on the caudal third of the urethra is innervated by fibers of the pudendal nerve, whereas three layers of smooth muscle on the superior two-thirds of the urethra receive thin fibers from the pelvic plexus. (Colleselli et al: The female urethral sphincter. J Urol 160:49-54, 1998.)

(use abbrevs.)

1_____ 8_____

2_____ 9_____

3_____ 10_____

4_____ 11_____

5_____

6_____

7_____

P-35 Female striated urethral sphincter II

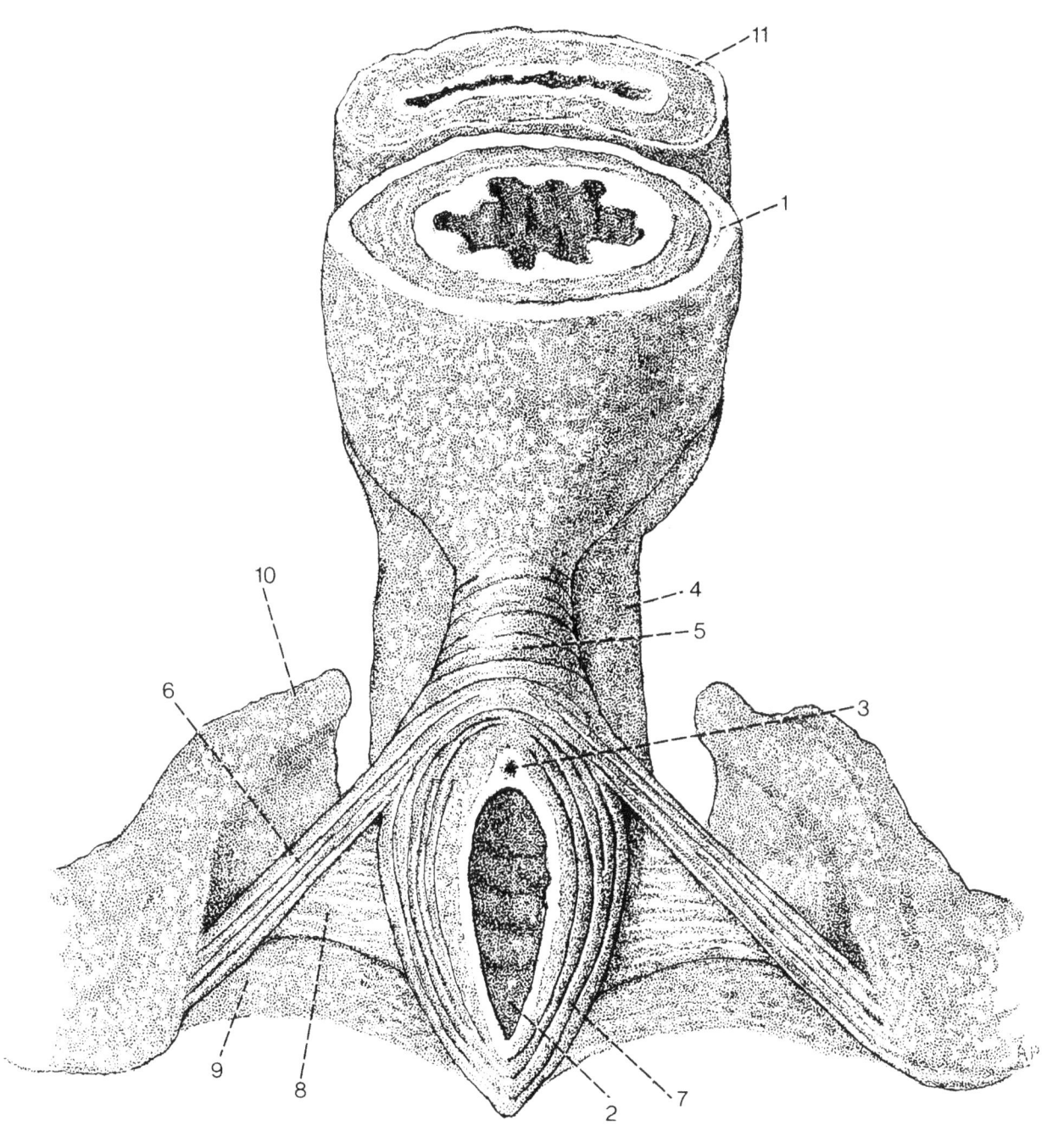

After Oelrich, 1983

P-36 Pelvis and ligaments
Anterior aspect

Color and label

1 Anterior superior iliac spine
2 Anterior inferior iliac spine
3 Iliopectineal eminence
4 Iliac fossa
5 Iliac crest
6 Ischial spine
7 Sacrospinous ligament
8 Sacrotuberous ligament
9 Greater sciatic foramen
10 Lesser sciatic foramen
11 Anterior longitudinal ligament
12 Anterior sacroiliac ligament
13 Iliolumbar ligament (superior band)
14 Iliolumbar ligament (inferior band)
15 Pectineal ligament
16 Superior pubic ligament
17 Interpubic disk (in pubic symphysis)

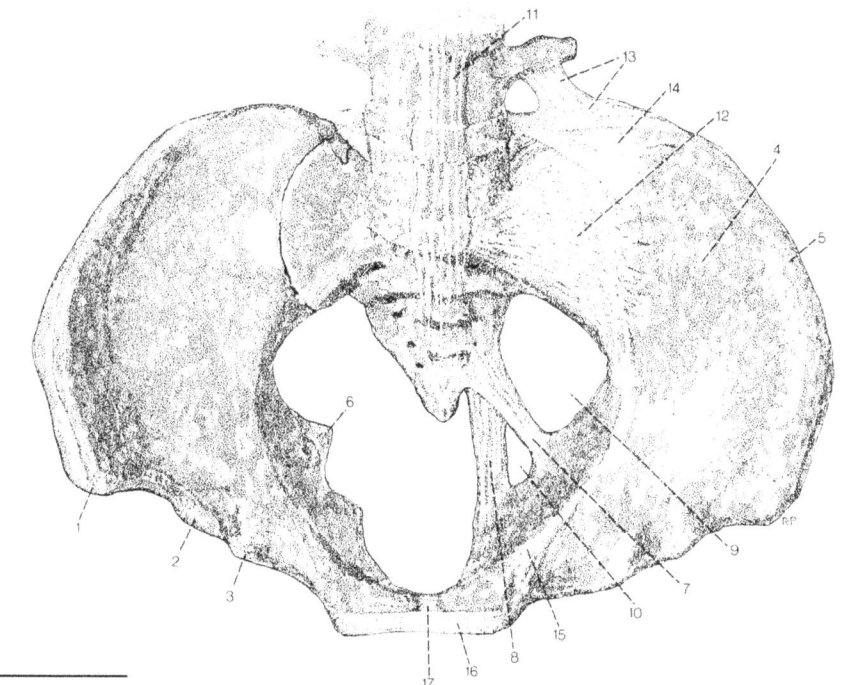

1 _____
2 _____
3 _____
4 _____
5 _____
6 _____
7 _____
8 _____
9 _____
10 _____
11 _____
12 _____
13 _____
14 _____
15 _____
16 _____
17 _____

www.ingramcontent.com/pod-product-compliance
Lightning Source LLC
Chambersburg PA
CBHW081214230426
43666CB00015B/2726